AMERICAN ACADEMY OF OPHTHALMOLOGY®
Protecting Sight. Empowering Lives.

MW01701676

10 | Glaucoma

Last major revision 2020–2021

2022–2023

BCSC

Basic and Clinical Science Course™

EBO Published after collaborative review with the European Board of Ophthalmology subcommittee

The American Academy of Ophthalmology is accredited by the Accreditation Council for Continuing Medical Education (ACCME) to provide continuing medical education for physicians.

The American Academy of Ophthalmology designates this enduring material for a maximum of 10 *AMA PRA Category 1 Credits*™. Physicians should claim only the credit commensurate with the extent of their participation in the activity.

CME expiration date: June 1, 2023. *AMA PRA Category 1 Credits*™ may be claimed only once between June 1, 2020, and the expiration date.

BCSC® volumes are designed to increase the physician's ophthalmic knowledge through study and review. Users of this activity are encouraged to read the text and then answer the study questions provided at the back of the book.

To claim *AMA PRA Category 1 Credits*™ upon completion of this activity, learners must demonstrate appropriate knowledge and participation in the activity by taking the posttest for Section 10 and achieving a score of 80% or higher. For further details, please see the instructions for requesting CME credit at the back of the book.

The Academy provides this material for educational purposes only. It is not intended to represent the only or best method or procedure in every case, nor to replace a physician's own judgment or give specific advice for case management. Including all indications, contraindications, side effects, and alternative agents for each drug or treatment is beyond the scope of this material. All information and recommendations should be verified, prior to use, with current information included in the manufacturers' package inserts or other independent sources, and considered in light of the patient's condition and history. Reference to certain drugs, instruments, and other products in this course is made for illustrative purposes only and is not intended to constitute an endorsement of such. Some material may include information on applications that are not considered community standard, that reflect indications not included in approved FDA labeling, or that are approved for use only in restricted research settings. **The FDA has stated that it is the responsibility of the physician to determine the FDA status of each drug or device he or she wishes to use, and to use them with appropriate, informed patient consent in compliance with applicable law.** The Academy specifically disclaims any and all liability for injury or other damages of any kind, from negligence or otherwise, for any and all claims that may arise from the use of any recommendations or other information contained herein.

Cover image: From BCSC Section 12, *Retina and Vitreous.* Confocal scanning laser ophthalmoscopy multicolor fundus image (30° field of view) of a healthy eye. *(Courtesy of Lucia Sobrin, MD.)*

FSC
www.fsc.org
MIX
Paper from responsible sources
FSC® C001701

Printed in China.

Basic and Clinical Science Course

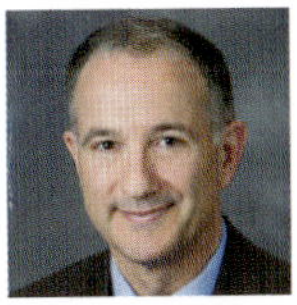

Christopher J. Rapuano, MD, Philadelphia, Pennsylvania
Senior Secretary for Clinical Education

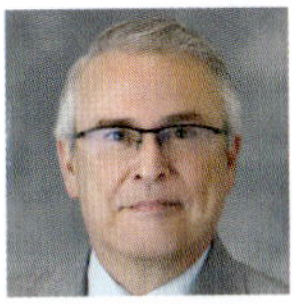

J. Timothy Stout, MD, PhD, MBA, Houston, Texas
Secretary for Lifelong Learning and Assessment

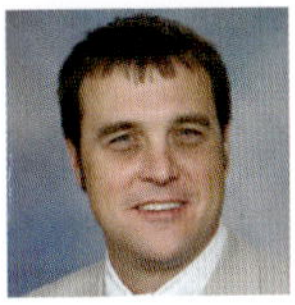

Colin A. McCannel, MD, Los Angeles, California
BCSC Course Chair

Section 10

Faculty for the Major Revision

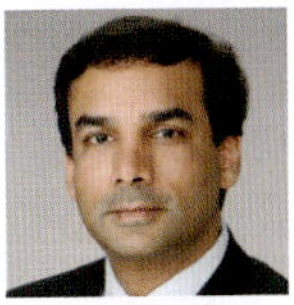

Angelo P. Tanna, MD
Chair
Chicago, Illinois

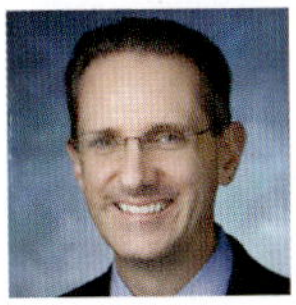

Michael V. Boland, MD, PhD
Baltimore, Maryland

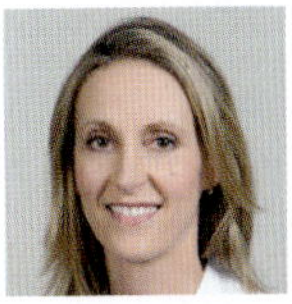

JoAnn A. Giaconi, MD
Los Angeles, California

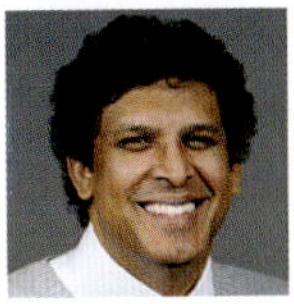

Chandrasekharan Krishnan, MD
Boston, Massachusetts

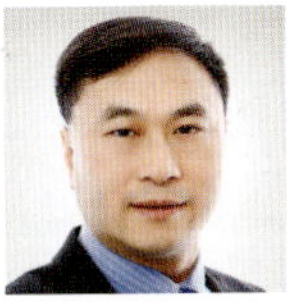

Shan C. Lin, MD
San Francisco, California

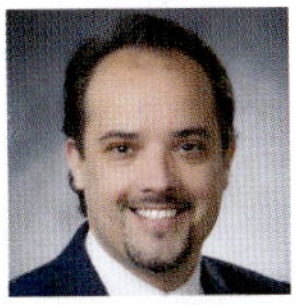

Felipe A. Medeiros, MD, PhD
Durham, North Carolina

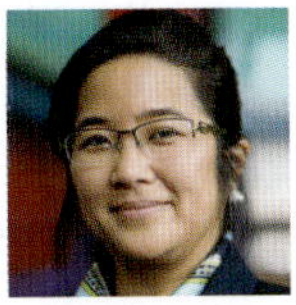

Sayoko E. Moroi, MD, PhD
Columbus, Ohio

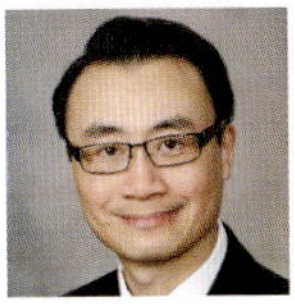

Arthur J. Sit, MD
Rochester, Minnesota

The Academy acknowledges the *American Glaucoma Society* for recommending faculty members to the BCSC Section 10 committee.

The Academy also acknowledges the following committees for review of this edition:

Committee on Aging: Joanna H. Queen, MD, Houston, Texas

Vision Rehabilitation Committee: Mona A. Kaleem, MD, PhD, Baltimore, Maryland

BCSC Resident/Fellow Reviewers: Sharon L. Jick, MD, *Chair*, Saint Louis, Missouri; Amar K. Bhat, MD; Mark P. Breazzano, MD; Shawn Lin, MD; Adam Rothman, MD

Practicing Ophthalmologists Advisory Committee for Education: Troy M. Tanji, MD, *Primary Reviewer*, Waipahu, Hawaii; Bradley D. Fouraker, MD, *Chair*, Tampa, Florida; Cynthia S. Chiu, MD, Oakland, California; George S. Ellis Jr, MD, New Orleans, Louisiana; Stephen R. Klapper, MD, Carmel, Indiana; Gaurav K. Shah, MD, Town and Country, Missouri; Rosa A. Tang, MD, MPH, MBA, Houston, Texas; Michelle S. Ying, MD, Ladson, South Carolina

In addition, the Academy acknowledges the following committee for assistance in developing Study Questions and Answers for this BCSC Section:

Resident Self-Assessment Committee: Robert A. Beaulieu, MD, Royal Oak, Michigan; Benjamin W. Botsford, MD, Pittsburgh, Pennsylvania; Olga M. Ceron, MD, Worcester, Massachusetts; Ian P. Conner, MD, PhD, Pittsburgh, Pennsylvania; Kimberly A. Crowder, MD, Jackson, Missouri; James Andrew David, MD, New Orleans, Louisiana; Claire E. Fraser, MD, PhD, Lexington, Kentucky; Kevin Halenda, MD, Augusta, Georgia; Rola N. Hamam, MD, Beirut, Lebanon; Amanda D. Henderson, MD, Baltimore, Maryland; Joshua Hendrix, MD, Dalton, Georgia; Matthew B. Kaufman, MD, Portland, Oregon; Sangeeta Khanna, MD, Saint Louis, Missouri; Chandrasekharan Krishnan, MD, Boston, Massachusetts; Ajay E. Kuriyan, MD, Pittsford, New York; Kevin E. Lai, MD, Indianapolis, Indiana; Kenneth C. Lao, MD, Temple, Texas; Ken Y. Lin, MD, Irvine, California; Kelly T. Mitchell, MD, Lubbock, Texas; Yasha S. Modi, MD, New York, New York; Matthew S. Pihlblad, MD, McDonald, Pennsylvania; Lorraine A. Provencher, MD, Cincinnati, Ohio; Jamie B. Rosenberg, MD, New York, New York; Syed Mahmood Shah, MD, Pittsburgh, Pennsylvania; Ann Shue, MD, Palo Alto, California; Misha F. Syed, MD, Galveston, Texas; Parisa Taravati, MD, Seattle, Washington; Sarah Van Tassel, MD, New York, New York; Evan L. Waxman, MD, PhD, Pittsburgh, Pennsylvania; Jules A. Winokur, MD, Great Neck, New York

EB

European Board of Ophthalmology: Carlo Traverso, MD, *Chair*, Genoa, Italy; Gordana Sunaric Mégevand, MD, FMH, FEBO, *Liaison*, Geneva, Switzerland; Augusto Azuara-Blanco, PhD, FRCS(Ed), FRCOphth, Belfast, Northern Ireland; Anders Heijl, MD, PhD, Malmö, Sweden; Gabor Hollo, MD, PhD, DSc, Budapest, Hungary; Anja Tuulonen, MD, PhD, Tampere, Finland

Financial Disclosures

Academy staff members who contributed to the development of this product state that within the 24 months prior to their contributions to this CME activity and for the duration of development, they have had no financial interest in or other relationship with any entity that produces, markets, resells, or distributes health care goods or services consumed by or used in patients, or with any competing commercial product or service.

The authors and reviewers state that within the 24 months prior to their contributions to this CME activity and for the duration of development, they have had the following financial relationships:*

Dr Boland: Alcon Laboratories (S), Carl Zeiss Meditec (C), Heidelberg Engineering (L), W.L. Gore and Associates (C)

Dr Conner: Ocugenix (C, O, P)

Dr Crowder: Gore (C), Medtronic (C), Phillips (C)

Dr Fouraker: Addition Technology (C, L), Alcon Laboratories (C, L), OASIS Medical (C, L)

Dr Giaconi: Allergan (L), New World Medical (C)

Dr Hamam: Abbvie (C, L, S)

Dr Heijl: Allergan (C, L), Santen (L), Zeiss (C, L, P)

Dr Hollo: Alcon Laboratories (C, L), Allergan (L), Santen (C, L)

Dr Klapper: AdOM Advanced Optical Technologies (O)

Dr Kuriyan: Alimera Sciences (C), Allergan (C), Regeneron (C), Second Sight (S) Valeant (C)

Dr Ken Lin: Johnson & Johnson (C)

Dr Shan Lin: Aerie Pharmaceuticals (C, L), AlEyegn (C), Allergan (C), Bausch + Lomb (C, L), Eyenovia (C), IRIDEX (C), Tomey Corporation (C)

Dr Medeiros: Carl Zeiss (C, S), Heidelberg Engineering (C, S), NGoggle (P)

Dr Mégevand: Alcon Laboratories (C), Allergan (C)

Dr Modi: Alimera (C), Allergan (C), Genentech (C), Novartis (C)

Dr Moroi: Aerie Pharmaceuticals (S), Allergan (S), Bausch + Lomb (L), MedForce (L), Icare USA (S),

Dr Gaurav Shah: Allergan (C, S), Bausch + Lomb (L), DORC International, bv/Dutch Ophthalmics, USA (S), Johnson & Johnson (L), QLT Phototherapeutics (C, L), Regeneron (C, L)

Dr Syed Shah: Quantum Analytics (O), Quantum Ophthalmics (O), Quantum Vision (O)

Dr Sit: Aerie Pharmaceuticals (C, S), Allergan (C), Glaukos Corporation (S), Inject-Sense (C, O), PolyActiva, Pty (C)

Dr Tanna: Aeon Astron B. V., Leiden (C), Alcon Laboratories (C), Apotex (C), Bausch + Lomb (C), Carl Zeiss Meditec (C), ForSight VISION5 (C), Ivantis (C), Lynntech (C), Par Pharmaceuticals (C), Sandoz (C), Watson Laboratories (C)

Dr Tang: EMD Serono (L), Horizon (C, S), Immunovant (S), Quark (C, S), Regenera (S), Sanofi (L), Zeiss (L)

Dr Traverso: Alcon Laboratories (C, L), Allergan (C), Santen (C, L), Théa (C)

Dr Van Tassel: New World Medical (L)

The other authors and reviewers state that within the 24 months prior to their contributions to this CME activity and for the duration of development, they have had no financial interest in or other relationship with any entity that produces, markets, resells, or distributes health care goods or services consumed by or used in patients, or with any competing commercial product or service.

*C = consultant fee, paid advisory boards, or fees for attending a meeting; E = employed by or received a W2 from a commercial company; L = lecture fees or honoraria, travel fees or reimbursements when speaking at the invitation of a commercial company; O = equity ownership/stock options in publicly or privately traded firms, excluding mutual funds; P = patents and/or royalties for intellectual property; S = grant support or other financial support to the investigator from all sources, including research support from government agencies, foundations, device manufacturers, and/or pharmaceutical companies

Recent Past Faculty

Anjali M. Bhorade, MD
Jonathan G. Crowston, MBBS, PhD
Christopher A. Girkin, MD

In addition, the Academy gratefully acknowledges the contributions of numerous past faculty and advisory committee members who have played an important role in the development of previous editions of the Basic and Clinical Science Course.

American Academy of Ophthalmology Staff

Dale E. Fajardo, EdD, MBA, *Vice President, Education*
Beth Wilson, Director, *Continuing Professional Development*
Denise Evenson, *Director, Brand & Creative*
Ann McGuire, *Acquisitions and Development Manager*
Stephanie Tanaka, *Publications Manager*
Susan Malloy, *Acquisitions Editor and Program Manager*
Jasmine Chen, *Manager, E-Learning*
Lana Ip, *Senior Designer*
Beth Collins, *Medical Editor*
Eric Gerdes, *Interactive Designer*
Lynda Hanwella, *Publications Specialist*
Debra Marchi, *Permissions Assistant*

American Academy of Ophthalmology
655 Beach Street
Box 7424
San Francisco, CA 94120-7424

Contents

Introduction to the BCSC

The Basic and Clinical Science Course (BCSC) is designed to meet the needs of residents and practitioners for a comprehensive yet concise curriculum of the field of ophthalmology. The BCSC has developed from its original brief outline format, which relied heavily on outside readings, to a more convenient and educationally useful self-contained text. The Academy updates and revises the course annually, with the goals of integrating the basic science and clinical practice of ophthalmology and of keeping ophthalmologists current with new developments in the various subspecialties.

The BCSC incorporates the effort and expertise of more than 100 ophthalmologists, organized into 13 Section faculties, working with Academy editorial staff. In addition, the course continues to benefit from many lasting contributions made by the faculties of previous editions. Members of the Academy Practicing Ophthalmologists Advisory Committee for Education, Committee on Aging, and Vision Rehabilitation Committee review every volume before major revisions, as does a group of select residents and fellows. Members of the European Board of Ophthalmology, organized into Section faculties, also review volumes before major revisions, focusing primarily on differences between American and European ophthalmology practice.

Organization of the Course

The Basic and Clinical Science Course comprises 13 volumes, incorporating fundamental ophthalmic knowledge, subspecialty areas, and special topics:

1 Update on General Medicine
2 Fundamentals and Principles of Ophthalmology
3 Clinical Optics and Vision Rehabilitation
4 Ophthalmic Pathology and Intraocular Tumors
5 Neuro-Ophthalmology
6 Pediatric Ophthalmology and Strabismus
7 Oculofacial Plastic and Orbital Surgery
8 External Disease and Cornea
9 Uveitis and Ocular Inflammation
10 Glaucoma
11 Lens and Cataract
12 Retina and Vitreous
13 Refractive Surgery

References

Readers who wish to explore specific topics in greater detail may consult the references cited within each chapter and listed in the Additional Materials and Resources section at the back of the book. These references are intended to be selective rather than exhaustive, chosen by the BCSC faculty as being important, current, and readily available to residents and practitioners.

Multimedia

This edition of Section 10, *Glaucoma,* includes videos related to topics covered in the book. Selected by members of the BCSC faculty, the videos are available to readers of the print and electronic versions of Section 10 (www.aao.org/bcscvideo_section10). Mobile-device users can scan the QR code below (you may need to install a QR-code reader on the device) to access the video content.

Self-Assessment and CME Credit

Each volume of the BCSC is designed as an independent study activity for ophthalmology residents and practitioners. The learning objectives for this volume are given on page 1. The text, illustrations, and references provide the information necessary to achieve the objectives; the study questions allow readers to test their understanding of the material and their mastery of the objectives. Physicians who wish to claim CME credit for this educational activity may do so by following the instructions given at the end of the book.*

Conclusion

The Basic and Clinical Science Course has expanded greatly over the years, with the addition of much new text, numerous illustrations, and video content. Recent editions have sought to place greater emphasis on clinical applicability while maintaining a solid foundation in basic science. As with any educational program, it reflects the experience of its authors. As its faculties change and medicine progresses, new viewpoints emerge on controversial subjects and techniques. Not all alternate approaches can be included in this series; as with any educational endeavor, the learner should seek additional sources, including Academy Preferred Practice Pattern Guidelines.

The BCSC faculty and staff continually strive to improve the educational usefulness of the course; you, the reader, can contribute to this ongoing process. If you have any suggestions or questions about the series, please do not hesitate to contact the faculty or the editors.

The authors, editors, and reviewers hope that your study of the BCSC will be of lasting value and that each Section will serve as a practical resource for quality patient care.

*This activity meets the Self-Assessment CME requirements defined by the American Board of Ophthalmology (ABO). Please be advised that the ABO is not an accrediting body for purposes of any CME program. ABO does not sponsor this or any outside activity, and ABO does not endorse any particular CME activity. Complete information regarding the ABO Self-Assessment CME Maintenance of Certification requirements is available at https://abop.org/maintain-certification/cme-self-assessment/.

Objectives

Upon completion of BCSC Section 10, *Glaucoma*, the reader should be able to

- state the epidemiologic features of glaucoma, including the social and economic impacts of the disease
- list recent advances in the understanding of hereditary and genetic factors in glaucoma
- describe the physiology of aqueous humor dynamics and the control of intraocular pressure (IOP)
- describe the clinical evaluation of the glaucoma patient, including history and general examination, gonioscopy, optic nerve examination, and visual field
- list the clinical features of the patient considered a glaucoma suspect
- describe the clinical features, evaluation, and treatment of primary open-angle glaucoma and normal-tension glaucoma
- list the various clinical features of and therapeutic approaches for the secondary open-angle glaucomas
- state the underlying causes of the increased IOP in various forms of secondary open-angle glaucoma and the impact that these underlying causes have on disease management
- describe the mechanisms and pathophysiology of primary angle-closure glaucoma
- describe the pathophysiology of secondary angle-closure glaucoma, both with and without pupillary block
- describe the pathophysiology of and therapy for primary congenital and juvenile-onset glaucomas

- describe the various classes of medical therapy for glaucoma, including efficacy, mechanism of action, and safety
- state the indications for, techniques used in, and complications of various laser and incisional surgical procedures for glaucoma

CHAPTER 1

Introduction to Glaucoma: Terminology, Epidemiology, and Genetics

Highlights

- The term *glaucoma* refers to a group of optic neuropathies characterized by optic disc excavation, or cupping, and corresponding patterns of vision loss.
- Glaucomas are classified by age of onset (childhood vs adult onset), etiology (primary vs secondary), and gonioscopic assessment of the iridocorneal angle (open vs closed).
- Elevated intraocular pressure (IOP) is a major risk factor for glaucoma; however, a large proportion of patients with primary open-angle glaucoma have IOP in the statistically normal range.
- Glaucoma is a major public health problem and is the leading cause of irreversible blindness worldwide.
- Many genes and genomic regions have been found to be associated with various types of glaucoma.

Definition

The term *glaucoma* refers to a group of progressive optic neuropathies characterized by an excavated appearance of the optic disc, often described as *cupped* (Fig 1-1), together with loss of retinal ganglion cells and their axons and corresponding vision loss. The primary site of injury is thought to be the lamina cribrosa, which has been shown to be structurally damaged in eyes with glaucomatous optic neuropathy, leading to the appearance of optic disc excavation. The causes of glaucoma are multifactorial and include genetic and environmental factors.

IOP is a continuous risk factor for the development of glaucoma over its entire range; however, it is not elevated above the statistically normal range in a substantial proportion of patients with primary open-angle glaucoma (POAG) and is not a defining characteristic of the disease. *Ocular hypertension (OHT)* is defined as the presence of statistically elevated IOP in the absence of glaucomatous visual field or optic disc damage. A large proportion of patients with OHT do not go on to develop glaucoma.

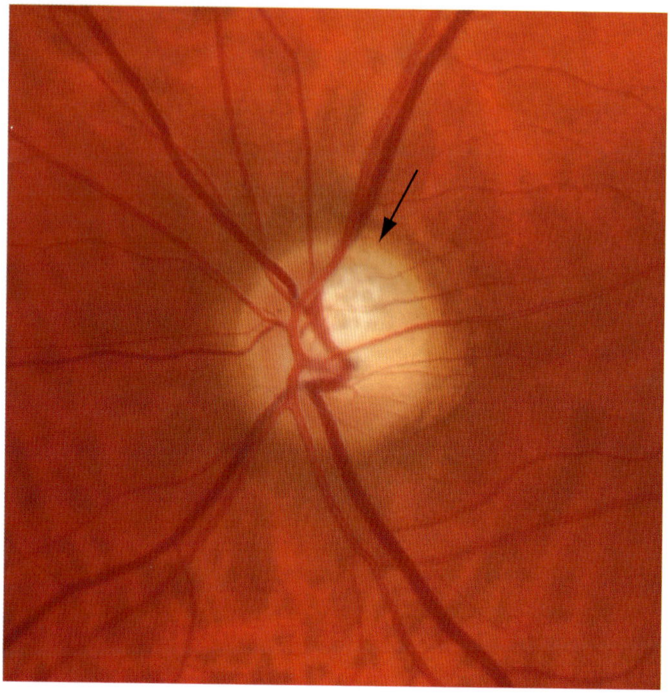

Figure 1-1 Optic disc photograph demonstrating optic disc excavation, or "cupping." Note the focal neural rim loss *(arrow)* and exposed laminar pores superiorly. *(Courtesy of Angelo P. Tanna, MD.)*

In patients with glaucoma, the IOP at baseline—regardless of its actual level—is too high for retinal ganglion cell function and survival. It has been shown that in most patients with glaucoma, lowering the IOP will stop or slow visual field loss. In some eyes, however, optic nerve damage may progress despite treatment to lower the IOP. Clinicians often imprecisely use the word *glaucoma* in describing conditions in which the IOP is elevated in the absence of known glaucomatous neuropathy. Although this is common parlance, it should be avoided.

Quigley HA. Glaucoma. *Lancet.* 2011;377(9774):1367–1377.

Classification

Open-Angle, Angle-Closure, Primary, and Secondary Glaucomas

Adult forms of glaucoma are classified as open angle or angle closure and as primary or secondary (Table 1-1). Pediatric forms of glaucoma are described in Chapter 11. Distinguishing open-angle glaucoma from angle-closure disease is essential from a therapeutic standpoint.

Open angle

In *open-angle glaucoma (OAG),* no obstruction of the trabecular meshwork is visible on gonioscopic examination of the anterior chamber angle. The condition is further classified as *primary open-angle glaucoma (POAG)* when no underlying abnormality known to cause

Table 1-1 Classification of Glaucoma and Related Conditions[a]

I. Open Angle

- A. Primary open-angle glaucoma
  1. Normal-tension glaucoma
  2. Juvenile open-angle glaucoma
- B. Secondary open-angle glaucoma
  1. Pseudoexfoliation syndrome
  2. Pigmentary glaucoma
  3. Traumatic glaucoma (in patients with angle recession, traumatic hyphema, or other evidence of trauma)
  4. Steroid-induced glaucoma
  5. Glaucoma associated with intraocular inflammation
  6. Hemolytic glaucoma (hemoglobin-laden macrophages obstruct TM)
  7. Ghost cell glaucoma (degenerated RBCs obstruct TM)
  8. Glaucoma associated with intraocular tumors (neoplastic cells, cellular material, debris, or RBCs obstruct outflow)
  9. Glaucomatocyclitic crisis (Posner-Schlossman syndrome)
  10. Fuchs uveitis syndrome
  11. Uveitis-glaucoma-hyphema syndrome
  12. Lens associated
      - a. Phacolytic glaucoma (leaked lens proteins obstruct TM)
      - b. Lens particle glaucoma (retained lens material after surgery or trauma)
      - c. Phacoantigenic glaucoma (inflammatory response after surgical or accidental lens trauma)
  13. Glaucoma associated with elevated episcleral venous pressure
  14. Glaucoma associated with siderosis
  15. Schwartz syndrome (IOP elevation caused by photoreceptor outer segment release in association with rhegmatogenous retinal detachment)
  16. IOP elevation associated with anti-VEGF therapy

II. Angle Closure

- A. Primary angle closure[b]
  1. Primary angle-closure suspect (≥180° iridotrabecular contact without IOP elevation, PAS, or glaucomatous optic neuropathy)
  2. Primary angle closure (≥180° iridotrabecular contact with IOP elevation and/or PAS in the absence of glaucomatous optic neuropathy)
  3. Primary angle-closure glaucoma (≥180° iridotrabecular contact with IOP elevation and/or PAS and evidence of glaucomatous optic neuropathy)
  4. Acute angle-closure crisis (closed angle with symptomatic IOP elevation)
  5. Plateau iris configuration (persistent iridotrabecular contact after a patent laser peripheral iridotomy without IOP elevation after pupil dilation)
  6. Plateau iris syndrome (persistent iridotrabecular contact after a patent laser peripheral iridotomy with IOP elevation after pupil dilation)
- B. Secondary angle-closure glaucoma
  1. With pupillary block
      - a. Lens-induced
          - i. Phacomorphic[c]
          - ii. Ectopia lentis

(Continued)

Table 1-1 *(continued)*

- iii. Pseudophakic pupillary block (especially with ACIOL)
- b. Aphakic pupillary block
- c. Posterior synechiae
- 2. Without pupillary block
  - a. Anterior pulling mechanism
    - i. Neovascular glaucoma
    - ii. Iridocorneal endothelial syndrome
    - iii. Posterior polymorphous dystrophy
    - iv. Consolidation of inflammatory material
    - v. Anterior synechiae due to trauma
  - b. Posterior pushing mechanism
    - i. Malignant glaucoma
    - ii. Uveal effusion
    - iii. Anterior rotation of ciliary body (eg, due to CRVO, scleral buckle, PRP)
    - iv. Phacomorphic[c]
    - v. Cysts of iris or ciliary body
    - vi. Persistent fetal vasculature
    - vii. Retinopathy of prematurity

III. Combined-Mechanism Glaucoma

ACIOL = anterior chamber intraocular lens; CRVO = central retinal vein occlusion; IOP = intraocular pressure; PAS = peripheral anterior synechiae; PRP = panretinal photocoagulation; RBCs = red blood cells; TM = trabecular meshwork; VEGF = vascular endothelial growth factor.

[a]For childhood glaucomas, see Chapter 11.

[b]The mechanism of primary angle closure usually involves pupillary block. Plateau iris configuration and syndrome are also usually accompanied by some degree of pupillary block. Those conditions can only be reliably diagnosed after an iridotomy is performed (see Chapter 9).

[c]Phacomorphic glaucoma can be caused by pupillary block and non–pupillary block mechanisms.

IOP elevation is seen on clinical examination; and IOP elevation, if present, cannot be attributed to the use of corticosteroids. OAG is classified as *secondary* when an abnormality is identified that has a putative role in the pathogenesis of the glaucoma.

In eyes that have POAG with elevated IOP, the etiology of the outflow obstruction is thought to be an abnormality in the extracellular matrix of the trabecular meshwork and in trabecular cells in the juxtacanalicular region or an abnormality in the function of the endothelial cells lining the inner wall of Schlemm canal (see Chapter 2). The term *normal-tension glaucoma* is often used for eyes with POAG without known IOP elevation. The conceptual basis for this distinction and for the terminology itself is controversial and is discussed in greater detail in Chapter 7.

Angle closure

In *angle closure,* the peripheral iris partially or completely obstructs the trabecular meshwork. The obstruction may be caused either by appositional iridotrabecular contact or by adhesions, known as *peripheral anterior synechiae (PAS),* between the iris and the trabecular meshwork. When angle closure is present in association with glaucomatous optic neuropathy, it is known as *angle-closure glaucoma.* Angle closure is classified as *primary* in the absence of an underlying disorder to explain the mechanism of iridotrabecular contact or *secondary* when the angle closure can be attributed to certain disease processes (see Table 1-1). Globally, primary angle closure is a major public health problem.

Normal aqueous humor flow in the anterior segment is illustrated in Figure 1-2A. In primary angle closure (and in some forms of secondary angle closure), the flow of aqueous humor from the posterior to the anterior chamber is obstructed at the pupil (Fig 1-2B). The resulting pressure gradient pushes the peripheral iris forward into the anterior chamber angle. This is known as *pupillary block angle closure.*

In some forms of secondary angle closure and in plateau iris, the peripheral iris or the entire lens–iris interface is pushed forward, narrowing the iridocorneal angle (see Chapter 9 in this volume). This can result from an abnormality of the ciliary body, posterior segment tumors, hemorrhage, or other causes described in Chapter 10. In other forms of secondary angle closure, the peripheral iris is pulled forward, typically by contraction of a cellular, fibrovascular, or inflammatory membrane. These conditions are called *non-pupillary block angle closure.*

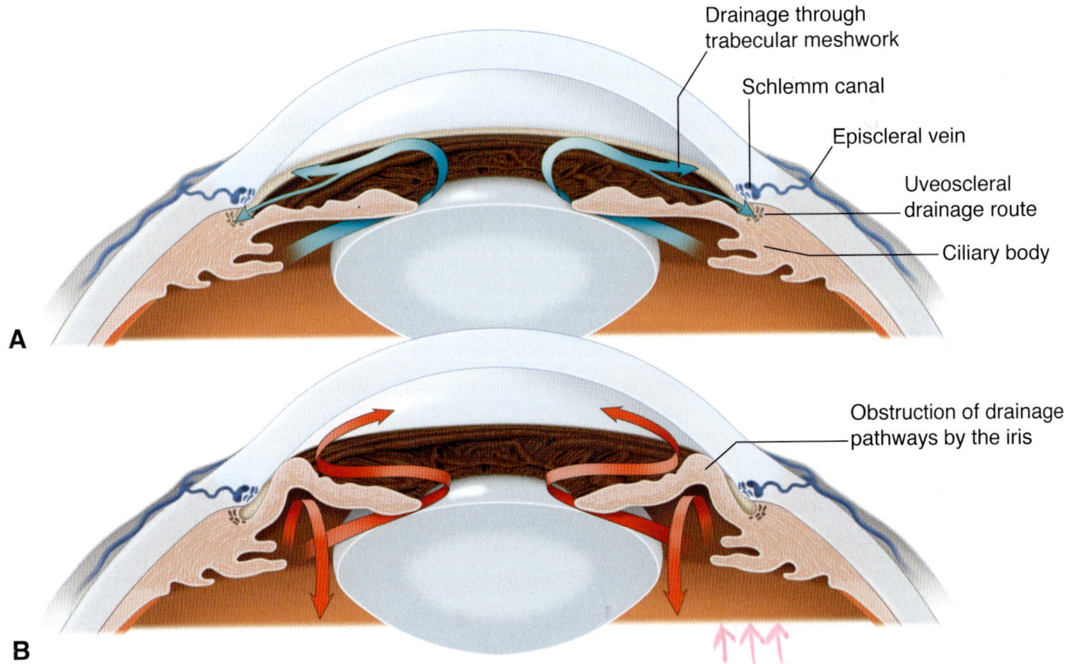

Figure 1-2 Aqueous humor flow. **A,** Normal flow of aqueous humor from the posterior chamber, through the pupil, and into the anterior chamber. Aqueous humor exits the eye through 2 pathways in the iridocorneal angle: the trabecular meshwork and the uveoscleral pathway. **B,** In primary angle closure due to pupillary block, the flow of aqueous through the pupil is obstructed, resulting in a positive pressure gradient between the posterior and anterior chambers, anterior displacement of the peripheral iris, and closure of the anterior chamber angle. *(Illustration by Mark Miller.)*

Combined mechanism

Combined-mechanism glaucoma refers to the condition in which an eye with glaucomatous optic neuropathy that has undergone successful treatment for angle closure with either laser iridotomy or removal of the crystalline lens continues to demonstrate reduced outflow facility and elevated IOP in the absence of PAS. This term can also be used when secondary causes of glaucoma play a role in the disease process in an eye with previously diagnosed POAG or primary angle-closure glaucoma, for example, when a patient with POAG develops a central retinal vein occlusion and subsequent neovascular glaucoma. IOP elevation associated with uveitis may occur due to a combination of mechanisms, including inflammation of the trabecular meshwork, increased viscosity of aqueous humor due to the presence of cells and protein, corticosteroid use, and the presence of PAS.

Epidemiology

As the leading cause of irreversible blindness in the world, glaucoma poses a significant public health problem. It has been estimated that by 2020, approximately 80 million people worldwide will have glaucoma, with 11.2 million bilaterally blind as a result. A meta-analysis estimated that the global prevalence is about 3.5% in the population aged 40–80 years. Because older age is a major risk factor for glaucoma and because life expectancies are increasing in most populations, the prevalence of glaucoma is expected to increase sharply in the coming decades. (Note: The confidence intervals have been omitted around the estimated prevalence and incidence values in this chapter.)

Bourne RR, Taylor HR, Flaxman SR, et al. Number of people blind or visually impaired by glaucoma worldwide and in world regions 1990–2010: a meta-analysis. *PLoS One.* 2016;11(10):e0162229.

Tham YC, Li S, Wong TY, Quigley HA, Aung T, Cheng CY. Global prevalence of glaucoma and projections of glaucoma burden through 2040: a systematic review and meta-analysis. *Ophthalmology.* 2014;121(11):2081–2090.

Primary Open-Angle Glaucoma

Prevalence and incidence

The prevalence (total number of individuals with a disease at a specific time) and incidence (number of new cases that develop during a specific period) of POAG vary widely across population-based samples owing to differences in ethnic and racial representation (Fig 1-3). In the Baltimore Eye Survey, the prevalence of POAG among White individuals ranged from 0.9% in those aged 40–49 years to 2.2% in those aged ≥80 years, whereas the prevalence among Black individuals ranged from 1.2% to 11.3%, respectively. The overall population-based prevalence was 4–5 times higher among Black individuals than White individuals.

In the Rotterdam Study, a longitudinal population-based study of northern Europeans, the observed prevalence was 1.1% among subjects ≥55 years of age. In the same study cohort, the incident risk of developing glaucoma at 10 years was 2.8%. In both the Baltimore Eye Survey and the Rotterdam Study, half of the subjects with glaucoma were unaware of their diagnosis.

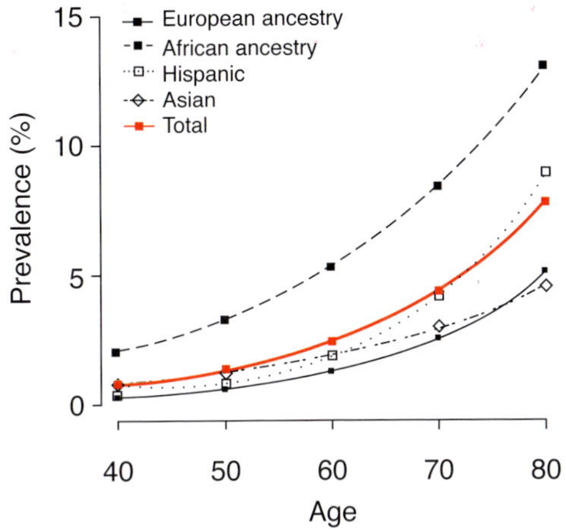

Figure 1-3 The prevalence of primary open-angle glaucoma as a function of age and ethnicity. *(Courtesy of Tham YC, Li X, Wong TY, Quigley HA, Aung T, Cheng CY. Global prevalence of glaucoma and projections of glaucoma burden through 2040: a systematic review and meta-analysis.* Ophthalmology. *2014;121[11]:2081–2090.)*

The prevalence of glaucoma in the Barbados Eye Study (a predominantly African Caribbean population) was 7% in individuals ≥40 years, and the 4-year incidence of glaucoma was 2.2%. Again, older age was found to be a major risk factor for the prevalence and incidence of glaucoma.

The observed prevalence of OAG in the Los Angeles Latino Eye Survey (LALES), a longitudinal population-based study of Latinos (mostly Mexican ancestry) ≥40 years of age, was 4.7%, with 75% unaware of their diagnosis at baseline. The prevalence among those 80 years or older was nearly 22%. The 4-year incidence rate of OAG was 2.3%.

In the Tajimi Study (Japan), the prevalence of POAG among subjects ≥40 years was 3.9%. The IOP was ≤21 mm Hg in 92% of those with POAG. The mean IOP in the nonglaucomatous eyes was 14.5 ± 2.5 mm Hg, about 2 mm Hg lower than observed in European-derived populations.

A meta-analysis estimated the global prevalence of POAG in 2013 to be 3.0% among persons 40–80 years of age. In this age group, the highest prevalence of POAG, an estimated 4.2%, is found in Africa. The same study estimated the prevalence of POAG in North America to be approximately 3.3%.

Leske MC, Connell AM, Wu SY, et al. Incidence of open-angle glaucoma: the Barbados Eye Studies. The Barbados Eye Studies Group. *Arch Ophthalmol.* 2001;119(1):89–95.

Tham YC, Li X, Wong TY, Quigley HA, Aung T, Cheng CY. Global prevalence of glaucoma and projections of glaucoma burden through 2040: a systematic review and meta-analysis. *Ophthalmology.* 2014;121(11):2081–2090.

Tielsch JM, Sommer A, Katz J, Royall RM, Quigley HA, Javitt J. Racial variations in the prevalence of primary open-angle glaucoma. The Baltimore Eye Survey. *JAMA.* 1991;266(3):369–374.

Varma R, Ying-Lai M, Francis BA, et al; Los Angeles Latino Eye Study Group. Prevalence of open-angle glaucoma and ocular hypertension in Latinos: the Los Angeles Latino Eye Study. *Ophthalmology.* 2004;111(8):1439–1448.

Risk factors

Population-based studies and prospective glaucoma clinical trials have identified a number of risk factors that are associated with POAG diagnosis and progression. The most widely accepted risk factors include higher IOP; lower ocular perfusion pressure; older age; lower central corneal thickness (thinner cornea); high myopia; and racial, ethnic, and genetic susceptibility. Other possible risk factors are discussed in Chapter 7.

Leske MC, Heijl A, Hyman L, Bengtsson B, Dong L, Yang Z; EMGT Group. Predictors of long-term progression in the Early Manifest Glaucoma Trial. *Ophthalmology.* 2007;114(11):1965–1972.

Primary Angle-Closure Glaucoma

Prevalence

The prevalence of primary angle-closure glaucoma (PACG) varies among racial and ethnic groups. A meta-analysis estimated the prevalence in Asia to be 1.1% among individuals aged 40–80 years; however, it is even higher in east Asia. Among people of European ancestry >40 years, the prevalence is estimated to between 0.1% and 0.4%. The estimated prevalence in African populations ranges from 0.1% to 0.6%. The highest-known prevalence, estimated to be between 2.5% and 4.8%, is found in Inuit populations >40 years in Alaska and Greenland.

Estimates of the prevalence of PACG vary among different Asian populations. Among those ≥50 years in Guangzhou, China, the prevalence of PACG was 1.5%; and the proportion of these subjects with unilateral blindness was 43% compared with 17% for those with POAG in the same population-based survey. In the Tajimi Study, the prevalence of PACG was 0.6%.

Risk factors

Age, race, and ethnicity are risk factors for PACG. The prevalence of PACG may vary by sex, with a significantly higher prevalence observed in women in most studies. Hyperopia and a family history of angle closure are also important risk factors. Other anatomic risk factors are discussed in Chapter 9.

American Academy of Ophthalmology Glaucoma Panel. Preferred Practice Pattern® Guidelines. *Primary Angle Closure.* American Academy of Ophthalmology; 2015. www.aao.org/ppp

Cho HK, Kee C. Population-based glaucoma prevalence studies in Asians. *Surv Ophthalmol.* 2014;59(4):434–447.

Genetics

In general, the early-onset forms of glaucoma are rare and often follow patterns of simple Mendelian inheritance with mutations that are highly penetrant. Previously, genes with such disease-causing mutations were identified by linkage analysis in large, multigenerational families that show either autosomal dominant or autosomal recessive patterns of inheritance. Current approaches using whole-exome sequencing can successfully identify disease genes using smaller families without evidence of linkage. Genetic regions associated with glaucoma are named according to the type of glaucoma—*GLC1* for open-angle glaucoma, *GLC2* for angle-closure glaucoma, and *GLC3* for congenital glaucoma—followed by a letter to indicate the sequence of discovery: *GLC1A, GLC1B, GLC1C,* and so on. Table 1-2 lists the important genes associated with glaucoma, for which genetic testing may be of clinical utility.

Table 1-2 Clinically Important Glaucoma Loci

Phenotype	Locus	Gene Name (Abbreviation)	Inheritance Pattern
Juvenile open-angle glaucoma	*GLC1A*	Myocilin *(MYOC);* formerly known as trabecular meshwork–induced glucocorticoid response protein *(TIGR)*	Autosomal dominant
Normal-tension glaucoma	*GLC1E*	Optineurin *(OPTN)*	Autosomal dominant
	GLC1P	TANK-binding kinase 1 *(TBK1)*	Autosomal dominant
Primary congenital glaucoma	*GLC3A*	Cytochrome P-450 subfamily 1 B member 1 *(CYP1B1)*	Autosomal recessive
	GLC3D	Latent transforming growth factor β-binding protein 2 *(LTBP2)*	Autosomal recessive
	GLC3E	Tunica interna endothelial cell kinase *(TEK,* also known as *TIE2)*	Autosomal dominant
		Angiopoietin 1 *(ANGPT1)*	Autosomal dominant
Axenfeld-Rieger syndrome	*IRID1*	Forkhead box C1 *(FOXC1)*	Autosomal dominant
	RIEG1	Paired-like homeodomain transcription factor 2 *(PITX2)*	Autosomal dominant
		Complement component 3- and pregnancy zone protein-like alpha-2-macroglobulin domain-containing protein 8 *(CPAMD8)*	Autosomal recessive
Nail-patella syndrome	*NPS*	LIM homeobox transcription factor 1 β *(LMX1B)*	Autosomal dominant
Aniridia		Paired box gene 6 *(PAX6)*	Autosomal dominant

Juvenile Open-Angle Glaucoma

Juvenile open-angle glaucoma (JOAG) is defined by having an onset before 40 years of age, an open anterior chamber angle, and an absence of secondary features. The myocilin gene (*MYOC*, formerly known as trabecular meshwork–inducible glucocorticoid response, or *TIGR*, within the initial larger chromosomal region of *GLC1A*) was the first glaucoma gene discovered. Autosomal dominant disease-causing mutations in *MYOC* account for up to 36% of cases of JOAG and 4% of POAG. There is evidence that mutant myocilin accumulates in cells rather than being secreted, possibly resulting in toxicity to the trabecular meshwork.

Familial Normal-Tension Glaucoma

Familial normal-tension glaucoma (NTG) is associated with mutations in optineurin *(OPTN)* and copy number variations involving TANK-binding kinase 1 *(TBK1)*. These genes encode proteins that interact with each other and are involved in autophagy. These genetic abnormalities are associated with early-onset autosomal dominant familial NTG and account for approximately 2%–3% of cases.

Primary Congenital Glaucoma

Primary congenital glaucoma (PCG) is rare, but it represents the most common form of childhood glaucoma, with an incidence ranging from 1:1250 to 1:10,000 depending on the population studied. Although most cases are sporadic, a large proportion is inherited. Disease-causing mutations have been identified in 4 genes. Recessive mutations in the gene encoding cytochrome P-450 1B1 *(CYP1B1)* are the most common cause of PCG identified to date. Cytochrome P-450 1B1 appears to be required for trabecular meshwork development and function. Recessive mutations in latent transforming growth factor β-binding protein 2 *(LTBP2)* also cause PCG. The gene encodes a protein associated with microfibrils, cell adhesion, and maintenance of the extracellular matrix. Other ophthalmic diseases associated with *LTBP2* mutations include Weill-Marchesani syndrome, microspherophakia, and ectopia lentis. Disease-causing mutations in tunica interna endothelial cell kinase *(TEK,* also known as *TIE2)* and angiopoietin 1 *(ANGPT1)* genes result in maldevelopment of the Schlemm canal in mouse models and are inherited as a dominant trait with variable expressivity in some patients with PCG.

Axenfeld-Rieger Syndrome

Axenfeld-Rieger syndrome includes a spectrum of abnormalities of ocular and systemic development, often associated with glaucoma. Linkage analysis has led to the discovery of autosomal dominant mutations in 2 genes, paired-like homeodomain transcription factor 2 *(PITX2)* and forkhead box C1 *(FOXC1)*. Both genes encode transcription factors that regulate embryonic development.

Aniridia

Aniridia, another ocular developmental disorder, is frequently associated with glaucoma. It occurs in an autosomal dominant inheritance pattern or sporadically. The autosomal dominant form is associated with missense mutations in paired box gene 6 *(PAX6)*, whereas the sporadic form is associated with large deletions or rearrangements involving the same gene, which encodes a transcription factor important for ocular development. Sporadic cases of aniridia caused by large deletions of chromosome 11p13, which includes *PAX6*, can cause a syndrome comprising Wilms tumor, aniridia, genitourinary anomalies, and mental retardation (WAGR syndrome). Patients with large deletions that involve the closely linked Wilms tumor suppressor gene *(WT1)* are at risk for developing Wilms tumor. Therefore, persons with sporadic aniridia should be tested for 11p13 deletions to determine if screening for Wilms tumor is required.

Genome-Wide Association Studies

The more common adult-onset forms of glaucoma are generally associated with complex genetic inheritance patterns. Genome-wide association studies (GWAS) have been used to identify 127 genetic loci associated with POAG and many others associated with PACG and pseudoexfoliation syndrome. GWAS have also led to the discovery of genetic risk alleles for IOP and certain glaucomatous optic nerve features.

Gharahkhani P, Jorgenson E, Hysi P, et al. Genome-wide meta-analysis identifies 127 open-angle glaucoma loci with consistent effect across ancestries. *Nat Commun.* 2021;12(1):1258.

Pseudoexfoliation Syndrome

Pseudoexfoliation syndrome is characterized by the presence of an abnormal fibrillar material that can be visualized on various structures in the anterior segment. Disease-associated genetic variants in lysyl oxidase like 1 (*LOXL1*) are present in up to 99% of cases and 80% of controls. This enzyme is involved in elastin metabolism. The abnormal fibrillar material may impair aqueous humor outflow. In addition, elastin is an important component of the lamina cribrosa, where an abnormality in elastin function may result in increased susceptibility to injury. Other factors, including environmental factors such as sun exposure and low ambient temperature, are thought to contribute to the risk of developing the disease.

Genetic Testing

Genetic counseling and diagnostic testing are important for patients with early-onset glaucoma or ocular developmental abnormalities associated with a high risk of developing glaucoma. Testing for disease-causing mutations in the genes listed in Table 1-2 can be useful to determine patterns of inheritance, identify children at risk early in the disease course, and estimate risk to future offspring.

Lewis CJ, Hedberg-Buenz A, DeLuca AP, Stone EM, Alward WLM, Fingert JH. Primary congenital and developmental glaucomas. *Hum Mol Genet.* 2017;26(R1):R28–R36.

Wiggs JL, Pasquale LR. Genetics of glaucoma. *Hum Mol Genet.* 2017;26(R1):R21–R27.

Environmental Factors

Evidence that environmental factors can play a role in the etiology of glaucoma arises from studies of twins in which the disease was not uniformly manifest in monozygotic twins. These data suggest that while genetic factors contribute to the development of glaucoma, environmental and behavioral factors are also important. Through the use of longitudinal epidemiologic studies (eg, the TwinsUK Registry, the United States Department of Veterans Affairs Normative Aging Study, and the Nurses' Health Study), a number of environmental factors have been identified that possibly modulate the risk for glaucoma. These factors include sun and low ambient temperature exposure (for pseudoexfoliation syndrome), estrogen exposure, cholesterol levels and statin use, and lead exposure.

Kang JH, Loomis, Wiggs JL, Stein JD, Pasquale LR. Demographic and geographic features of exfoliation glaucoma in 2 United States–based prospective cohorts. *Ophthalmology.* 2012;119(1):27–35.

Stein JD, Pasquale LR, Talwar N, et al. Geographic and climatic factors associated with exfoliation syndrome. *Arch Ophthalmol.* 2011;129(8):1053–1060.

CHAPTER 2

Intraocular Pressure and Aqueous Humor Dynamics

This chapter includes a related video. Go to www.aao.org/bcscvideo_section10 or scan the QR code in the text to access this content.

Highlights

- An understanding of aqueous humor dynamics is essential for the evaluation and management of glaucoma.
- Aqueous humor is produced in the ciliary processes at 2–3 µL/min diurnally (and approximately 50% less nocturnally) and drains through the trabecular and uveoscleral pathways.
- The parameters that contribute to intraocular pressure (IOP) are modeled by the modified Goldmann equation; they include outflow facility, aqueous humor production rate, episcleral venous pressure, and uveoscleral outflow rate.
- IOP is found in the population in a skewed distribution, and glaucoma can occur at any pressure level.
- Various tonometry methods can be used to estimate IOP, but all of the devices have inherent sources of measurement error.

Aqueous Humor Production and Outflow

Aqueous Humor Production

As shown in Figure 1-2 in Chapter 1, aqueous humor is produced by the ciliary processes in the posterior chamber and flows through the pupil into the anterior chamber. The average rate of aqueous humor production is 2–3 µL/min while awake, decreasing by about 50% during sleep. Because the anterior segment volume is approximately 200–300 µL, the eye's total volume of aqueous humor is turned over about every 100 minutes. The ciliary body contains approximately 80 ciliary processes, each of which is composed of a double layer of epithelium over a core of stroma and a rich supply of fenestrated capillaries (Fig 2-1). These capillaries are supplied mainly by branches of the major arterial circle of the iris. The apical surfaces of both the outer pigmented and the inner nonpigmented layers of epithelium face each other and are joined by tight junctions, which are an important

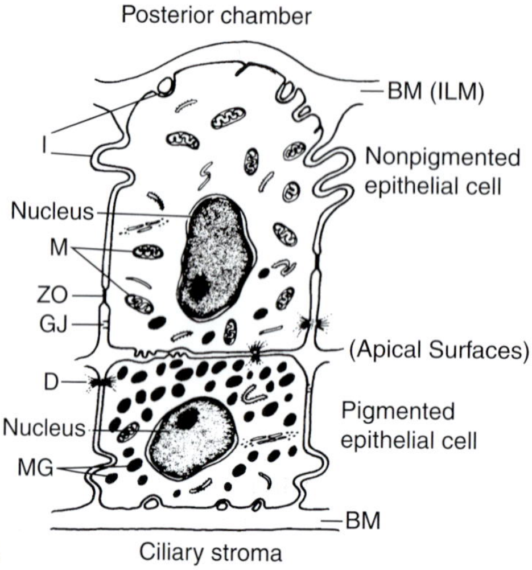

A

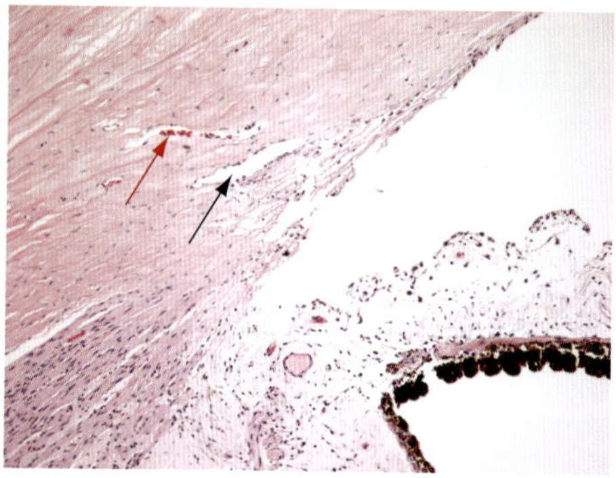

B

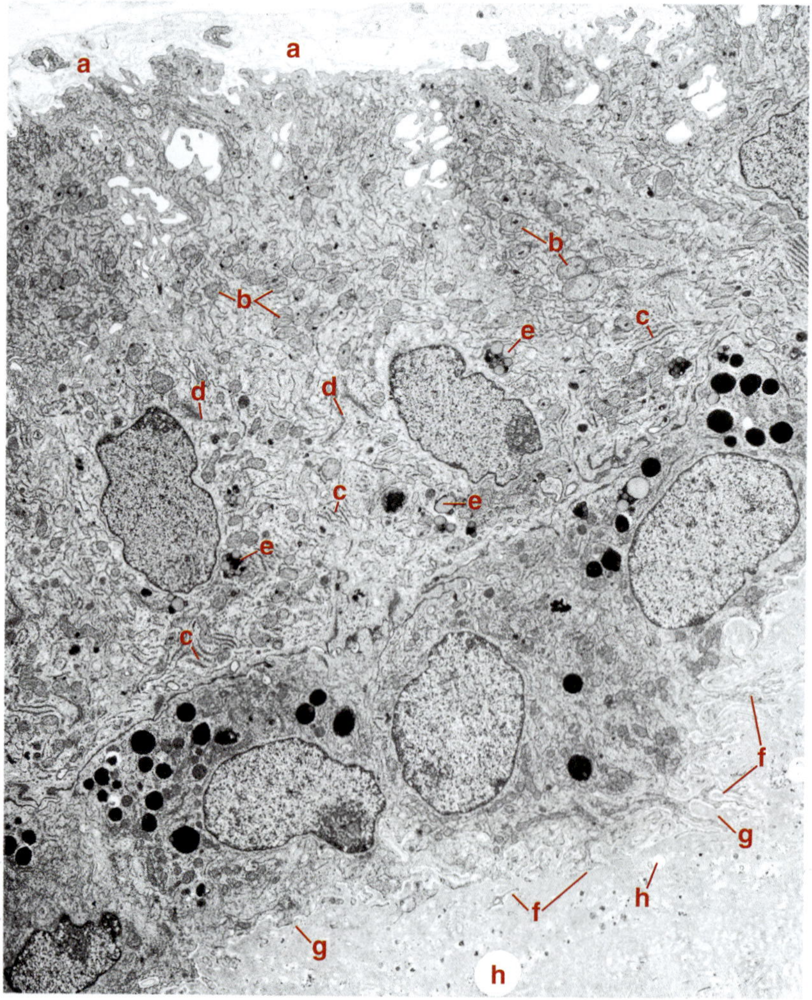

C

(Continued)

component of the blood–aqueous barrier. The inner nonpigmented epithelial cells, which protrude into the posterior chamber, contain numerous mitochondria and microvilli; these cells are thought to be the site of aqueous production. The ciliary processes provide a large surface area for secretion.

Aqueous humor enters the posterior chamber by the following physiologic mechanisms:

- active secretion, which takes place in the double-layered ciliary epithelium
- ultrafiltration
- simple diffusion

Active secretion refers to transport that requires energy to move sodium, chloride, bicarbonate, and other ions (currently unknown) against an electrochemical gradient. Active secretion is independent of pressure and accounts for the majority of aqueous humor production. It involves, at least in part, activity of the enzyme carbonic anhydrase II. *Ultrafiltration* refers to a pressure-dependent movement along a pressure gradient. In the ciliary processes, the hydrostatic pressure difference between capillary pressure and IOP favors fluid movement into the eye, whereas the oncotic gradient between the two resists fluid movement. The relationship between secretion and ultrafiltration is not known. *Diffusion* involves the passive movement of ions, based on charge and concentration, across a membrane.

In humans, aqueous humor has a higher concentration of hydrogen and chloride ions, a higher concentration of ascorbate, and a lower concentration of bicarbonate compared with plasma. In the normal eye, the blood–aqueous barrier keeps the aqueous humor essentially protein-free (1/200–1/500 of the protein found in plasma), allowing for optical clarity. Albumin accounts for approximately half of the total protein. Other

Figure 2-1 *(continued)* Anatomic details of the anterior chamber angle and ciliary body. **A,** The 2 layers of the ciliary epithelium, showing apical surfaces in apposition to each other. Basement membrane (BM) lines the double layer and constitutes the internal limiting membrane (ILM) on the inner surface. The nonpigmented epithelium is characterized by large numbers of mitochondria (M), zonula occludens (ZO), and lateral and surface interdigitations (I). The pigmented epithelium contains numerous melanin granules (MG). Additional intercellular junctions include desmosomes (D) and gap junctions (GJ). **B,** Light micrograph of the anterior chamber angle shows the Schlemm canal *(black arrow),* adjacent to the trabecular meshwork in the sclera. One of the external collector vessels can be seen *(red arrow)* adjacent to the Schlemm canal. **C,** Pars plicata of the ciliary body showing the 2 epithelial layers in the eye of an older person. The nonpigmented epithelial cells measure approximately 20 µm high by 12 µm wide. The cuboidal pigmented epithelial cells are approximately 10 µm high. The thickened ILM *(a)* is laminated and vesicular; such thickened membranes are characteristic of older eyes. The cytoplasm of the nonpigmented epithelium is characterized by its numerous mitochondria *(b)* and the cisternae of the rough-surfaced endoplasmic reticulum *(c).* A poorly developed Golgi apparatus *(d)* and several lysosomes and residual bodies *(e)* are shown. The pigmented epithelium contains many melanin granules, measuring about 1 µm in diameter, located mainly in the apical portion. The basal surface is irregular, with many fingerlike processes *(f).* The basement membrane of the pigmented epithelium *(g)* and a smooth granular material containing vesicles *(h)* and coarse granular particles are seen at the bottom of the figure. The appearance of the basement membrane is typical of older eyes and can be discerned with the light microscope (×5700). *(Part A reproduced with permission from Shields MB.* Textbook of Glaucoma. *3rd ed. Williams & Wilkins; 1992. Part B courtesy of Nasreen A. Syed, MD. Part C modified with permission from Hogan MJ, Alvarado JA, Weddell JE.* Histology of the Human Eye. *Saunders; 1971:283.)*

components of aqueous humor include growth factors; several enzymes such as carbonic anhydrase, lysozyme, diamine oxidase, plasminogen activator, dopamine β-hydroxylase, and phospholipase A_2; and prostaglandins, cyclic adenosine monophosphate (cAMP), catecholamines, steroid hormones, and hyaluronic acid. The composition of the aqueous humor is altered as it flows from the posterior chamber, through the pupil, and into the anterior chamber. This alteration occurs across the hyaloid face of the vitreous, the surface of the lens, the blood vessels of the iris, and the corneal endothelium; and it is secondary to other dilutional exchanges and active processes. See BCSC Section 2, *Fundamentals and Principles of Ophthalmology,* for further discussion of aqueous humor composition and production.

Suppression of Aqueous Humor Formation

Various classes of drugs can suppress formation of aqueous humor. The mechanisms of action of these drugs are discussed in Chapter 12.

Inhibition of the enzyme carbonic anhydrase suppresses aqueous humor formation. However, the precise role of carbonic anhydrase has been debated vigorously. Its function may be to provide the bicarbonate ion, which, evidence suggests, is actively secreted in human eyes. Carbonic anhydrase may also provide bicarbonate or hydrogen ions for an intracellular buffering system.

Blockade of β_2-receptors, the most prevalent adrenergic receptors in the ciliary epithelium, may reduce aqueous humor formation and affect active secretion by causing a decrease either in the efficiency of Na^+,K^+-ATPase or in the number of pump sites. For additional discussion of the sodium-potassium pump and the pump–leak mechanism, see BCSC Section 2, *Fundamentals and Principles of Ophthalmology.* Stimulation of α_2-receptors also reduces aqueous humor formation, possibly by means of a decrease in ciliary body blood flow mediated through inhibition of cAMP; the exact mechanism is unclear.

Aqueous Humor Outflow

Aqueous humor outflow occurs by 2 major mechanisms: (1) the pressure-sensitive *trabecular* (or *conventional*) pathway and (2) the pressure-insensitive *uveoscleral* (or *unconventional*) pathway.

Trabecular outflow

Aqueous humor exiting the eye through the trabecular pathway first crosses the trabecular meshwork, enters the Schlemm canal, passes through collector channels in the outer wall of the Schlemm canal, which drain either directly into aqueous veins or into the vessels of the intrascleral plexus, which then drain into aqueous veins. From there, aqueous humor returns to the systemic circulation via the episcleral venous system, which connects to the anterior ciliary and superior ophthalmic veins, ultimately draining into the cavernous sinus.

The *trabecular meshwork* is classically divided into 3 layers: (1) uveal, (2) corneoscleral, and (3) juxtacanalicular (Fig 2-2). The *uveal trabecular meshwork* is adjacent to the anterior chamber and is arranged in bands that extend from the iris root and the ciliary body

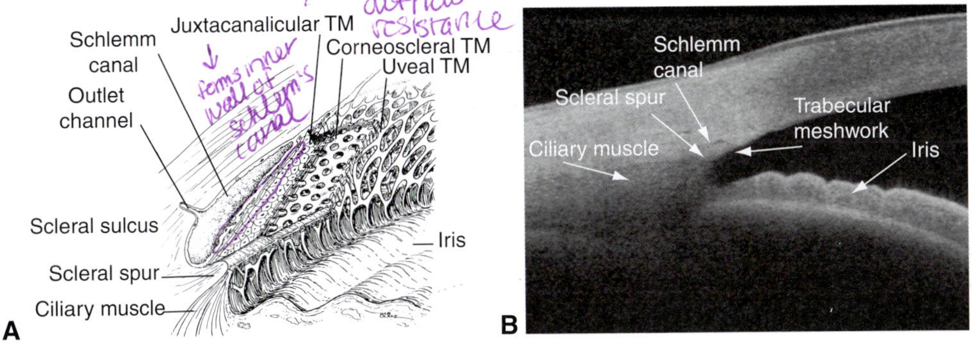

Figure 2-2 Trabecular meshwork and Schlemm canal. **A,** Three layers of the trabecular meshwork (TM; shown in cutaway views): uveal, corneoscleral, and juxtacanalicular. **B,** Anterior segment optical coherence tomography image of the TM and Schlemm canal. *(Part A modified with permission from Shields MB.* Textbook of Glaucoma. *3rd ed. Williams & Wilkins; 1992; part B courtesy of Syril K. Dorairaj, MD.)*

to the peripheral cornea. The *corneoscleral meshwork* consists of sheets of trabeculum that extend from the scleral spur to the lateral wall of the scleral sulcus. The *juxtacanalicular meshwork,* which is thought to be the major site of outflow resistance, is adjacent to and actually forms the inner wall of the Schlemm canal. Aqueous humor moves both across and between the endothelial cells lining the inner wall of the Schlemm canal.

The trabecular meshwork is composed of multiple layers, each of which consists of a collagenous connective tissue core covered by a continuous endothelial layer. The trabecular meshwork is the site of pressure-sensitive aqueous humor outflow and functions as a 1-way valve, permitting aqueous humor to leave the eye by bulk flow but limiting flow in the other direction, independent of energy. The cells of the trabecular meshwork are phagocytic, and this function may increase in the presence of inflammation and after laser trabeculoplasty.

In most older adults, the trabecular cells contain a large number of pigment granules in their cytoplasm, giving the entire meshwork a pigmented appearance, the degree of which can vary with position in the meshwork and among individuals. There are approximately 200,000–300,000 trabecular cells per eye. With age, the number of trabecular cells decreases, and the basement membrane beneath them thickens, potentially increasing outflow resistance. An interesting effect of all types of laser trabeculoplasty is that it induces division of trabecular cells and causes a change in the production of cytokines and other structurally important elements of the extracellular matrix. The extracellular matrix material is found throughout the dense portions of the trabecular meshwork.

The *Schlemm canal* is completely lined with an endothelial layer that rests on a discontinuous basement membrane. The canal is a single channel, typically with a diameter of about 200–300 μm, although there is significant variability, and it is traversed by tubules. The exact path of aqueous flow across the inner wall of the Schlemm canal is uncertain. Intracellular and intercellular pores suggest bulk flow, while so-called *giant vacuoles* that have direct communication with the intertrabecular spaces suggest active transport; however, these vacuoles may be artifacts of tissue preparation and microscopy. The outer wall of the Schlemm canal is formed by a single layer of endothelial cells that do not contain pores.

A complex system of *collector channels* connects the Schlemm canal to the aqueous veins, which in turn drain into the episcleral veins, forming the *distal portion* of the trabecular outflow system (Video 2-1). The episcleral veins subsequently drain into the anterior ciliary and superior ophthalmic veins. These, in turn, ultimately drain into the cavernous sinus.

VIDEO 2-1 Aqueous humor flow through the distal outflow system as seen using indocyanine green aqueous angiography.
Courtesy of Alex Huang, MD, PhD.
Go to www.aao.org/bcscvideo_section10 to access all videos in Section 10.

The trabecular outflow pathway is dynamic. With increasing IOP, the cross-sectional area of the Schlemm canal decreases, while the trabecular meshwork expands. Similarly, in the distal outflow system, the amount of aqueous humor flow through individual vessels appears to vary dynamically. The effect of these changes on outflow resistance is unclear.

Johnson M. What controls aqueous humour outflow resistance? *Exp Eye Res.* 2006;82(4):545–557.

Uveoscleral outflow

In the normal eye, any nontrabecular outflow is termed *uveoscleral,* or *unconventional, outflow.* Uveoscleral outflow is also referred to as *pressure-insensitive outflow.* Although it is pressure insensitive, uveoscleral outflow is bulk flow that depends on a pressure gradient that remains relatively constant with changes in IOP. Various mechanisms are probably involved in uveoscleral outflow, but the predominant one is passage of aqueous humor from the anterior chamber into the interstitial spaces between the ciliary muscle bundles and then into the supraciliary and suprachoroidal spaces. From there, the exact path of the aqueous humor exiting the eye is unclear. It may include passage through the intact sclera or along the nerves and vessels that penetrate it or may involve absorption into the vortex veins. Lymphatic vessels have also been identified in the ciliary body, and aqueous humor drainage through a uveolymphatic pathway has also been proposed.

Johnson M, McLaren JW, Overby DR. Unconventional aqueous humor outflow: a review. *Exp Eye Res.* 2017;158:94–111.

Aqueous Humor Dynamics

An understanding of aqueous humor dynamics is essential for the evaluation and management of glaucoma. Aqueous humor dynamics involves the measurement of parameters that affect IOP. The modified *Goldmann equation* is a mathematical model of the relationship between IOP and the parameters that contribute to its level in the eye at steady state:

$$P_0 = (F - U)/C + P_v$$

where P_0 is the IOP in mm Hg, F is the rate of aqueous humor production in microliters per minute (μL/min), U is the rate of aqueous humor drainage through the pressure-insensitive uveoscleral pathway in microliters per minute (μL/min), C is the facility of

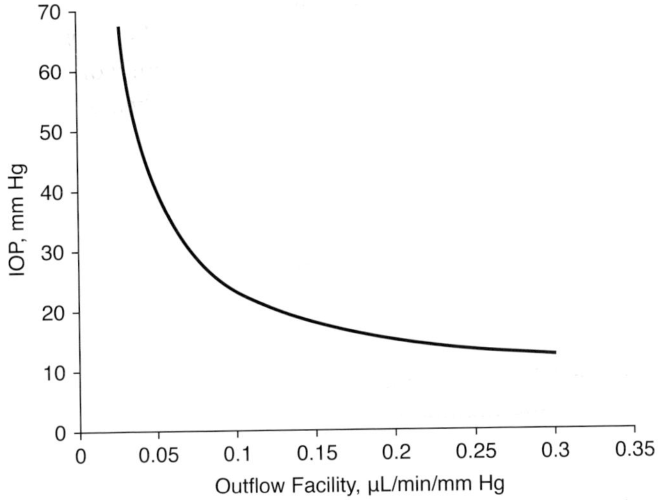

Figure 2-3 The effect of outflow facility on intraocular pressure (IOP), based on the modified Goldmann equation (assuming a constant aqueous humor production rate of 2.5 μL/min, uveoscleral outflow rate of 35%, and episcleral venous pressure of 7 mm Hg). *(Courtesy of Arthur J. Sit, MD.)*

outflow through the pressure-sensitive trabecular pathway in microliters per minute per mm Hg (μL/min/mm Hg), and P_v is the episcleral venous pressure in mm Hg. Although there are 5 parameters in the equation, only 4 need to be measured—the fifth parameter can then be calculated. Resistance to outflow *(R)* is the inverse of facility *(C)*. Figure 2-3 illustrates the effect of reduced outflow facility *(C)* on IOP.

Measurement of Aqueous Humor Production

The rate of aqueous humor production by the ciliary processes cannot be measured noninvasively, but it is assumed to be equal to the aqueous humor outflow rate in an eye at steady state. The most common method used to measure the rate of aqueous humor outflow is *fluorophotometry*. For this test, fluorescein is administered topically, its gradual dilution in the anterior chamber is measured optically, and the change in fluorescein concentration over time is then used to calculate aqueous flow. As previously noted, the normal flow rate is approximately 2–3 μL/min while awake, and the aqueous volume is turned over at a rate of approximately 1% per minute.

The rate of aqueous humor formation varies diurnally and is reduced by approximately half during sleep. It also decreases with age. The rate is affected by a variety of factors, including the following:

- integrity of the blood–aqueous barrier
- blood flow to the ciliary body
- neurohumoral regulation of vascular tissue and the ciliary epithelium

Aqueous humor production may decrease after trauma or intraocular inflammation and after the administration of certain systemic drugs (eg, general anesthetics and some systemic hypotensive agents), as well as aqueous humor suppressants used for treatment of glaucoma. Carotid occlusive disease may also decrease aqueous humor production.

Brubaker RF. Flow of aqueous humor in humans [The Friedenwald Lecture]. *Invest Ophthalmol Vis Sci.* 1991;32(13):3145–3166.

Measurement of Outflow Facility

The facility of outflow (*C* in the Goldmann equation) is the mathematical inverse of outflow resistance and varies widely in normal eyes, with a mean ranging from 0.22 to 0.30 μL/min/mm Hg. Outflow facility decreases with age and is affected by surgery, trauma, medications, and endocrine factors. Patients with glaucoma and elevated IOP typically have decreased outflow facility. In normal eyes, approximately 50% of conventional outflow resistance is in the trabecular meshwork, while the remainder is in the distal outflow system. However, in primary open-angle glaucoma with elevated IOP or ocular hypertension, most of the pathologic change occurs in the juxtacanalicular tissue of the trabecular meshwork and inner wall of the Schlemm canal.

Tonography is a method used to measure the facility of aqueous humor outflow. In this technique, a weighted Schiøtz tonometer or pneumatonometer is placed on the cornea, acutely elevating the IOP. Outflow facility in μL/min/mm Hg can be computed from the rate at which the pressure declines with time, reflecting the ease with which aqueous humor leaves the eye.

However, tonography depends on a number of assumptions (eg, ocular rigidity, stability of aqueous humor formation, and constancy of ocular blood volume) and is subject to many sources of error, such as poor patient fixation and eyelid squeezing. These problems reduce the accuracy and reproducibility of tonography for an individual patient. In general, tonography is best employed as a research tool and is rarely used clinically.

Kazemi A, McLaren JW, Lin SC, et al. Comparison of aqueous outflow facility measurement by pneumatonography and digital Schiøtz tonography. *Invest Ophthalmol Vis Sci.* 2017;58(1):204–210.

Rosenquist R, Epstein D, Melamed S, Johnson M, Grant WM. Outflow resistance of enucleated human eyes at two different perfusion pressures and different extents of trabeculotomy. *Curr Eye Res.* 1989;8(12):1233–1240.

Vahabikashi A, Gelman A, Dong B, et al. Increased stiffness and flow resistance of the inner wall of Schlemm's canal in glaucomatous human eyes. *Proc Natl Acad Sci USA.* 2019;116(52):26555–26563.

Measurement of Episcleral Venous Pressure

The episcleral veins are the ultimate destination for aqueous humor draining through the trabecular pathway. Thus, the pressure in these veins, the *episcleral venous pressure (EVP)*, represents the lowest possible IOP in an intact eye with normal aqueous humor production. It is a dynamic parameter that varies with alterations in body position and systemic blood pressure. EVP is often increased in syndromes with facial hemangiomas (eg, Sturge-Weber), carotid-cavernous sinus fistulas, and cavernous sinus thrombosis; and it may be partially responsible for the elevated IOP seen in thyroid eye disease. EVP may also be altered by some medications, including topical Rho kinase inhibitors.

EVP can be measured noninvasively by *venomanometry,* in which a transparent flexible membrane is placed against the sclera and the pressure is slowly increased. The pressure that begins to collapse an episcleral vein corresponds to EVP; however, visualizing this endpoint can be difficult. The use of automated pressure measurements, video recording of the vein collapse, and image analysis software can help to precisely identify the endpoint and associated EVP. The usual range of values is 6–9 mm Hg, but higher values have been reported when different endpoints and measurement techniques are used. According to the Goldmann equation, IOP acutely rises approximately 1 mm Hg for every 1 mm Hg increase in EVP. However, elevation of EVP can cause reflux of blood into the Schlemm canal, altering the normal outflow of aqueous humor. As a result, the change in IOP may be greater or less than that predicted by the Goldmann equation.

Sit AJ, McLaren JW. Measurement of episcleral venous pressure. *Exp Eye Res.* 2011; 93(3):291–298.

Measurement of Uveoscleral Outflow Rate

Uveoscleral outflow rate cannot be measured noninvasively and, therefore, is usually calculated from the Goldmann equation after determination of the other parameters. There is evidence that outflow via the uveoscleral pathway is significant in human eyes, accounting for up to 45% of total aqueous outflow, although invasive studies using tracers tend to report lower values. Some studies indicate that uveoscleral outflow decreases with age and is reduced in patients with glaucoma. It is increased by cycloplegia, adrenergic agents, and prostaglandin $F_{2\alpha}$ analogues but decreased by miotics. It is also increased by suprachoroidal stents and by cyclodialysis clefts.

Bill A, Phillips CI. Uveoscleral drainage of aqueous humour in human eyes. *Exp Eye Res.* 1971;12(3):275–281.
Brubaker RF. Measurement of uveoscleral outflow in humans. *J Glaucoma.* 2001;10(5 Suppl 1): S45–S48.

Intraocular Pressure

IOP Distribution and Relation to Glaucoma

Pooled data from large epidemiologic studies indicate that the mean IOP in the general population of European ancestry is approximately 15.5 mm Hg, with a standard deviation of 2.6 mm Hg. IOP has a non-Gaussian distribution with a skew toward higher pressures, especially in individuals older than 40 years (Fig 2-4). IOP is also genetically influenced. The value 21 mm Hg (2 standard deviations above the mean) was traditionally used both to separate normal from abnormal pressures and to define which patients required ocular hypotensive therapy. However, it is now understood that glaucoma is a multifactorial disease process for which IOP is an important risk factor. Many patients with glaucoma consistently have IOPs ≤21 mm Hg, and most individuals with IOP >21 mm Hg do not

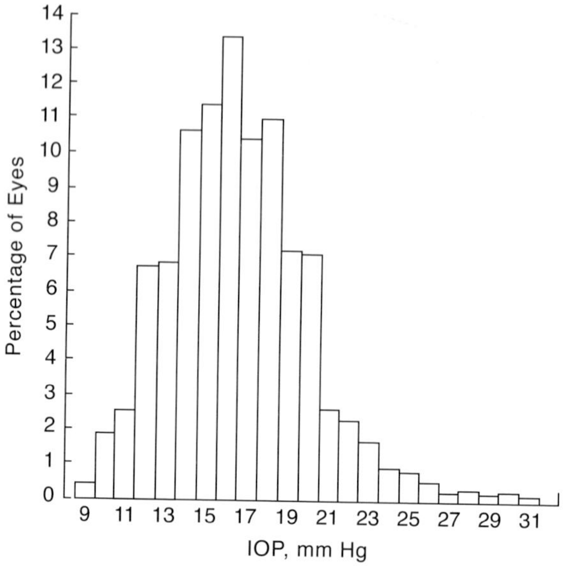

Figure 2-4 Frequency distribution of IOP: 5220 eyes in the Framingham Eye Study. *(Modified from Colton T, Ederer F. The distribution of intraocular pressures in the general population.* Surv Ophthalmol. *1980;25[3]: 123–129.)*

develop glaucoma. Further, the cutoff value of 21 mm Hg is statistically flawed, given the non-Gaussian distribution of IOP values in the population. Consequently, screening for glaucoma based solely on the criterion of IOP >21 mm Hg misses up to half of the people with glaucoma and optic nerve damage in the screened population.

General agreement has been reached that, for the population as a whole, there is no clear level below which IOP can be considered "normal" or safe and above which IOP can be considered "elevated" or unsafe. IOP is a continuous risk factor across its entire range: the higher the IOP, the greater the risk for glaucoma. Although other risk factors affect an individual's susceptibility to glaucoma, all current treatments are designed to reduce IOP.

Sommer A, Tielsch JM, Katz J, et al. Relationship between intraocular pressure and primary open-angle glaucoma among white and black Americans. The Baltimore Eye Survey. *Arch Ophthalmol.* 1991;109(8):1090–1095.

Variations in IOP

Intraocular pressure varies with a number of factors, including the time of day (see the section "Circadian variation"), heartbeat, respiration, exercise, fluid intake, systemic medications, and topical medications (Table 2-1).

Body position has a significant effect on IOP, and the lowest IOP measurements are obtained when a person is seated with the neck in neutral position. IOP is higher when an individual is recumbent rather than upright, predominantly because of an increase in the EVP. Some people have an exaggerated rise in IOP when recumbent; this tendency may be important in the pathogenesis of certain forms of glaucoma. Alcohol consumption causes

Table 2-1 Factors That Affect Intraocular Pressure

Factors that may increase intraocular pressure

- Elevated episcleral venous pressure
  - Bending over or being in a supine position
  - Breath holding
  - Elevated central venous pressure
  - Intubation
  - Orbital venous outflow obstruction
  - Playing a wind instrument
  - Valsalva maneuver
  - Wearing a tight collar or tight necktie
- Pressure on the eye
  - Blepharospasm
  - Eyelid squeezing and crying, especially in young children
- Elevated body temperature (associated with increased aqueous humor production)
- Hormonal influences
  - Hypothyroidism
  - Thyroid eye disease
- Drugs unrelated to glaucoma therapy
  - Anticholinergics: may precipitate angle closure
  - Corticosteroids
  - Ketamine
  - Lysergic acid diethylamide (LSD)
  - Topiramate

Factors that may decrease intraocular pressure

- Aerobic exercise
- Anesthetic drugs
  - Depolarizing muscle relaxants such as succinylcholine
- Metabolic or respiratory acidosis (decreases aqueous humor production)
- Hormonal influences
  - Pregnancy
- Drugs unrelated to glaucoma therapy
  - Alcohol
  - Heroin
  - Marijuana (cannabis)
  - Ketamine

a transient decrease in IOP. Cannabis also decreases IOP but has not proved clinically useful because of its short duration of action and its side effects. In most studies, caffeine has not been shown to have an appreciable effect on IOP. There is little variation in IOP with age in healthy individuals.

Circadian variation

In individuals without glaucoma, IOP varies by 2–6 mm Hg over a 24-hour period, as aqueous humor production, outflow facility, and uveoscleral outflow rate change. Higher mean IOP is associated with wider fluctuation in pressure. The time at which peak IOP occurs varies among individuals. However, 24-hour IOP measurement performed with individuals in their habitual body positions (standing or sitting during the daytime and supine at night) indicates that most people (with or without glaucoma) have peak pressures during sleep, in the early-morning hours, corresponding with a decrease in aqueous humor production, outflow facility, and uveoscleral outflow. During the waking hours, peak pressure often occurs soon after awakening. In selected patients, measurement of IOP outside office hours may be useful in determining why optic nerve damage continues to occur despite apparently adequately controlled pressure.

Liu JH, Zhang X, Kripke DF, Weinreb RN. Twenty-four-hour intraocular pressure pattern associated with early glaucomatous changes. *Invest Ophthalmol Vis Sci.* 2003;44(4):1586–1590.

Nau CB, Malihi M, McLaren JW, Hodge DO, Sit AJ. Circadian variation of aqueous humor dynamics in older healthy adults. *Invest Ophthalmol Vis Sci.* 2013;54(12):7623–7629.

IOP fluctuation and glaucoma

A significant body of literature demonstrates an association between IOP fluctuation and the risk of glaucoma progression. However, the data are largely retrospective, based on post hoc analyses of IOP variations between visits in large clinical trials. IOP fluctuation is also closely correlated with the level of mean IOP and appears to be a more important risk factor in certain groups of patients, including those with low IOP. Surgery results in less IOP fluctuation than medical therapy, but the clinical significance of this finding has not been demonstrated. Moreover, the specific measures of variability that may best predict glaucoma progression are not known, and the technology to effectively measure IOP fluctuation in a short time frame is currently limited.

Caprioli J, Coleman AL. Intraocular pressure fluctuation a risk factor for visual field progression at low intraocular pressures in the Advanced Glaucoma Intervention Study. *Ophthalmology.* 2008;115(7):1123–1129.

Musch DC, Gillespie BW, Niziol LM, Lichter PR, Varma R; CIGTS Study Group. Intraocular pressure control and long-term visual field loss in the Collaborative Initial Glaucoma Treatment Study. *Ophthalmology.* 2011;118(9):1766–1773.

Clinical Measurement of IOP

Tonometry is the noninvasive measurement of IOP. Many different methods of tonometry have been developed, and each has advantages and disadvantages. All currently used methods have sources of error, and no device can accurately measure intracameral pressure in all eyes.

Applanation tonometry

Applanation tonometry, the most widely used method, is based on the Imbert-Fick principle, which states that the pressure inside an ideal dry, infinitely thin-walled sphere equals the force necessary to flatten its surface divided by the area of the flattening:

$$P = F/A$$

where P = pressure, F = force, and A = area. In applanation tonometry, the cornea is flattened, and IOP is determined by measuring the applanating force and the area flattened.

The *Goldmann applanation tonometer* (Fig 2-5) measures the force necessary to flatten an area of the cornea 3.06 mm in diameter. At this diameter, the material resistance of the cornea to flattening is counterbalanced by the capillary attraction of the tear film meniscus to the tonometer head. Furthermore, the IOP (in mm Hg) equals the flattening

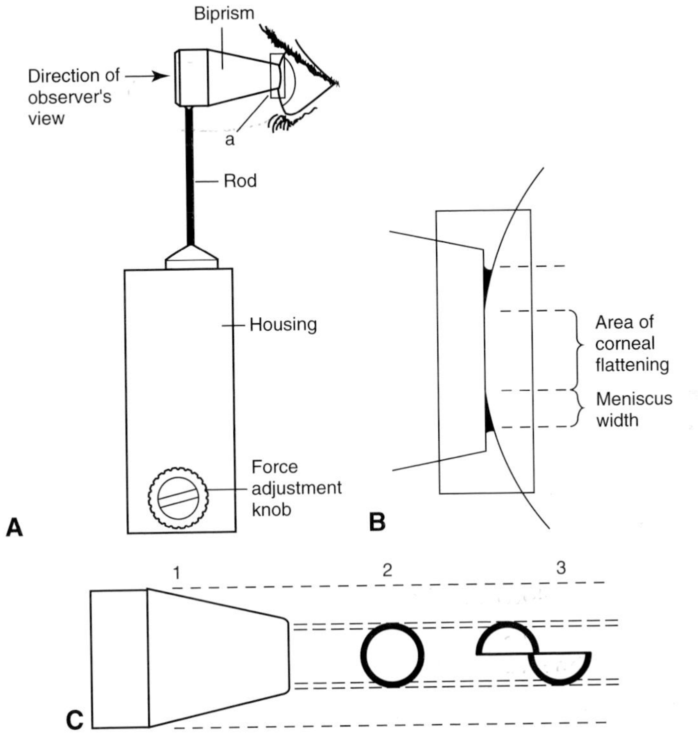

Figure 2-5 Goldmann-type applanation tonometry. **A,** Basic features of the tonometer, shown in contact with the patient's cornea. **B,** The enlargement shows the tear film meniscus created by contact of the split-image prism and cornea. **C,** The view through the split-image prism *(1)* reveals a circular meniscus *(2)*, which is converted into 2 semicircles *(3)* by the prisms. *(Redrawn with permission from Shields MB.* Textbook of Glaucoma. *3rd ed. Williams & Wilkins; 1992.)*

force (in gram-force) multiplied by 10. A split-image prism allows the examiner to determine the flattened area with great accuracy. Topical anesthetic and fluorescein dye are instilled in the tear film to outline the area of flattening. Fluorescein semicircles, or *mires,* visible through the split-image prism move with the ocular pulse, and the endpoint is reached when the inner edges of the semicircles touch each other at the midpoint of their excursion (Fig 2-6). By properly aligning the mires, the examiner can ensure the appropriate area of corneal applanation to obtain the most accurate IOP reading.

The *Perkins tonometer* is a counterbalanced applanation tonometer that, like the Goldmann tonometer, uses a split-image prism and requires instillation of fluorescein dye in the tear film. It is portable and can be used with the patient either upright or supine.

Applanation measurements are safe, easy to perform, and relatively accurate in most clinical situations. Of the currently available devices, the Goldmann applanation tonometer is the most widely used in clinical practice and research. Because applanation does not displace much fluid (approximately 0.5 μL) or substantially increase the pressure in the eye, IOP measurement by this method is relatively unaffected by ocular rigidity, compared with indentation tonometry (see the section “Indentation tonometry”).

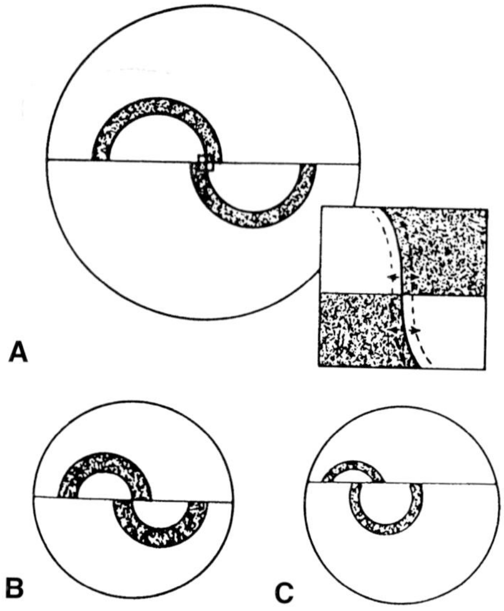

Figure 2-6 Mires viewed through the split-image prism of the Goldmann-type applanation tonometer. **A,** Proper width and position. The enlargement depicts excursions of the mires, which are caused by ocular pulsations. **B,** The mires are too wide. **C,** Improper vertical and horizontal alignment. *(Reproduced with permission from Shields MB.* Textbook of Glaucoma. *3rd ed. Williams & Wilkins; 1992.)*

The accuracy of applanation tonometry can be reduced in certain situations (see Table 2-2, which lists possible sources of error in tonometry). An inadequate amount of fluorescein can lead to poor visualization of the mires and the measurement endpoint, resulting in inaccurate readings. Tear film thickness can also affect accuracy. A common misconception is that a thick tear film leads to erroneous readings because of excessively thick mires, which require greater force to reach the measurement endpoint. However, this is incorrect, as the inner edges of the mires will touch when an area 3.06 mm in diameter is applanated, regardless of the mire thickness. Rather, the error occurs because the surface tension changes with tear film thickness. Because the cornea is curved, an increasing tear film thickness will form a meniscus with a larger radius of curvature, which has a lower surface tension. The low surface tension inadequately counterbalances the corneal resistance, resulting in an artificially high IOP reading. Conversely, a very thin tear film has a small radius of curvature with a high surface tension that exceeds the corneal resistance, yielding a falsely low IOP reading.

Marked corneal astigmatism can also produce inaccuracy, as the fluorescein pattern seen by the clinician through the instrument appears elliptical, and the IOP may be artificially high or low. To obtain an accurate reading in an astigmatic eye, the clinician should rotate the prism so that the red mark on the prism holder is set at the least-curved meridian of the cornea (along the negative axis). Alternatively, 2 pressure readings taken 90° apart can be averaged. Corneal edema predisposes to inaccurately low readings, whereas pressure measurements taken over a corneal scar will be falsely high. Tonometry performed over a soft contact lens gives artificially low values. Central corneal thickness is another factor that can affect the accuracy of tonometry; see the following section.

Whitacre MM, Stein R. Sources of error with use of Goldmann-type tonometers. *Surv Ophthalmol.* 1993;38(1):1–30.

Table 2-2 Possible Sources of Error in Tonometry

Factors That May Cause Artificially Low IOP	Factors That May Cause Artificially High IOP
Corneal biomechanical properties (eg, rigidity)	Breath holding or Valsalva maneuver
Corneal edema	Corneal biomechanical properties (eg, rigidity)
Corneal irregularity (eg, ectasia)	Corneal irregularity (eg, ectasia)
High corneal astigmatism	Corneal scarring or band keratopathy
Inaccurately calibrated tonometer	Excessively thick tear film
Inadequate amount of fluorescein in tear film	Extraocular muscle force applied to a restricted globe
Measurement done over a soft contact lens	High corneal astigmatism
Technician errors	Inaccurately calibrated tonometer
Thin central cornea	Obesity or straining to reach slit lamp
	Pressure on the globe
	Squeezing of the eyelids
	Technician errors
	Thick central cornea
	Tight collar or tight necktie

IOP = intraocular pressure.

Tonometry and central corneal thickness

Measurements obtained with the most common types of tonometers are affected by central corneal thickness (CCT). Goldmann tonometer readings are most accurate when the CCT is 520 µm. Thicker corneas resist the deformation inherent in most methods of tonometry, resulting in an overestimation of IOP, while thinner corneas may give an artificially low reading. IOP may also be underestimated after laser or other types of keratorefractive surgery if these procedures resulted in a CCT significantly less than that assumed for Goldmann tonometry.

The relationship between measured IOP and CCT is not linear, so correction factors are only estimates at best. In addition, the biomechanical properties of individual corneas may vary, and the stiffness or elasticity of the cornea may affect IOP measurement. Currently, there is no validated correction factor for the effect of CCT on applanation tonometers; therefore, the correction methods proposed in the literature are not applicable to clinical use. A thin central cornea is a known risk factor for progression from ocular hypertension to glaucoma. However, it has not been determined whether this increased risk of glaucoma is attributable only to underestimation of IOP or whether a thin central cornea is a biomarker for another risk factor independent of IOP measurement (see Chapter 4).

Gordon MO, Beiser JA, Brandt JA, et al. The Ocular Hypertension Treatment Study: baseline factors that predict the onset of primary open-angle glaucoma. *Arch Ophthalmol.* 2002; 120(6):714–720.

Mackay-Marg–type tonometers

Mackay-Marg–type tonometers use an annular ring to gently flatten a small area of the cornea. As the area of flattening increases, the pressure in the center of the ring increases as well and is measured with a transducer. The IOP is equivalent to the pressure when the center of the ring is just covered by the flattened cornea.

Portable electronic devices of the Mackay-Marg type (eg, Tono-Pen, Reichert Technologies; Fig 2-7A) contain a strain gauge to measure the pressure at the center of an annular ring placed on the cornea. The instrument tip is tapped against the surface of the cornea, obtaining several measurements that are then used by the device to provide an IOP measurement along with the coefficient of variation. These devices are particularly useful in patients with corneal scars or edema, as the measurement tip is small enough to be applied only on areas of normal cornea. It also can be used to obtain measurements regardless of the patient's body position. However, some studies suggest that the Tono-Pen tends to overestimate low IOPs and underestimate high IOPs.

Eisenberg DL, Sherman BG, McKeown CA, Schuman JS. Tonometry in adults and children. A manometric evaluation of pneumatonometry, applanation, and TonoPen in vitro and in vivo. *Ophthalmology.* 1998;105(7):1173–1181.

Mackay RS, Marg E. Fast, automatic, electronic tonometers based on an exact theory. *Acta Ophthalmol (Copenh).* 1959;37:495–507.

Pneumatonometer

The *pneumatic tonometer,* or *pneumatonometer,* is an applanation tonometer that shares some characteristics with the Mackay-Marg–type devices (Fig 2-7B). It has a cylindrical air-filled chamber and a probe tip covered with a flexible, inert silicone elastomer (Silastic membrane) diaphragm. Because of the constant flow of air through the chamber, there is a small gap between the diaphragm and the probe edge. As the probe tip touches and applanates the cornea, the air pressure increases until this gap is completely closed, at which point the IOP is equivalent to the air pressure. Similar to the Tono-Pen, this instrument makes contact with only a small area of the cornea and is especially useful in eyes with corneal scars or edema and can be used with the patient in sitting, lateral decubitus, or supine body positions. In addition, measurements obtained by placing the probe on the sclera appear to correlate well with those obtained with the probe placed on the cornea, suggesting that it can be used to monitor IOP in patients with keratoprostheses. The pneumatonometer can also record IOP continuously while the probe is on the eye and can be used for tonography.

Durham DG, Bigliano RP, Masino JA. Pneumatic applanation tonometer. *Trans Am Acad Ophthalmol Otolaryngol.* 1965;69(6):1029–1047.

Kapamajian MA, de la Cruz J, Hallak JA, Vajaranant TS. Correlation between corneal and scleral pneumatonometry: an alternative method for intraocular pressure measurement. *Am J Ophthalmol.* 2013;156(5):902–906.e1.

Noncontact tonometers

Noncontact (air-puff) tonometers determine IOP by measuring the force of air required to indent and flatten the cornea, thereby avoiding contact with the eye. IOP is measured when the amount of corneal indentation corresponds with the maximum amount of light reflection from the cornea. Readings obtained with these instruments vary widely, and IOP is often overestimated. Noncontact tonometers are often used in large-scale glaucoma-screening programs or by nonmedical health care providers.

The *Ocular Response Analyzer* (ORA; Reichert Technologies; Fig 2-7C) is a type of noncontact tonometer that uses correction algorithms so that its IOP readings more

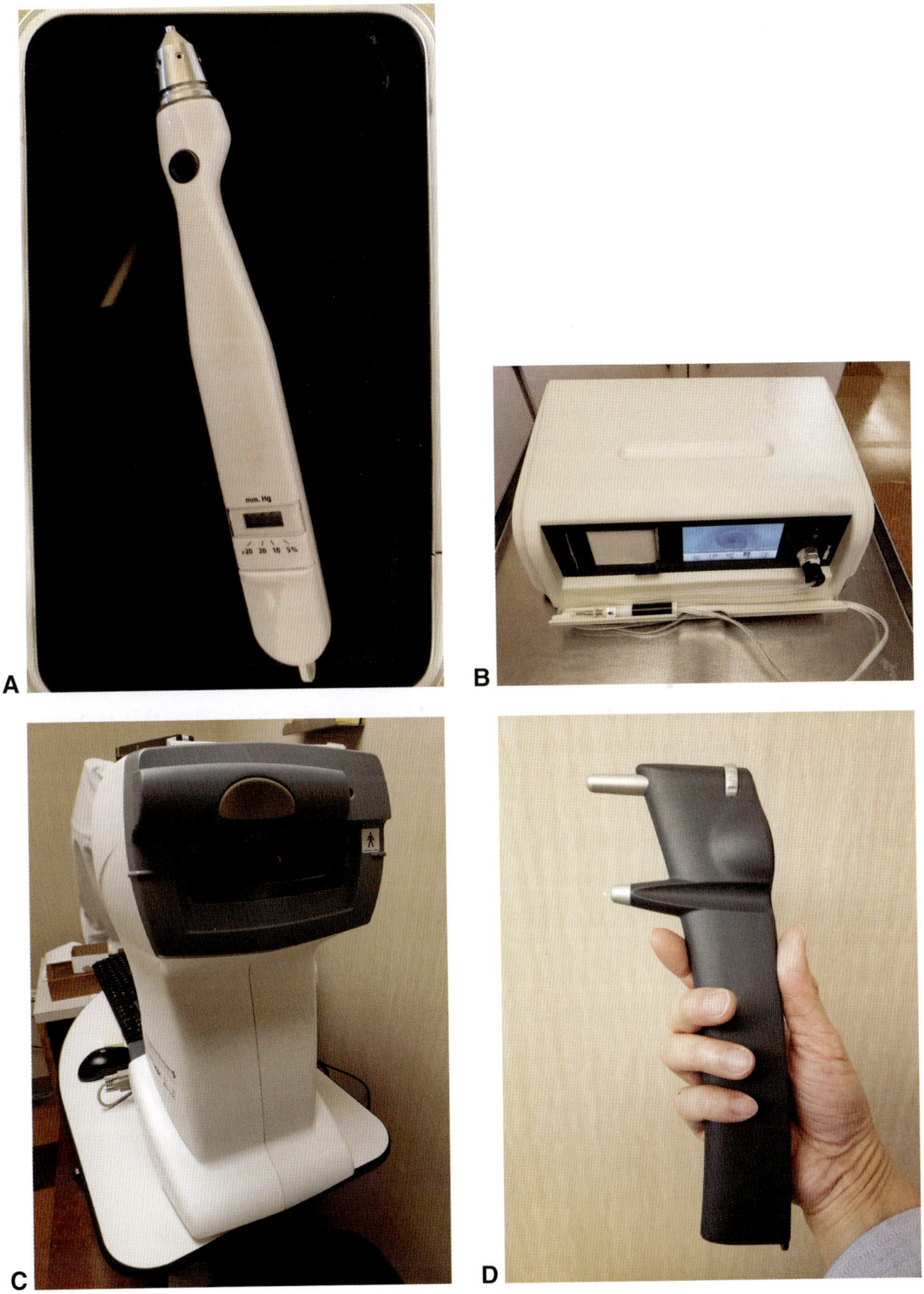

Figure 2-7 Nonapplanation tonometers in common use offer advantages and disadvantages compared with Goldmann applanation tonometry. **A,** Tono-Pen. **B,** Pneumatonometer. **C,** Ocular Response Analyzer. **D,** Rebound tonometer. *(Courtesy of Arthur J. Sit, MD.)*

closely match those obtained with applanation techniques, and the effect of corneal biomechanical properties on pressure measurement is reduced. One study reported that the corneal compensated IOP (IOPcc) has a stronger correlation with glaucoma progression than does IOP measured with Goldmann or rebound tonometry. In addition, indicators of ocular biomechanical properties are calculated, including *corneal hysteresis*. During the measurement process, the cornea is indented beyond the IOP measurement point. Corneal hysteresis is the difference between IOP measured during the initial corneal indentation and IOP measured during corneal rebound. Reduced corneal hysteresis has been associated with an increased risk of developing visual field defects in glaucoma suspects and with disease progression in patients with confirmed glaucoma.

Medeiros FA, Meira-Freitas D, Lisboa R, Kuang TM, Zangwill LM, Weinreb RN. Corneal hysteresis as a risk factor for glaucoma progression: a prospective longitudinal study. *Ophthalmology.* 2013;120(8):1533–1540.

Susanna BN, Ogata NG, Daga FB, Susanna CN, Diniz-Filho A, Medeiros FA. Association between rates of visual field progression and intraocular pressure measurements obtained by different tonometers. *Ophthalmology.* 2019;126(1):49–54.

Susanna CN, Diniz-Filho A, Daga FB, et al. A prospective longitudinal study to investigate corneal hysteresis as a risk factor for predicting development of glaucoma. *Am J Ophthalmol.* 2018;187:148–152.

Rebound tonometers

Rebound tonometry determines IOP by measuring the speed at which a small probe propelled against the cornea decelerates and rebounds after impact (Fig 2-7D). Rebound tonometers are portable, and topical anesthesia is not required; these characteristics make them particularly suitable for use in pediatric populations and for home tonometry in some patients. However, rebound tonometry is strongly influenced by central corneal thickness, even when compared with applanation tonometry. Thus, care must be taken in the interpretation of IOP measurements in eyes with thick or thin corneas.

Kontiola AI. A new induction-based impact method for measuring intraocular pressure. *Acta Ophthalmol Scand.* 2000;78(2):142–145.

Rao A, Kumar M, Prakash B, Varshney G. Relationship of central corneal thickness and intraocular pressure by iCare rebound tonometer. *J Glaucoma.* 2014;23(6):380–384.

Dynamic contour tonometer

The *dynamic contour tonometer,* a newer type of nonapplanation contact tonometer, is based on the principle that when the surface of the cornea is aligned with the surface of the instrument tip, the pressure in the tear film between these surfaces is equal to the IOP and can be measured by a pressure transducer. The tip is similar in shape and size to an applanation tonometer tip, with a pressure transducer placed in the center, and enables measurement of ocular pulse amplitude in addition to IOP. Evidence suggests that IOP measurements obtained with dynamic contour tonometry may be more independent of corneal biomechanical properties and thickness than those obtained with applanation.

Schneider E, Grehn F. Intraocular pressure measurement-comparison of dynamic contour tonometry and Goldmann applanation tonometry. *J Glaucoma.* 2006;15(1):2–6.

Indentation tonometry

Schiøtz tonometry determines IOP by measuring the amount of corneal indentation produced by a known weight. Measurements are taken with the patient supine, and the amount of indentation is read on a linear scale on the instrument and converted to IOP by a calibration table. However, indentation of the cornea results in a significant volume change in the globe, the amount of which depends on the IOP and the ocular rigidity. The assumption of average ocular rigidity in the calibration tables makes the accuracy of Schiøtz tonometry highly dependent on ocular biomechanical properties. Although Schiøtz tonometry is now rarely used in the developed world, it remains the only form of tonometry that does not require electrical power.

Tactile tension

It is possible to estimate IOP by *digital pressure* on the globe, referred to as *tactile tension.* This test may be useful in uncooperative patients; however, the results may be inaccurate even when the test is performed by very experienced clinicians. In general, tactile tensions are useful only for detecting large differences in IOP between a patient's 2 eyes.

Infection control in clinical tonometry

Many infectious agents—including HIV, hepatitis C virus, and adenovirus—can be recovered from tears. Tonometers must be cleaned after each use to prevent the transfer of such pathogens. For Goldmann-type and Perkins tonometers, the tonometer tips (prisms) should be cleaned immediately after use. The ideal method for disinfection is controversial. Sodium hypochlorite (dilute bleach) offers effective disinfection against adenovirus and herpes simplex virus, the viruses commonly associated with nosocomial outbreaks in eye care. In contrast, alcohol wipes or soaks do not appear to be effective at eradicating all infectious virions. The efficacy of other disinfection protocols has not been adequately evaluated. The prism head should be rinsed with water and dried before reuse to prevent damage to the corneal epithelium. Single-use disposable applanation tonometer tips may be a useful alternative to cleaning. For cleaning other tonometers, refer to the manufacturer's recommendations.

Junk AK, Chen PP, Lin SC, et al. Disinfection of tonometers: a report by the American Academy of Ophthalmology. *Ophthalmology.* 2017;124(12):1867–1875.

CHAPTER 3

Clinical Evaluation: History

Highlights

- Appropriate management of glaucoma is based on accurate diagnosis, assessment of severity, and likelihood of progression, as established by means of clinical evaluation.
- Clinical evaluation of a patient with, or suspected of having, glaucoma begins with a thorough ocular and medical history as well as a review of available pertinent records.
- Relevant factors include the individual's age, race or ethnicity, and family history of glaucoma.
- The patient's past and present ocular and systemic conditions and use of medications are important considerations in both the diagnosis and management of glaucoma.
- Evaluation of a patient with glaucoma also includes assessment of the effects of the disease on the patient's quality of life, with referral to a low vision specialist if warranted.

Importance of Patient History

Appropriate management of glaucoma depends on the clinician's ability to diagnose the specific form of the disease in a given patient, to determine the severity of the condition, to predict the likelihood of progression, and to detect progression when it occurs. Clinical evaluation of the glaucoma patient or suspect begins with taking a thorough history of the current condition, including symptoms, onset, duration, and severity. Also important are the past ocular history and a general medical history, including the patient's medications and allergies.

Relevant Factors

The following points are relevant in the assessment of all glaucoma patients. However, the clinician will tailor the evaluation to the individual patient by inquiring about other factors, as appropriate.

Demographics

- *Age.* Although glaucoma can occur in any age group, the most common forms are more prevalent in older individuals.
- *Race and ethnicity.* Individuals of African descent or Hispanic ethnicity are at increased risk for primary open-angle glaucoma, while persons of Asian descent are at increased risk for angle-closure glaucoma. In individuals from Scandinavian countries, pseudoexfoliation syndrome accounts for a high proportion of glaucoma cases.

- *Family history of glaucoma.* If there is a family history of glaucoma, the disease severity and outcomes experienced by other family members, including vision loss and blindness, should be obtained during initial evaluation.

Symptoms

Although the most common forms of glaucoma are usually asymptomatic until relatively late stages, some conditions, such as acute angle closure, are generally accompanied by pain, redness, and decreased vision. Patients with anatomically narrow angles and intermittent angle closure may report a history of having headaches and seeing halos, especially colored halos, around lights. Patients with pigment dispersion syndrome may sometimes report blurred vision, pain, or halos around lights after exercise; these symptoms may be related to active pigment dispersion and acute intraocular pressure (IOP) elevation.

Ocular history

Certain aspects of the patient's ocular history may be pertinent to glaucoma, including:

- *Refractive error.* High myopia is a risk factor for primary open-angle glaucoma, while hyperopia is a risk factor for angle closure.
- *Trauma.* Ocular trauma can be associated with angle recession and traumatic glaucoma. Of note, it is common for patients with traumatic glaucoma to report a history of ocular trauma that occurred decades before the development of IOP elevation.
- *Ocular surgery.* A history of complicated cataract surgery, corneal transplant, or vitrectomy may all be associated with increased risk for glaucoma. Although refractive surgery is generally not associated with an increased risk of glaucoma, keratorefractive procedures such as laser in situ keratomileusis (LASIK) or photorefractive keratotomy may result in thin corneas and artificially low IOP measurement on Goldmann applanation tonometry.

Systemic disorders

A patient's systemic conditions can affect both the diagnosis of glaucoma and the choice of medications to treat it. Systemic diseases of particular relevance include asthma, chronic obstructive pulmonary disease (COPD), migraine headache, vasospasm, sleep apnea, diabetes, cardiovascular disease, and thyroid disease. For example, β-blockers may be contraindicated in patients with asthma or COPD; therefore, a history of these conditions should be actively sought in all patients with glaucoma or suspected glaucoma for whom treatment with topical β-blockers is being considered.

A history of migraine or vasospasm (eg, Raynaud disease) may be more prevalent in patients with glaucoma occurring at relatively low IOP. Though controversial, sleep apnea has also been described as a risk factor for glaucoma. Patients with autoimmune thyroid disorders and thyroid eye disease may have elevated episcleral venous pressure. In addition, a history of systemic arterial hypertension and therapy is relevant; treatment-related hypotension may increase the risk of progression.

Medication use

Use of topical, inhaled, or systemic corticosteroids can be a risk factor for increased IOP. It is also important to inquire what, if any, ocular hypotensive medications the patient has previously used and reactions or allergies to them. If a patient is already taking systemic β-blockers for other conditions, topical β-blockers will have diminished IOP-lowering efficacy. The clinician should also inquire about a history of reaction or allergy to sulfonamide medications, including the type and severity of the reaction; patients with a known allergy to a sulfonamide agent may have a higher risk of a subsequent reaction to carbonic anhydrase inhibitors, although cross-reactivity between sulfonamide antibiotics and nonantibiotics may be as low as 10%. Certain systemic medications, such as topiramate, may be associated with increased risk for angle-closure glaucoma (see Chapter 10). In addition, the systemic use of drugs that have anticholinergic activity may increase the risk of angle-closure disease in persons with anatomically narrow anterior chamber angles.

sulfa allergy = NO CAIs

Review of records

A review of pertinent records, particularly those documenting past IOP levels, status of the optic nerve, and visual field, is useful in guiding current glaucoma management. Information on maximum recorded IOP levels is important in setting IOP goals for treatment. Records of optic nerve status and visual fields can be crucial in establishing whether changes have occurred over time, both for patients suspected of disease and for those with established glaucoma. In cases of suspected glaucoma, documentation of optic disc progression over time may establish the diagnosis even in the absence of visual field loss. In patients with previously diagnosed disease, records showing progressive optic nerve damage or visual field loss are indicative of uncontrolled disease. If the disease is not adequately controlled while the patient is on topical ocular hypotensive therapy, the clinician should actively seek to obtain a history of adherence to treatment.

Quality of Life

It is also important to ask patients with glaucoma about any effects of the disease on their quality of life, such as the ability to drive, walk, find objects, or maintain social interactions. Patients who report progressive decline in quality of life may require more aggressive interventions to control the disease and may benefit from evaluation by a low vision specialist. In patients with very severe glaucoma and advanced visual field loss, subjective changes in quality of vision may be the only indicator that the disease is not adequately controlled.

CHAPTER 4

Clinical Evaluation and Imaging of the Anterior Segment

Highlights

- Systematic examination of the anterior segment, including gonioscopy, is necessary to establish an accurate diagnosis for patients with glaucoma or ocular hypertension.
- Detection of angle closure and important secondary causes of ocular hypertension or glaucoma requires careful and complete assessment of the anterior segment anatomy.
- Various anterior segment imaging modalities can add important information to aid in the diagnosis of disease processes associated with glaucoma.

Refractive Error

Determining the refractive status of the eye is important in the evaluation of glaucoma. First, correcting any significant refractive error is necessary for accurate perimetry; and second, different refractive states can be associated with various types of glaucoma. For example, *myopia,* especially high myopia, is a risk factor for primary open-angle glaucoma. In addition, pigment dispersion syndrome is more common in moderately myopic eyes. Optic nerve head (also called *optic disc*) and peripapillary anomalies associated with myopia can confound the evaluation of the optic disc and retinal nerve fiber layer, both clinically and with optical coherence tomography (OCT) imaging (see Chapter 5). *Hyperopia* is associated with an increased risk of primary angle closure, and the hyperopic eye generally has a smaller optic nerve head.

Ocular Adnexa

Examination and assessment of the ocular adnexa are necessary to identify various conditions associated with secondary glaucomas as well as possible external effects of glaucoma therapy. The entities described in this section are discussed in greater depth and illustrated elsewhere in the BCSC series, particularly BCSC Sections 6, 7, and 8.

Examples of diseases associated with glaucoma that can also involve the ocular adnexa include tuberous sclerosis (Bourneville syndrome), juvenile xanthogranuloma, and oculodermal melanocytosis (nevus of Ota). In *tuberous sclerosis,* glaucoma may occur secondary to vitreous hemorrhage, anterior segment neovascularization, or retinal detachment. A typical external sign of tuberous sclerosis is pink to red-brown angiofibromas, which are often found on the face and chin. In *juvenile xanthogranuloma,* yellow or orange papules or nodules can be present on the eyelids or face. In *oculodermal melanocytosis,* blue to brown discoloration or darkening occurs on the periocular skin. It can be unilateral or bilateral, and it may be subtle, particularly in persons of African, Asian, or Hispanic ancestry.

The presence of subcutaneous eyelid plexiform neurofibromas is a hallmark of the type 1 variant of *neurofibromatosis (NF1,* or *von Recklinghausen disease).* Although glaucoma is generally uncommon in patients with NF1, it occurs in 25%–50% of those who have an eyelid plexiform neurofibroma. In these patients, glaucoma is usually unilateral and ipsilateral to the eyelid neurofibroma.

Several disease processes with ocular adnexal abnormalities are associated with elevated episcleral venous pressure (see Chapter 8). The presence of a facial cutaneous angioma *(nevus flammeus,* or *port-wine stain)* can indicate *encephalotrigeminal angiomatosis (Sturge-Weber syndrome).* The cutaneous hemangiomas of a closely related condition, *Klippel-Trénaunay-Weber syndrome,* extend over an affected limb and may also involve the face and eyes. Orbital varices, arteriovenous fistulas, and superior vena cava syndrome may also be associated with elevated episcleral venous pressure and secondary glaucoma. Intermittent unilateral proptosis and dilated eyelid veins are key external signs of *orbital varices. Carotid-cavernous, dural-cavernous,* and other *arteriovenous fistulas* can produce orbital bruits, restricted ocular motility, proptosis, and pulsating exophthalmos. *Superior vena cava syndrome* can cause proptosis and facial and eyelid edema, as well as conjunctival chemosis. *Thyroid eye disease* may also be associated with glaucoma; ocular adnexal features of this disease include exophthalmos, eyelid retraction, and motility disorders.

Long-term use of prostaglandin analogues may result in ocular adnexal abnormalities, including increased periocular pigmentation and hypertrichosis of the eyelashes. Other reported external abnormalities include orbital fat atrophy, enophthalmos, deepening of the upper eyelid sulcus, upper eyelid ptosis, inferior scleral show, and tightening of the eyelids (see Chapter 12).

Pupillary Function

Pupil diameter can be affected by parasympathomimetic agents and adrenergic agonists (see Chapter 12). A *relative afferent pupillary defect (RAPD)* is often seen in the presence of asymmetric glaucoma damage; however, if an RAPD cannot be reconciled with the overall clinical picture of glaucoma, the presence of a nonglaucomatous optic neuropathy must be ruled out. In some clinical situations, it is not possible to assess the pupils objectively for the presence of an RAPD, and a subjective comparison between the eyes of the perceived brightness of a test light may be helpful.

Slit-Lamp Biomicroscopy

Biomicroscopy of the anterior segment is performed to detect signs of underlying ocular conditions that may be associated with glaucoma or ocular hypertension, to evaluate the eye in preparation for glaucoma surgery, and to monitor the function of a previously performed glaucoma surgery. BCSC Section 8, *External Disease and Cornea,* discusses slit-lamp technique and the examination of the external eye in greater depth.

Conjunctiva

Eyes with acutely elevated intraocular pressure (IOP) may have conjunctival hyperemia. Long-term use of many ocular hypotensive medications may also cause conjunctival hyperemia. Allergic or hypersensitivity reactions to medications (especially α_2-adrenergic agonists) or their preservatives can result in a follicular conjunctivitis. Other potential adverse effects of topical hypotensive drugs include decreased tear production, foreshortening of the conjunctival fornices, and, in severe cases, pseudopemphigoid with conjunctival scarring. Prior to filtering surgery, the presence or absence of subconjunctival scarring or other conjunctival abnormalities is assessed. The presence or absence of any filtering bleb is noted. If a bleb is present, it is characterized as either cystic or diffuse, and its size, degree of elevation, amount of vascularization, and integrity are noted. A Seidel test is performed if a leak is suspected (Fig 4-1).

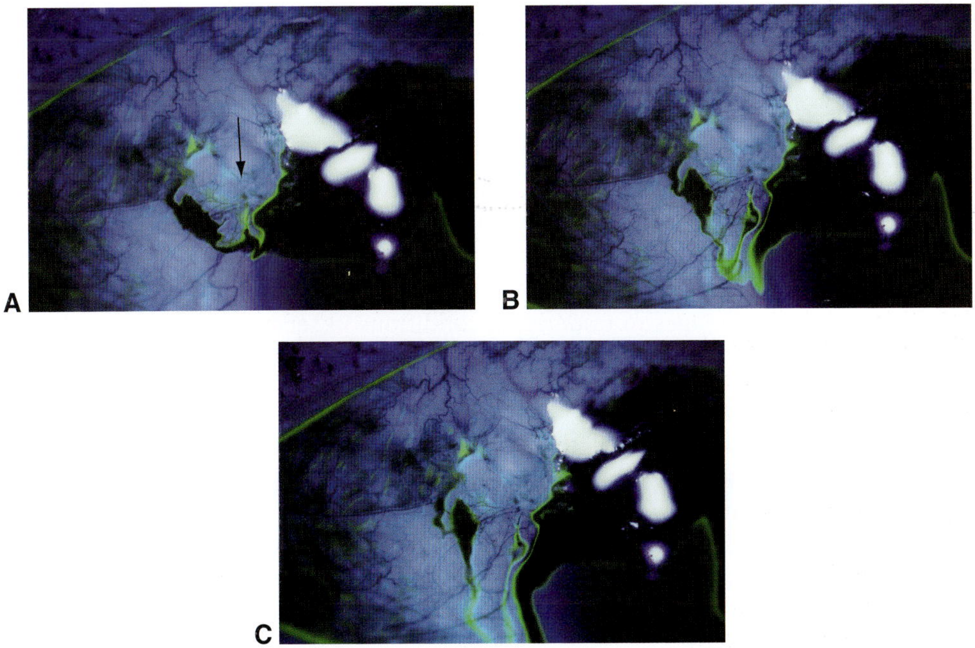

Figure 4-1 Seidel test. After application of a concentrated fluorescein solution, quenching will block fluorescence unless there is an aqueous humor leak that dilutes the fluorescein. The dark area on the right of these images represents an area of highly concentrated fluorescein. As aqueous humor leaks (*arrow,* **A**) the fluorescein is diluted, and an enlarging rivulet of fluorescence is detected **(A–C)**. *(Courtesy of Angelo P. Tanna, MD.)*

CLINICAL PEARL

The Seidel test is used to detect an aqueous humor leak. A sterile topical anesthetic solution is instilled to prevent a blinking response. Concentrated sodium fluorescein is applied to the area where the leak is suspected. A moistened fluorescein strip or 2% sodium fluorescein solution is used. Immediately after application of fluorescein, the examiner looks for fluorescence, using a slit-lamp microscope with a cobalt blue filter. When a high concentration of fluorescein is present, fluorescence is not seen due to quenching, but if the fluorescein is diluted by leakage of aqueous, fluorescence will be detected (see Fig 4-1).

Episclera and Sclera

Dilation of the episcleral vessels may indicate elevated episcleral venous pressure, which can be idiopathic or can occur in the secondary glaucomas associated with disease processes (see the previous section Ocular Adnexa and Chapter 8). Sentinel vessels may be seen in eyes harboring an intraocular tumor. The clinician should note any thinning or staphylomatous areas. Slate-gray patches of scleral pigmentation are present in oculodermal melanocytosis, and affected patients are at increased risk for developing glaucoma and ocular melanoma. Scleritis may also be associated with elevated IOP.

Cornea

Enlargement of the cornea associated with breaks in Descemet membrane *(Haab striae)* is commonly found in childhood glaucoma patients who had onset of IOP elevation before the age of 4 years. Glaucomas associated with other corneal abnormalities are described in Chapters 10 and 11. *Punctate epithelial defects*, especially in the inferonasal interpalpebral region, are often indicative of medication toxicity. *Microcystic epithelial edema* is commonly associated with severely elevated IOP, particularly when the IOP increase is acute. The following corneal endothelial abnormalities can provide important clues to underlying conditions in secondary IOP elevation or glaucoma:

- Krukenberg spindle in pigment dispersion syndrome
- deposition of exfoliation material in pseudoexfoliation syndrome
- keratic precipitates (KPs) in uveitis, especially pancorneal stellate KPs associated with herpesvirus infections
- irregular and vesicular lesions in posterior polymorphous dystrophy
- a "beaten bronze" appearance in iridocorneal endothelial syndrome

The clinician should note the presence of traumatic or surgical corneal scars. The central corneal thickness of all patients suspected of having glaucoma should be assessed by corneal pachymetry, as a thin central cornea is a risk factor for glaucoma and results in underestimation of IOP by most tonometers (see Chapters 2 and 7).

Anterior Chamber

When evaluating the anterior chamber, the examiner should note the uniformity of depth of the chamber. In the Van Herick method of estimating angle width, the examiner projects a narrow slit beam onto the cornea at approximately a 60° angle, just anterior to the limbus. However, the results can be misleading: this method is not sensitive enough to detect angle closure and is not a substitute for gonioscopy (discussed in detail in the Gonioscopy section).

Iris bombé and *plateau iris syndrome* can both result in an anterior chamber that is deep centrally and shallow or flat peripherally. In contrast, in *malignant glaucoma* and other forms of non–pupillary block angle closure with a posterior "pushing" mechanism, both the peripheral and central anterior chamber are shallow. In many circumstances, especially in the assessment of acute unilateral IOP elevation (when the cornea is often edematous, limiting the view of the anterior chamber and angle), examination of the fellow eye can provide useful information.

The anterior chamber is very deep and the iris configuration is often concave in *pigment dispersion syndrome.* In this condition, friction between the posteriorly bowed iris and the lens zonules causes pigment liberation from the iris epithelial cells.

The presence of white or red blood cells, circulating pigment, or inflammatory debris (such as fibrin) should be noted. The degree of inflammation (flare and cells) and presence of pigment should be determined before instillation of eyedrops.

Iris

The iris should be examined before pupillary dilation. The clinician should note heterochromia, iris atrophy, ectropion uveae (the presence of pigmented iris epithelial cells on the anterior iris surface), corectopia (displacement of the pupil), nevi, nodules, exfoliative material, transillumination defects, the presence and patency of an iridotomy or iridectomy, and any surgically induced iris abnormalities. Iris color should be noted, especially in patients being considered for treatment with a prostaglandin analogue.

Early stages of neovascularization of the anterior segment may appear as either fine tufts at the pupillary margin or a fine network of vessels on the surface of the iris adjacent to the iris root. The clinician should also examine the iris for evidence of ocular trauma, such as iris sphincter tears, iridodialysis (tear in the iris root), or iridodonesis (abnormal iris motion caused by poor or absent lens zonular support).

The contour of the iris can provide clues about the underlying mechanism of angle closure and the presence of pigment dispersion syndrome. Irregularities in the iris contour may suggest choroidal effusion or hemorrhage. Other conditions that can cause irregularity of the iris contour include an iris or ciliary body cyst or, rarely, uveal melanoma; ultrasonography is required to characterize such lesions, and either type can lead to IOP elevation.

Lens

The clinician should examine the lens both before and after pupillary dilation, evaluating its size, shape, clarity, and stability. Examination of the lens may help the clinician to determine the etiology and guide the management of lens-related glaucomas. Assessment prior to dilation provides useful information about the effect of lens opacity, posterior capsule opacification, or lens subluxation on visual function. A posterior subcapsular cataract may be indicative of prior long-term corticosteroid use. An intraocular foreign body with siderosis and glaucoma may result in a characteristic yellow-brown or rust-color discoloration of the lens epithelium.

Vitreous and Fundus

Dilated examination of the posterior segment allows the clinician to evaluate the vitreous for signs of inflammation, hemorrhage, or ghost cells. Careful stereoscopic evaluation of the optic nerve head should be performed, followed by examination of the fundus to detect pathology such as hemorrhages, effusions, masses, inflammatory lesions, retinal vascular occlusions, diabetic retinopathy, or retinal detachments that can be associated with glaucoma.

Gonioscopy

Gonioscopy is an essential diagnostic technique for examining the structures of the anterior chamber angle (Table 4-1). Unfortunately, this procedure is underutilized in clinical practice, potentially leading to incorrect diagnosis and management. Gonioscopy is necessary to visualize the anatomy of the angle because, under normal conditions, light reflected from the angle structures undergoes total internal reflection at the tear–air interface. At that interface, the critical angle (approximately 46°) is reached, and light is totally reflected back into the corneal stroma, which prevents direct visualization of the angle structures. During gonioscopy, the examiner eliminates the tear–air interface by placing a plastic or glass lens surface against the cornea. The small space between the lens and cornea is filled by the patient's tears, saline solution, or a clear viscous substance. Figures 4-2 and 4-3 show schematic and clinical views of the angle as seen with gonioscopy.

Direct and Indirect Gonioscopy

Gonioscopy techniques fall into 2 broad categories: (1) direct and (2) indirect (Fig 4-4). *Direct gonioscopy* is performed with a binocular microscope, fiber-optic illuminator, or slit-pen light

Table 4-1 Gonioscopic Examination

Tissue	Features and Pathologic Findings
Posterior cornea	Pigmentation, keratic precipitates
Schwalbe line	Thickening, anterior displacement
Trabecular meshwork	Pigmentation, peripheral anterior synechiae (PAS), inflammatory or neovascular membranes
Scleral spur	Iris processes
Ciliary body band	Angle recession, cyclodialysis cleft
Iris	Contour, rubeosis, atrophy, cysts, tumors, iridodonesis, iridodialysis
Zonular fibers	Pigmentation, rupture (can be visible after dilation)

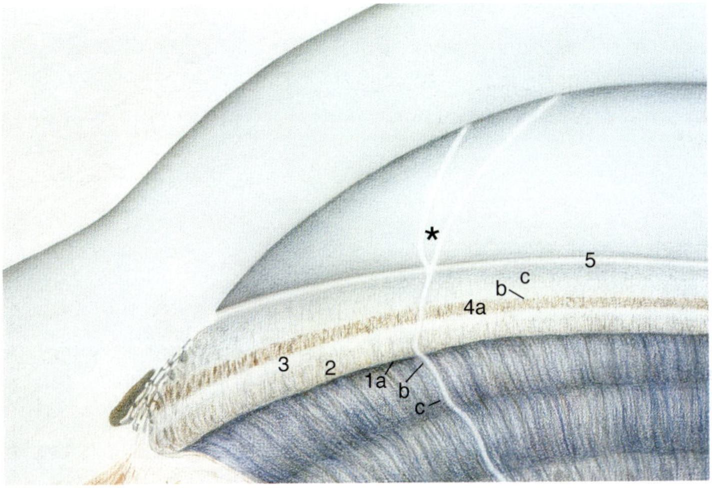

Figure 4-2 Gonioscopic appearance of a normal anterior chamber angle. *1,* Peripheral iris: *a,* insertion; *b,* curvature; *c,* angular approach. *2,* Ciliary body band. *3,* Scleral spur. *4,* Trabecular meshwork: *a,* posterior; *b,* mid; *c,* anterior. *5,* Schwalbe line. *Asterisk,* Corneal optical wedge (parallelepiped corneal wedge).

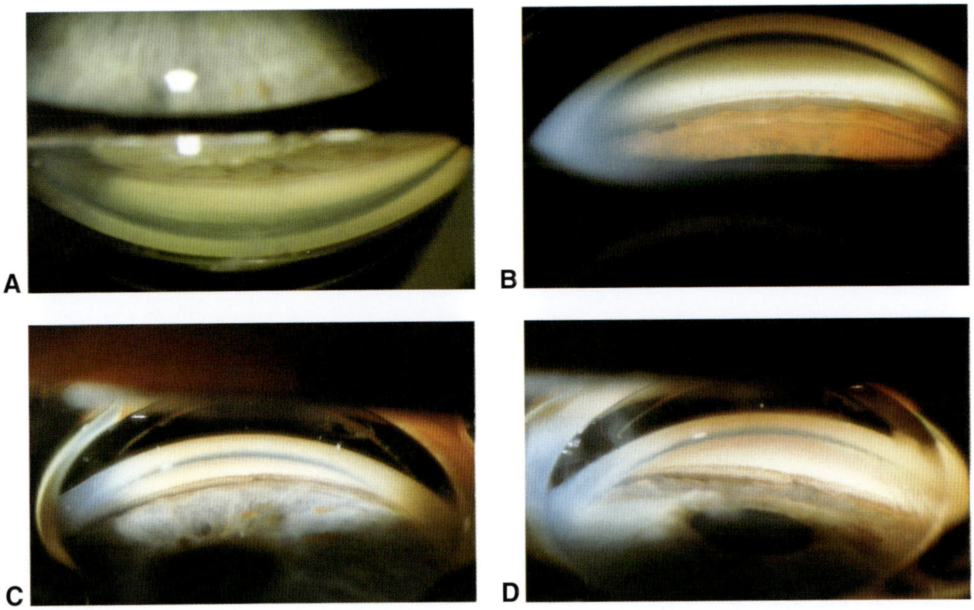

Figure 4-3 Normal and narrow angles. **A,** Normal open angle. Gonioscopic photograph shows trace pigmentation of the posterior trabecular meshwork and normal insertion of the iris into a narrow ciliary body band. The Goldmann lens was used. **B,** Normal open angle. This gonioscopic view using the Goldmann lens shows mild pigmentation of the posterior trabecular meshwork. A wide ciliary body band with posterior insertion of the iris can also be seen. **C,** Narrow angle. This gonioscopic view using the Zeiss lens without indentation shows pigment in the inferior angle but poor visualization of angle anatomy. **D,** Narrow angle. Gonioscopy with a Zeiss lens with indentation shows peripheral anterior synechiae (PAS) in the posterior trabecular meshwork. Pigment deposits on the Schwalbe line can also be seen. This is the same angle as shown in part C. *(Part A courtesy of Angelo P. Tanna, MD; parts B–D courtesy of Elizabeth A. Hodapp, MD.)*

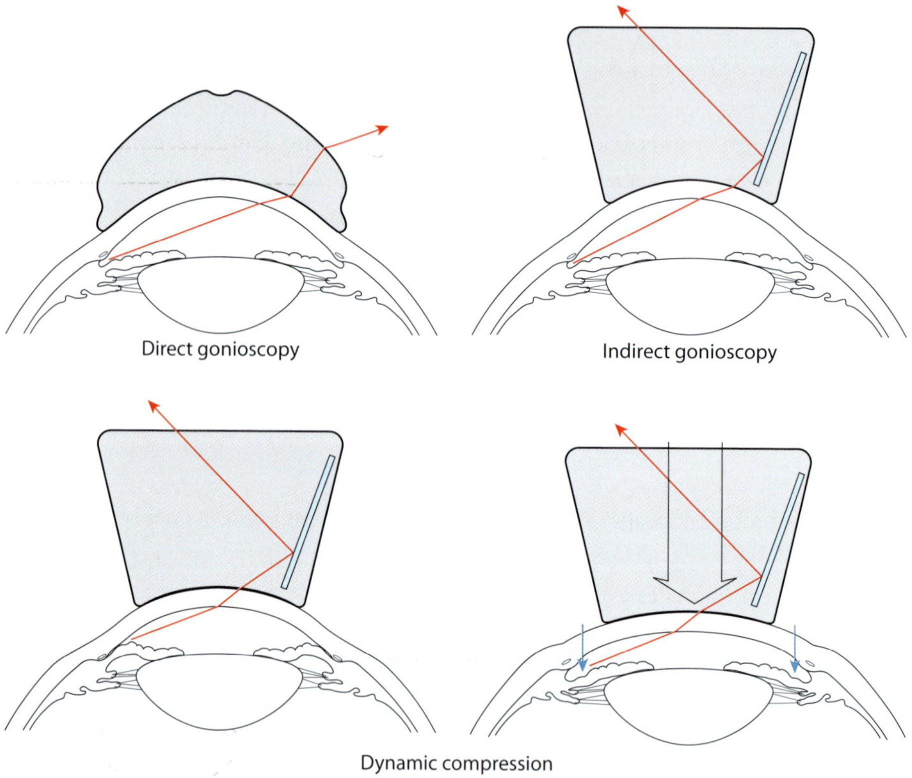

Figure 4-4 Direct and indirect gonioscopy. Gonioscopic lenses eliminate the tear–air interface and total internal reflection. With a direct lens, the light ray reflected from the anterior chamber angle is observed directly, whereas with an indirect lens, the light ray is reflected by a mirror within the lens. Posterior pressure with an indirect lens forces open an appositionally closed or narrow anterior chamber angle (dynamic gonioscopy). *(Illustration courtesy of Mark Miller.)*

together with a direct goniolens, such as the Koeppe, Swan-Jacob, Barkan, Wurst, or Richardson type. The lens is placed on the eye; and saline solution, methylcellulose, or an ophthalmic viscosurgical device is used to fill the space between the cornea and the lens, acting as an optical coupler between the 2 surfaces. The goniolens provides direct visualization of the anterior chamber angle (ie, light reflected directly from the angle is visualized). With direct gonioscopy, the clinician has an erect view of the angle structures, which is essential when angle surgery (eg, goniotomy or placement of a stent in the Schlemm canal) is performed. Direct gonioscopy is most easily accomplished with the patient in a supine position, and it is commonly used in the operating room for examining the eyes of infants under anesthesia.

Indirect gonioscopy is more frequently used in the clinician's office. Light reflected from the angle passes into the indirect gonioscopy lens and is reflected by 1 or more mirrors within the lens. This method may be used with the patient in an upright position, with illumination and magnification provided by a slit-lamp microscope. The indirect goniolens yields an inverted and slightly foreshortened image of the opposite angle. Although the image is inverted, the right–left orientation of a horizontal mirror and the up–down orientation of a vertical mirror remain unchanged. The foreshortening, combined with the upright position of the patient, makes the angle appear somewhat shallower than it does on direct gonioscopy. The Goldmann-type 1- or 3-mirror gonioscopy lens requires a viscous fluid such as methylcellulose for optical coupling with the cornea. Posterior pressure on the lens, especially if it is tilted, indents the sclera and may falsely narrow the angle. Among indirect gonioscopy lenses, these provide the clearest visualization of the anterior chamber angle structures, and they may be modified with antireflective coatings for use during laser procedures.

The Posner, Sussman, and Zeiss 4-mirror gonioscopy lenses allow all 4 quadrants of the anterior chamber angle to be visualized without rotation of the lens during examination. Because these lenses have approximately the same radius of curvature as the cornea, they are optically coupled by the patient's tears. The posterior diameter of these lenses is smaller than the corneal diameter, and thus posterior pressure can be used to force open a narrow angle by means of a technique called *dynamic gonioscopy* (also known as *compression* or *indentation gonioscopy*). With dynamic gonioscopy, the clinician puts gentle pressure on the cornea with the goniolens, which forces aqueous humor into the angle, causing it to open to a greater degree than its native state in the absence of peripheral anterior synechiae (PAS) (see Fig 4-4). With indirect gonioscopy, the observer can optimize the view of the anterior chamber angle by repositioning the patient's eye (having the patient look toward the mirror being viewed by the examiner) or by slightly tilting the lens. However, pressure on the cornea will artificially open a truly narrow or closed angle. The examiner can detect this pressure by noting the induced Descemet membrane folds.

When an area of the angle is closed, one cannot initially differentiate between appositional angle closure and angle closure due to PAS. The technique of dynamic gonioscopy is essential for distinguishing iridocorneal apposition from synechial closure. Many clinicians prefer these 4-mirror lenses because of their ease of use and the ability to perform dynamic gonioscopy.

Gonioscopic Assessment and Documentation

In performing both direct and indirect gonioscopy, the clinician must recognize the landmarks of the anterior chamber angle. It is important to perform gonioscopy with dim room lighting and a thin, short light beam in order to minimize the amount of light entering the pupil. An excessive amount of light can cause increased pupillary constriction that could falsely open the angle, changing the peripheral angle appearance and potentially preventing the identification of a narrow or occluded angle. The scleral spur and the Schwalbe line, 2 important angle landmarks, are most consistently identified. A convenient gonioscopic technique to determine the exact position of the Schwalbe line is the *parallelepiped,* or *corneal wedge, technique* (see www.aao.org/basic-skills/corneal-wedge-introduction and Fig 4-2). This technique allows the observer to determine the exact junction of the cornea and the trabecular meshwork. Using a narrow slit beam and sharp focus, the examiner sees 2 curvilinear reflections, 1 from the external surface of the cornea and its junction with the sclera and the other from the internal surface of the cornea. The 2 reflections meet at the Schwalbe line (see Fig 4-2). The scleral spur is a thin, pale stripe between the ciliary body face and the pigmented zone of the trabecular meshwork. The inferior portion of the angle is generally wider and is the easiest place in which to locate the landmarks. After verifying the landmarks, the clinician should examine the entire angle in an orderly manner (see Table 4-1).

Proper management of glaucoma requires the clinician to determine not only whether the angle is open or closed but also whether other pathologic findings, such as angle recession or PAS, are present. In angle closure, the peripheral iris obstructs the trabecular meshwork—that is, the meshwork is not visible on gonioscopy. The width of the angle is determined by the site of insertion of the iris on the ciliary face, the convexity of the iris, and the prominence of the peripheral iris roll. In many cases, the angle appears to be open but very narrow. It is often difficult to distinguish a narrow but open angle from an angle with partial closure; dynamic gonioscopy is useful in this situation (see Figs 4-3 and 4-4).

Grading

The best method for describing the angle is to use a standardized grading system or to draw the iris contour, the location of the iris insertion, and the angle between the iris and the trabecular meshwork. Various gonioscopic grading systems have been developed, all of which facilitate standardized description of angle structures and abbreviate that description. However, the clinician should keep in mind that some details about the angle structure will be eliminated with the use of abbreviated descriptions. The most commonly used gonioscopic grading systems are the Shaffer and Spaeth systems. A quadrant-by-quadrant narrative description of the chamber angle noting localized findings such as neovascular tufts, angle recession, or PAS may also be used to document serial gonioscopic findings. If a grading system is used, the clinician should specify which one.

The *Shaffer system* describes the angle between the trabecular meshwork and the iris as follows:

- *Grade 4:* The angle between the iris and the surface of the trabecular meshwork is 45°.
- *Grade 3:* The angle between the iris and the surface of the trabecular meshwork is greater than 20° but less than 45°.
- *Grade 2:* The angle between the iris and the surface of the trabecular meshwork is 20°. Angle closure is possible.
- *Grade 1:* The angle between the iris and the surface of the trabecular meshwork is 10°. Angle closure is probable over time.
- *Slit:* The angle between the iris and the surface of the trabecular meshwork is less than 10°. Angle closure is very likely.
- *Grade 0:* The iris is against the trabecular meshwork. Angle closure is present.

The *Spaeth gonioscopic grading system* expands on this schema to include a description of the peripheral iris contour, the insertion of the iris root, and the effects of dynamic gonioscopy on the angle configuration (Fig 4-5).

Blood and vessels

Ordinarily, the Schlemm canal cannot be seen on gonioscopy; however, it can easily be visualized if blood enters the canal. This can occur when episcleral venous pressure exceeds IOP, most commonly because of compression of the episcleral veins by the lip of the goniolens (Fig 4-6). Pathologic causes of blood in the canal include hypotony and elevated episcleral venous pressure, as in carotid-cavernous fistula or Sturge-Weber syndrome.

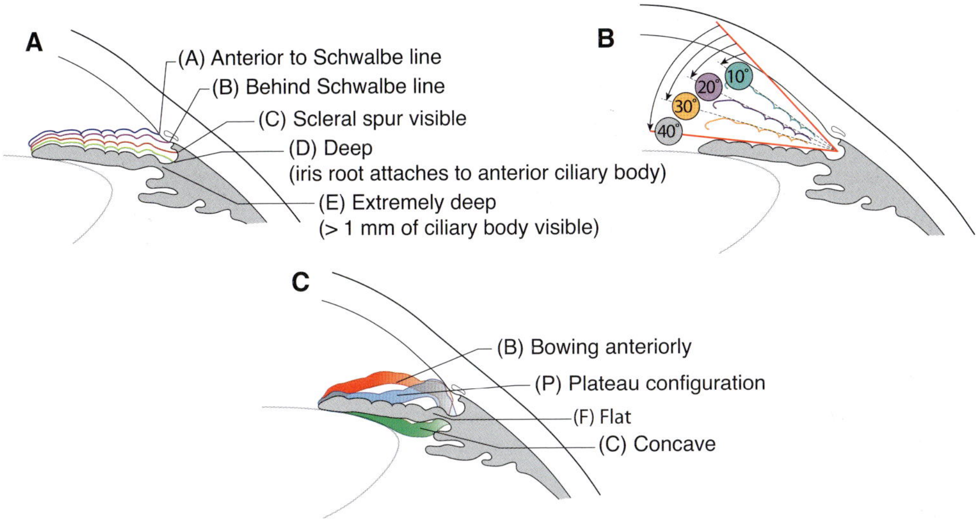

Figure 4-5 The Spaeth gonioscopic classification of the anterior chamber angle, based on 3 variables: **A,** site of iris attachment to the inner surface of the cornea, sclera, or ciliary body; **B,** angular width of the angle recess; **C,** configuration of the peripheral iris. *(Illustration courtesy of Mark Miller.)*

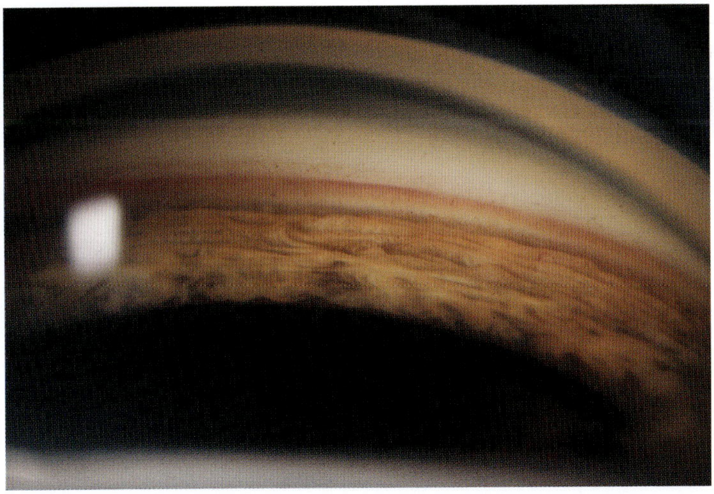

Figure 4-6 Goniophotograph showing blood in the Schlemm canal, visible through the semi-opaque trabecular meshwork. Elevated episcleral venous pressure resulted in blood reflux into the canal. *(Courtesy of G.A. Cioffi, MD.)*

Normal blood vessels in the angle include radial iris vessels, portions of the arterial circle of the ciliary body, and vertical branches of the anterior ciliary arteries. Normal vessels are oriented either radially along the iris or circumferentially (in a serpentine manner) in the ciliary body face. Vessels that cross the scleral spur to reach the trabecular meshwork are usually abnormal (Fig 4-7). The vessels seen in Fuchs uveitis syndrome are fine, branching, unsheathed, and meandering. Patients with neovascular glaucoma have vessels crossing the ciliary body and scleral spur and arborizing over the trabecular meshwork. Contraction of the myofibroblasts accompanying these vessels leads to PAS formation.

Iris processes and PAS

It is important to distinguish PAS from iris processes, which are open and lacy and follow the normal curve of the angle. The angle structures are visible in the open spaces between the iris processes. Synechiae are more solid or sheetlike (Fig 4-8). They are composed of iris stroma and obliterate the angle recess.

Pigmentation

Pigmentation of the trabecular meshwork increases with age and tends to be more marked in individuals with darkly pigmented irides. Pigmentation can be segmental and is usually

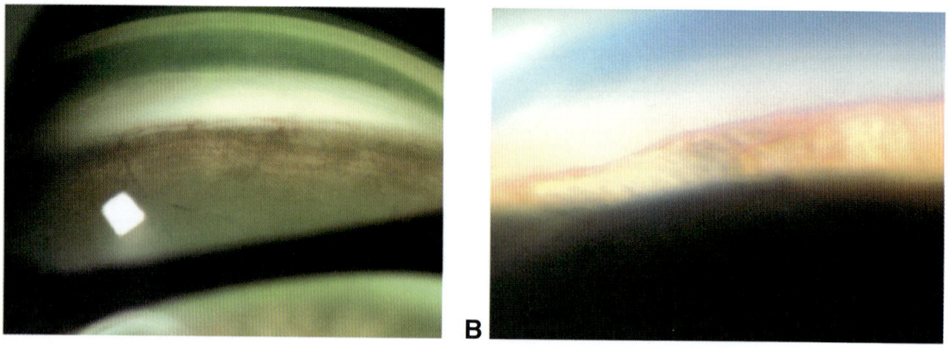
A B

Figure 4-7 Goniophotographs showing neovascularization of the angle. **A,** Anatomically open angle. **B,** Closed angle. *(Part A courtesy of Keith Barton, MD; part B courtesy of Ronald L. Gross, MD.)*

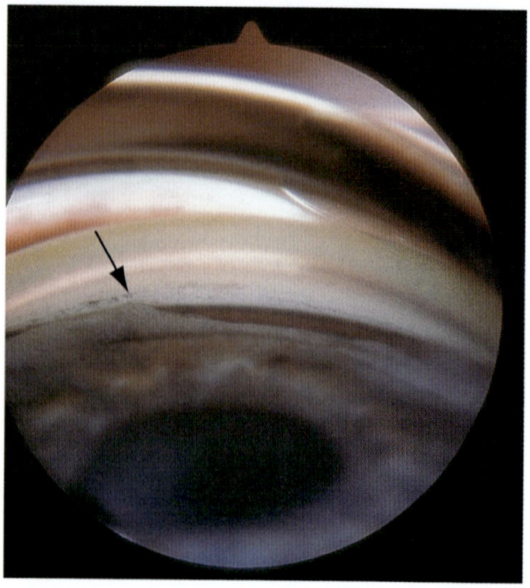

Figure 4-8 Goniophotograph showing both an area of sheetlike PAS *(arrow)* and an open angle *(right)*. *(Courtesy of Louis B. Cantor, MD.)*

most marked in the inferior angle. The pigmentation pattern of an individual angle is dynamic over time, especially in conditions such as *pigment dispersion syndrome.* Heavy pigmentation of the trabecular meshwork should suggest pigment dispersion or pseudoexfoliation syndrome. In pigment dispersion syndrome, over time, pigment may no longer be actively liberated, and the trabecular meshwork pigmentation dissipates. This occurs most rapidly in the inferior angle, resulting in relatively heavier pigmentation of the superior angle—sometimes the only remaining sign of previous pigment dispersion syndrome.

Pseudoexfoliation syndrome may be associated with pigment granules on the anterior surface of the iris and increased pigmentation in the anterior chamber angle, as iridolenticular friction in the peripupillary region is thought to cause pigment liberation from the iris epithelium and peripupillary transillumination defects. In addition, a line of pigment deposition, known as the *Sampaolesi line,* anterior to the Schwalbe line is often present in pseudoexfoliation syndrome. Other conditions that cause increased anterior chamber angle pigmentation include uveal melanoma, trauma, surgery, inflammation, angle closure, and hyphema.

Effects of trauma

Posttraumatic angle recession may be associated with monocular open-angle glaucoma. The gonioscopic criteria for diagnosing angle recession include

- an abnormally wide ciliary body band (Fig 4-9)
- increased prominence of the scleral spur
- torn iris processes
- marked variation of ciliary face width and angle depth in different quadrants of the same eye

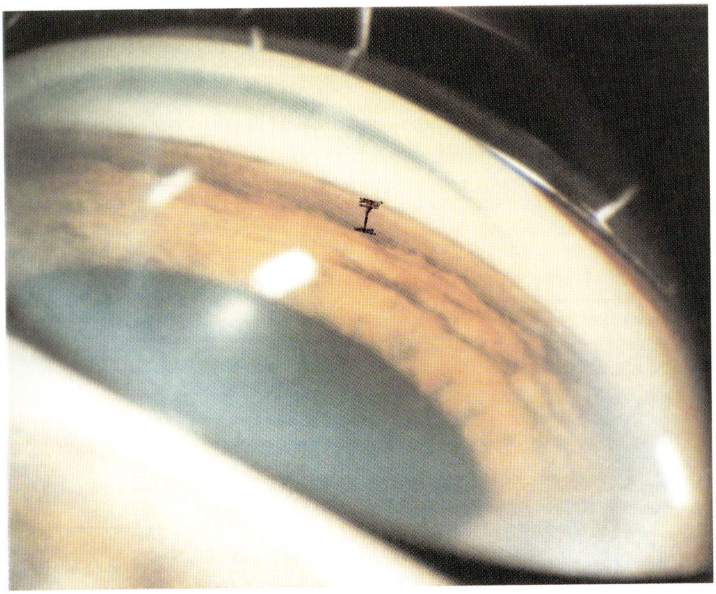

Figure 4-9 Goniophotograph showing angle recession. Note the widening of the ciliary body band. *(Reprinted with permission from Wright KW, ed.* Textbook of Ophthalmology. *Williams & Wilkins; 1997.)*

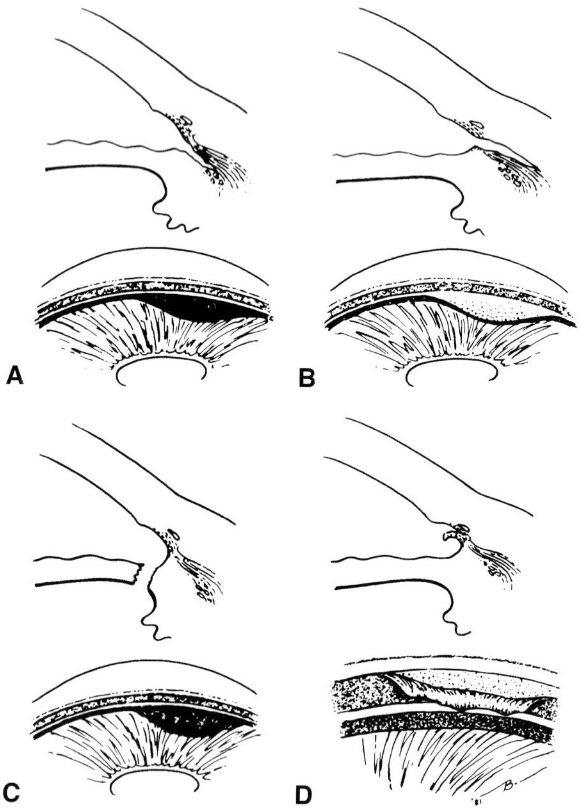

Figure 4-10 Forms of anterior chamber angle injury associated with blunt trauma, showing cross-sectional and corresponding gonioscopic appearance. **A,** Angle recession (tear between longitudinal and circular muscles of ciliary body). **B,** Cyclodialysis (separation of ciliary body from scleral spur) with widening of suprachoroidal space. **C,** Iridodialysis (tear in root of iris). **D,** Trabecular damage (tear in anterior portion of meshwork, creating a flap that is hinged at the scleral spur). *(Reproduced with permission from Shields MB.* Textbook of Glaucoma. *3rd ed. Williams & Wilkins; 1992.)*

In evaluating for angle recession, the clinician may find it helpful to compare one part of the angle to other areas in the same eye or to the same area in the fellow eye. Figure 4-10 illustrates a variety of gonioscopic findings caused by blunt trauma. If the ciliary body separates from the scleral spur *(cyclodialysis),* it will appear gonioscopically as a deep angle recess with a gap between the scleral spur and the ciliary body. Detection of a very small cleft may require ultrasound biomicroscopy.

Other findings

Various other findings that may be visible by gonioscopy include

- angle recession
- anteriorly rotated ciliary processes (sometimes visible after dilation)
- cyclodialysis cleft
- goniotomy or trabeculotomy cleft
- inflammatory angle precipitates (analogous to KPs)
- intraocular lens haptics
- iridodialysis
- iris or ciliary body tumors or cysts
- hyphema or hypopyon
- surgical devices such as aqueous drainage tubes and stents

- peripheral lens abnormalities such as severe zonular dehiscence (sometimes visible after dilation)
- retained anterior chamber foreign body or crystalline lens material
- sclerostomy site for trabeculectomy

Alward WLM, Longmuir RA. *Color Atlas of Gonioscopy.* 2nd ed. Foundation of the American Academy of Ophthalmology; 2008. Accessed October 6, 2021. www.aao.org/disease-review/color-atlas-of-gonioscopy

Anterior Segment Imaging

Ultrasound Biomicroscopy

Ultrasound biomicroscopy (UBM) is used to evaluate the anterior chamber angle and a variety of anterior segment structures and implanted devices that cannot be directly visualized or fully assessed with slit-lamp biomicroscopy. Similarly, UBM can be helpful in evaluating the anterior chamber angle of eyes with corneal opacities that prevent gonioscopic examination. UBM has also been used to assess the iris contour in pigment dispersion syndrome, helping to clarify the underlying mechanism of this condition (see Chapter 8).

Structures and conditions that can be evaluated by UBM include

- iris and ciliary body
  - plateau iris
  - choroidal effusion
  - tumors, cysts (Fig 4-11)
- position of implanted devices
  - drainage device tubes and stents
  - intraocular lens haptics
- foreign bodies or retained lens material

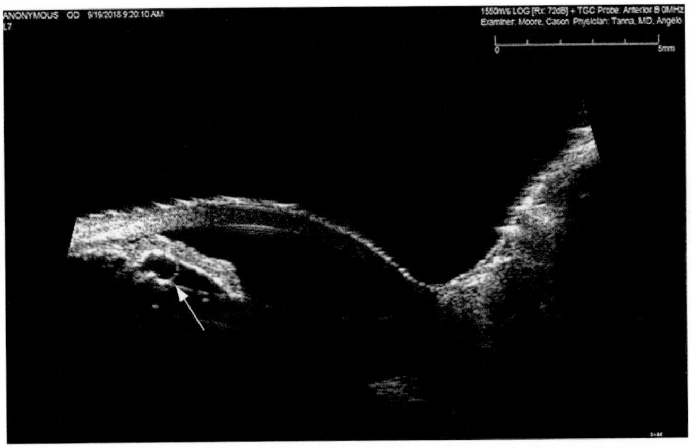

Figure 4-11 Ultrasound biomicroscopy b-scan demonstrating an area of angle closure as a result of a peripheral iris pigment epithelial cyst *(arrow)*. *(Courtesy of Angelo P. Tanna, MD.)*

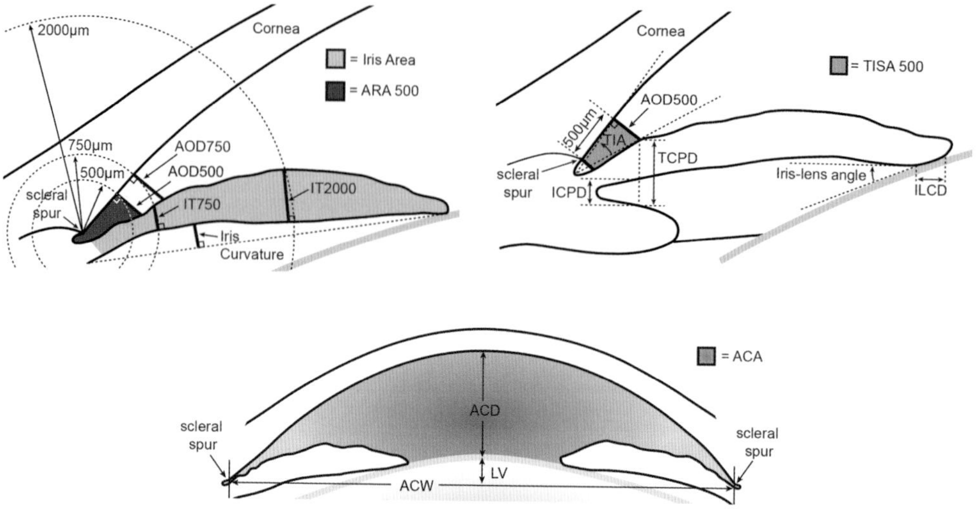

Figure 4-12 Schematic diagrams depicting anterior segment parameters captured by ultrasound biomicroscopy and anterior segment OCT. ACA = anterior chamber area; ACD = anterior chamber depth; ACW = anterior chamber width; AOD = angle opening distance; ARA = angle recess area; ICPD = iris–ciliary process distance; ILCD = iris–lens contact distance; LV = lens vault; TCPD = trabecular–ciliary process distance; TIA = trabecular iris angle; TISA = trabecular iris space. *(Courtesy of Chansangpetch S, Rojanapongpun P, Lin SC. Anterior segment imaging for angle closure.* Am J Ophthalmol. *2018;188:xvi–xxix.)*

Conventional ocular ultrasonography is typically performed using a transducer that operates at 10–20 MHz. Higher frequencies, however, are required to image anteriorly located structures and to provide sufficient resolution for meaningful evaluation of the anterior segment. Thus, anterior segment UBM is performed using 35–60 MHz (or higher frequency for imaging Schlemm canal) linear probes that must be positioned very close to the eye with a fluid interface (often contained within a disposable probe cover) for acoustic coupling. The high ultrasound frequency results in limited penetration—approximately 5 mm for a probe operating at 50 MHz.

The information provided by UBM is complementary to that obtained though gonioscopy and can help elucidate the underlying mechanism in some cases of angle closure (see Chapters 9 and 10). Assessment of UBM images for angle closure begins with identification of the scleral spur and determination of the degree of angle crowding. The mechanism(s) of angle closure can be inferred based on a qualitative assessment of the iris contour, peripheral iris thickness, ciliary body anatomy (size, position, and degree of rotation), anterior chamber depth, lens thickness, and lens vault (Fig 4-12; see also Chapter 9). Various quantitative parameters that characterize some of these anatomic features on UBM are also being investigated with OCT (see the following section). The most important ones are summarized in Table 4-2 and illustrated in Figure 4-12. Automated quantitative analysis is available on some commercially available UBM platforms; however, the operator must usually identify the scleral spur.

Anterior Segment Optical Coherence Tomography

Anterior segment OCT (AS-OCT) enables high-resolution imaging of the anterior segment, including the anterior chamber angle (Fig 4-13). Compared with UBM, a major limitation of

Table 4-2 Anterior Segment Parameters Obtained From Anterior Segment Imaging[a]

Parameters	Definition	Common Parameters[b]	Devices
Angle opening distance (AOD)	The distance between the cornea and iris along a line perpendicular to the cornea at a specified distance (μm) from the scleral spur	AOD 250 AOD 500 AOD 750	AS-OCT UBM
Angle recess area (ARA)	The triangular area lying between the line used for AOD, the anterior iris surface, and the inner corneoscleral wall	ARA 500 ARA 750	AS-OCT UBM
Trabecular iris space area (TISA)	The trapezoidal area lying between the line for AOD, the anterior iris surface, the inner corneoscleral wall, and the line drawn from the scleral spur perpendicular to the plane of the inner scleral wall to the opposing iris	TISA 500 TISA 750	AS-OCT
Iris thickness (IT)	The length of a perpendicular line drawn from the point of intersection at the anterior surface of the iris, where a circle with a specified radius (eg, 750 μm) centered at the scleral spur intersects with the anterior surface of the iris, to the posterior surface of the iris	IT 750 IT 2000 ITM (max iris thickness along the entire iris)	AS-OCT UBM
Iris curvature	The length of a perpendicular line extending from a line drawn from the most peripheral to the most central points of the posterior iris to the iris pigment epithelium at the point of greatest convexity	NA	AS-OCT
Iris area	The cross-sectional area of the full length of the iris from the scleral spur to the pupil margin	NA	AS-OCT
Iris volume	The entire iris volume, calculated from the summation of 8 partial volumes mathematically estimated from 4 iris cross-sectional areas at 45° intervals	NA	AS-OCT
Lens vault	The perpendicular distance between the anterior pole of the crystalline lens and a horizontal line joining the 2 scleral spurs	NA	AS-OCT
Anterior chamber width (ACW)	The length of the horizontal line connecting scleral spur to scleral spur	NA	AS-OCT
Anterior chamber depth (ACD)	The axial distance from the internal corneal surface to the lens surface	NA	AS-OCT UBM
Anterior chamber area (ACA)	The cross-sectional area whose boundaries are the corneoscleral inner surface and the anterior iris and lens surfaces (within the pupil)	NA	AS-OCT

(Continued)

Table 4-2 *(continued)*

Parameters	**Definition**	**Common Parameters**[b]	**Devices**
Anterior chamber volume (ACV)	The sum of partial volumes of every 15° meridional section that is calculated from the whole chamber volume, which is based on a mathematical calculation from 12 cross-sectional images of the anterior chamber	NA	AS-OCT
Trabecular–ciliary process distance (TCPD)	The distance between the trabecular meshwork and the ciliary process at 500 μm anterior to the scleral spur	NA	UBM

AS-OCT = anterior segment optical coherence tomography; NA = not applicable; UBM = ultrasound biomicroscopy.
[a] See Fig 4-12 for an illustration of many of these features.
[b] The number indicates the distance (μm) measured anterior to the scleral spur; for example, AOD 500 is the distance between the cornea and iris along a line perpendicular to the cornea at a distance of 500 μm from the scleral spur.

Modified with permission from Chansangpetch S, Rojanapongpun P, Lin SC. Anterior segment imaging for angle closure. *Am J Ophthalmol.* 2018;188:xix.

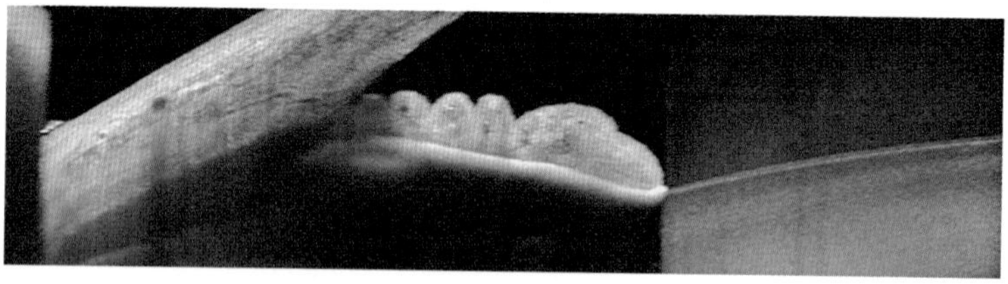

Figure 4-13 An example of an anterior segment OCT scan that demonstrates iridotrabecular contact. *(Courtesy of Angelo P. Tanna, MD.)*

AS-OCT is that it does not allow visualization of the ciliary sulcus and ciliary body. As with UBM, AS-OCT does not always yield images that allow reliable identification of angle landmarks. Moreover, neither modality can differentiate between appositional and synechial angle closure—a distinction that is possible only with dynamic gonioscopy. In contrast, AS-OCT is a noncontact modality that can be performed relatively rapidly.

Gonioscopy remains the reference standard method for evaluating the anterior chamber angle, but it has limitations. A skilled examiner and patient cooperation are required, and the results are inherently subjective. The illumination required to obtain an adequate view of the angle structures can cause miosis, resulting in the relative opening of the angle compared to its status at lower levels of ambient light. These limitations are largely obviated with AS-OCT; however, correct identification of the scleral spur is not always possible, complicating the interpretation of the degree of angle crowding.

AS-OCT has the potential to add meaningful information to aid in the detection of angle-closure disease. Both time-domain and spectral-domain OCT, operating at various wavelengths, have been studied and seem to have similar diagnostic performance. The principles for evaluation of the angle are similar to those previously described for UBM, as are many of the quantitative parameters (see Table 4-2 and Fig 4-12). As with UBM, automated quantitative analysis is available on some platforms.

Chansangpetch S, Rojanapongpun P, Lin SC. Anterior segment imaging for angle closure. *Am J Ophthalmol.* 2018;188:xvi–xxix.

Specular Microscopy

Specular microscopy (Fig 4-14B) is discussed in BCSC Section 8, *External Disease and Cornea.* The technique allows noncontact, noninvasive imaging of the corneal endothelial cell layer. Most commercially available devices automatically identify the endothelial cells and analyze the images to provide the user with quantitative assessments of the endothelial cell density (ECD) and morphology. ECD is often monitored in the context of clinical trials of surgically implanted devices such as aqueous drainage devices and stents. The US Food and Drug Administration (FDA) has advised monitoring ECD in eyes with the CyPass Micro-Stent, a suprachoroidal stent that was recalled by the FDA (see Chapter 13).

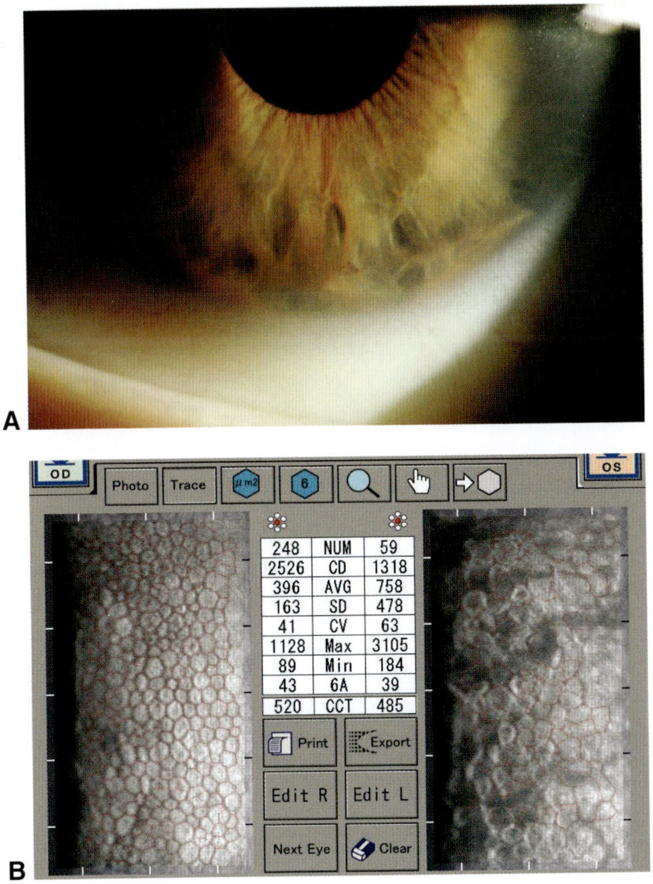

Figure 4-14 Iridocorneal endothelial syndrome. **A,** Slit-lamp view, with mild distortion of the inferior iris and peripheral anterior synechiae. **B,** Specular microscopy images of the same patient. The right-eye image discloses tightly packed endothelial cells with a normal hexagonal shape, while the left-eye images reveal endothelial cells that are reduced in number and pleomorphic. Many cells exhibit a dark specular reflex. *(Courtesy of Angelo P. Tanna, MD.)*

Specular microscopy is useful for the diagnosis and monitoring of various posterior corneal disorders such as posterior polymorphous dystrophy and iridocorneal endothelial syndrome. The latter is a rare condition in which corneal endothelial cells proliferate and migrate beyond the Schwalbe line and anterior chamber angle, onto the iris. Secondary angle-closure glaucoma ensues as this cellular membrane contracts (see Chapter 10). In this disease the endothelial cell count is reduced, and the cells lose their normal hexagonal shape (see Fig 4-14).

CHAPTER 5

Clinical Evaluation and Imaging of the Posterior Segment: Optic Nerve, Retinal Nerve Fiber Layer, and Macula in Glaucoma

Highlights

- Glaucomatous damage tends to preferentially affect the inferior and superior poles of the optic disc, especially in the early stages of the disease.
- Funduscopic determination of the cup–disc ratio is an insufficient and generally inaccurate way of documenting the amount of optic nerve damage in glaucoma. It is preferable to obtain objective documentation of the appearance of the optic disc by photographs or imaging whenever possible.
- Optical coherence tomography (OCT) is the most commonly used imaging technique. OCT provides quantitative measurements of the peripapillary retinal nerve fiber layer thickness, optic nerve head topography, and macular thickness, which can help discriminate glaucomatous eyes from healthy eyes.
- Glaucomatous damage frequently affects the macular region, leading to central visual field losses that can go undetected with conventional perimetry. This damage may be detectable by OCT imaging of the macula.
- It is important to consider the possible effects of aging on longitudinal changes of OCT parameters over time.

Optic Nerve Anatomy

The entire visual pathway is described and illustrated in BCSC Section 5, *Neuro-Ophthalmology*. For further discussion of retinal involvement in the visual process, see Section 12, *Retina and Vitreous*.

An understanding of the normal and pathologic appearance of the optic nerve allows the clinician to detect and monitor glaucoma. The optic nerve is composed of the axons of retinal ganglion cells (RGCs), glial tissue, extracellular matrix, and blood vessels. The human optic nerve consists of approximately 1.2–1.5 million RGC axons, although

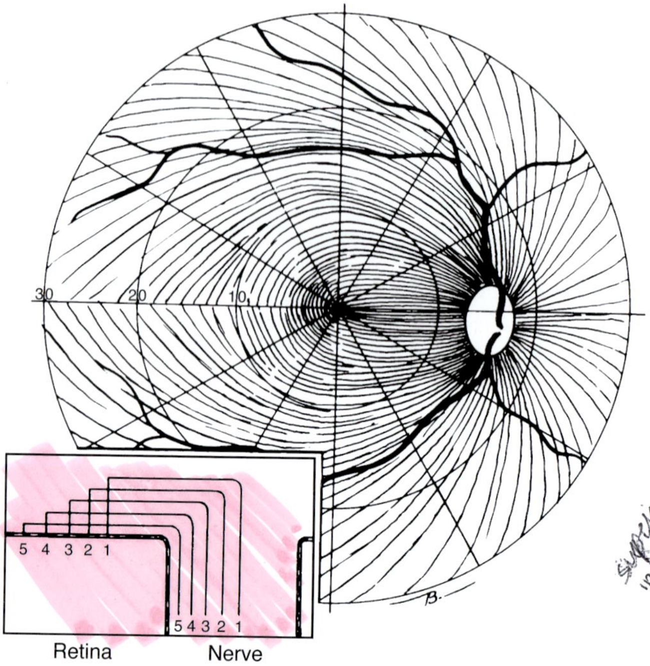

Figure 5-1 Anatomy of retinal nerve fiber distribution. Inset depicts cross-sectional view of axonal arrangement. Peripheral fibers run closer to the choroid and exit in the periphery of the optic nerve, whereas fibers originating closer to the nerve head are situated closer to the vitreous and occupy a more central portion of the nerve. In this schematic, the fovea is depicted as being located along the horizontal meridian through the center of the optic disc. In most eyes, however, the fovea is located inferior to the horizontal meridian. *(Reproduced with permission from Shields MB.* Textbook of Glaucoma. *3rd ed. Williams & Wilkins; 1992.)*

there is significant individual variability. The cell bodies of the RGCs lie in the ganglion cell layer of the retina, and their axons synapse in the lateral geniculate nucleus. The intraorbital portion of the optic nerve has 2 components: the anterior optic nerve and the posterior optic nerve. The anterior optic nerve extends from the retinal surface to the retrolaminar region, where the nerve exits the posterior aspect of the globe.

The average diameter of the optic nerve head (ONH)* is approximately 1.5–1.7 mm as measured with planimetry, but it varies widely among individuals and ethnic groups. Immediately upon exiting the globe, the optic nerve expands to approximately 3–4 mm. This increase in size is accounted for by axonal myelination, glial tissue, and the beginning of the leptomeninges (optic nerve sheath). The axons are separated into fascicles within the optic nerve, with the intervening spaces occupied by astrocytes.

Figure 5-1 shows the distribution of nerve fibers as they enter the ONH. The arcuate nerve fibers entering the superior and inferior poles of the optic disc are more susceptible to glaucomatous damage, possibly because of the larger size of the pores of the lamina cribrosa in these regions. This susceptibility explains the frequent occurrence of arcuate

*Note: The terms *optic disc* and *optic nerve head* are used interchangeably in the literature and in this book.

visual field defects in eyes with glaucoma. The arrangement of the axons in the ONH and their differential susceptibility to damage determine the patterns of visual field loss in glaucoma, which are described and illustrated in Chapter 6 in this volume.

The anterior optic nerve can be divided into 4 layers:

- nerve fiber
- prelaminar
- laminar
- retrolaminar

The most anterior zone is the *superficial nerve fiber layer region,* which is continuous with the nerve fiber layer (NFL) of the retina. This region is composed primarily of the axons of the RGCs in transition from the superficial retina to the neuronal component of the optic nerve. The NFL can best be visualized with slit-lamp biomicroscopy or in fundus photographs with a red-free (green) filter. Immediately posterior to the NFL is the *prelaminar region,* which lies adjacent to the peripapillary choroid. More posteriorly, the *laminar region* is continuous with the sclera and is composed of the lamina cribrosa, a structure consisting of fenestrated connective tissue lamellae that allow the transit of neural fibers through the scleral coat. Finally, the *retrolaminar region* posterior to the lamina cribrosa is marked by the beginning of axonal myelination and is surrounded by the leptomeninges of the central nervous system.

The lamina cribrosa provides the main structural support for the optic nerve as it exits the eye. It consists of a reticulated network of connective tissue beams that are composed primarily of collagen (Fig 5-2). Other extracellular matrix components include elastin, laminin, and fibronectin. The laminar beams also contain the capillaries that nourish this critical region. Neural components of the optic nerve pass through these connective tissue beams. In addition, relatively large central fenestrations allow transit of the central retinal artery and central retinal vein. Scanning electron microscopy of the normal lamina cribrosa discloses a lower density of connective tissue and extracellular matrix material at its inferior and superior poles, where the laminar pores are larger in comparison to the nasal and temporal regions. This difference may explain the greater susceptibility to damage of the inferior and superior regions of the optic nerve. The pores of the lamina cribrosa may often be seen by ophthalmoscopy at the base of the optic disc cup. Between the optic nerve and the adjacent choroidal and scleral tissue lies a rim of connective tissue called the ring of Elschnig.

Downs JC. Optic nerve head biomechanics in aging and disease. *Exp Eye Res.* 2015;133:19–29.

Blood Supply to the Optic Nerve

The vascular anatomy of the anterior optic nerve and peripapillary region has been studied extensively (Fig 5-3). The arterial supply of the anterior optic nerve is derived entirely from branches of the ophthalmic artery via 1–5 posterior ciliary arteries. Typically, between 2 and 4 posterior ciliary arteries course anteriorly before dividing into approximately 10–20 short posterior ciliary arteries prior to entering the posterior globe. Often,

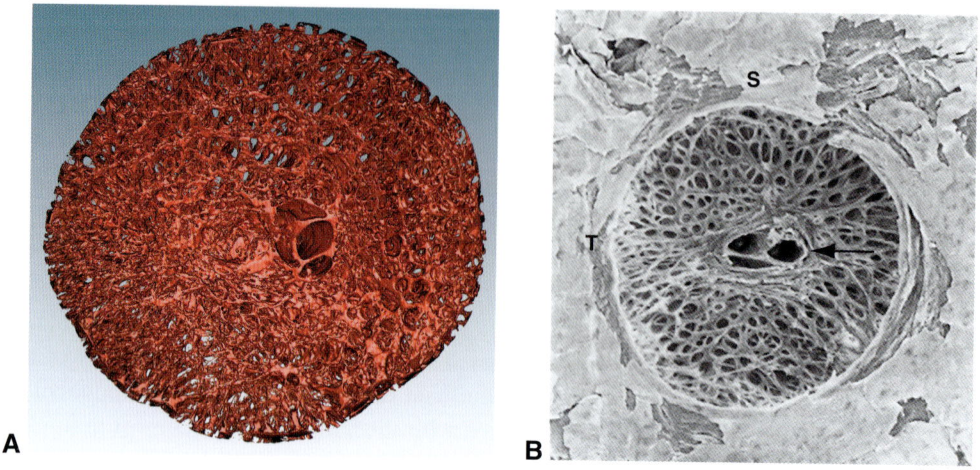

Figure 5-2 Imaging of the lamina cribrosa, which consists of a reticulated network of connective tissue beams. **A,** Anterior view of the human lamina cribrosa from a healthy donor, obtained from 3-dimensional episcopic autofluorescent reconstruction illustrating the reticular network of supportive connective tissue. **B,** A scanning electron micrograph of a nonglaucomatous human lamina cribrosa after trypsin digestion viewed en face. The *arrow* points to the central retinal vessels. *S* and *T* indicate the superior and temporal regions of the lamina cribrosa, respectively. The density of the connective tissue and the size of the laminar pores vary by region. The lamina cribrosa is thought to be more structurally vulnerable to damage in the inferior and superior poles of the optic nerve head (ONH) because of the larger pores in these locations. *(Part A courtesy of Crawford Downs, PhD, and Christopher Girkin, MD; part B courtesy of Harry A. Quigley, MD.)*

the posterior ciliary arteries separate into a medial and a lateral group before branching into the short posterior ciliary arteries. These arteries penetrate the perineural sclera of the posterior globe to supply the peripapillary choroid, as well as most of the anterior optic nerve. Some short posterior ciliary arteries course, without branching, through the sclera directly into the choroid; others divide within the sclera to provide branches to both the choroid and the optic nerve. Often a discontinuous arterial circle, the *circle of Zinn-Haller,* exists within the perineural sclera. The central retinal artery, also a posterior orbital branch of the ophthalmic artery, penetrates the optic nerve approximately 10–15 mm posterior to the globe. The central retinal artery has few, if any, intraneural branches; the exception is an occasional small branch within the retrolaminar region, which may anastomose with the pial system. The central retinal artery courses adjacent to the central retinal vein within the central portion of the optic nerve.

The superficial NFL is supplied principally by recurrent retinal arterioles branching from the central retinal artery. These small vessels, referred to as *epipapillary vessels,* originate in the peripapillary NFL and run toward the center of the ONH. The capillary branches from these vessels are continuous with the retinal capillaries at the ONH margin, but they also have posterior anastomoses with the prelaminar capillaries of the optic nerve. The temporal NFL may have an arterial contribution from the cilioretinal artery, when it is present.

The prelaminar region is principally supplied by direct branches of the short posterior ciliary arteries and by branches of the circle of Zinn-Haller, when it is present. In eyes

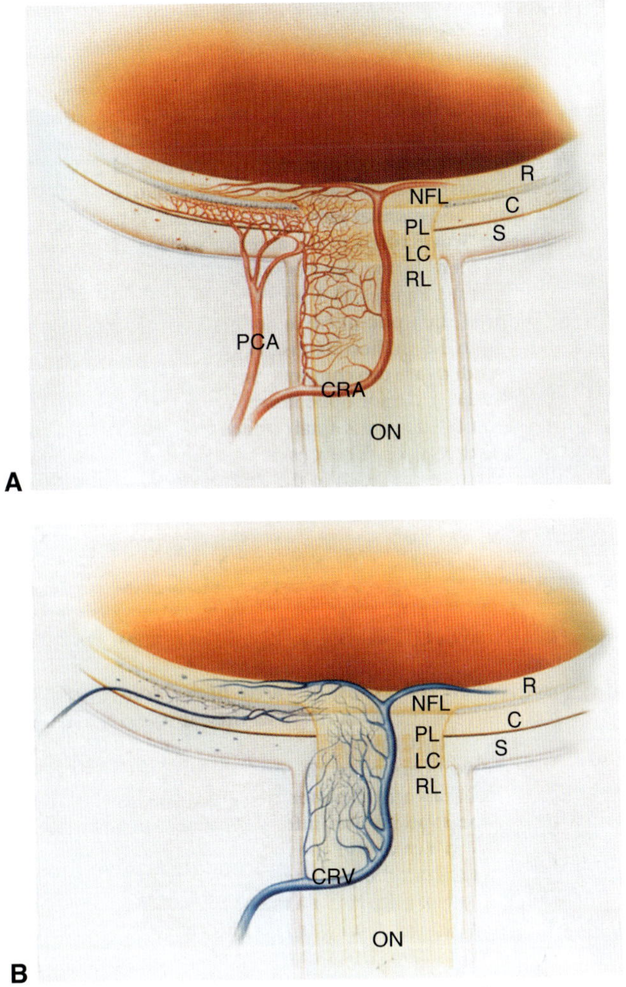

Figure 5-3 Anterior optic nerve vasculature. **A,** Arterial supply to the anterior optic nerve and peripapillary choroid. **B,** Venous drainage of the anterior optic nerve and peripapillary choroid. C=choroid; CRA=central retinal artery; CRV=central retinal vein; LC=lamina cribrosa; NFL=nerve fiber layer; ON=optic nerve; PCA=posterior ciliary artery; PL=prelamina; R=retina; RL=retrolamina; S=sclera. *(Reprinted with permission from Cioffi GA. In Ritch R, Shields MB, Krupin T, eds.* The Glaucomas. *2nd ed. Mosby; 1996:178, 183, Figs 8-2, 8-12.)*

with a well-developed circle of Zinn-Haller, arterial branches emerge to supply both the prelaminar and laminar regions. Similar to the prelaminar region, the lamina cribrosa region receives its blood supply from branches of the short posterior ciliary arteries or from branches of the circle of Zinn-Haller. These precapillary branches perforate the outer aspects of the lamina cribrosa before branching into an intraseptal capillary network. Arterioles also branch from the short posterior ciliary arteries and the circle of Zinn-Haller and course posteriorly to supply the pial arteries. These pial arteries often contribute to the laminar region. As in the prelaminar region, the larger vessels of the peripapillary choroid may contribute occasional small arterioles to this region, although there is no connection between the peripapillary choriocapillaris and the capillaries of the optic nerve.

The retrolaminar region is also supplied by branches from the short posterior ciliary arteries, as well as by the pial arterial branches coursing adjacent to the retrolaminar optic nerve region. The pial arteries originate both from the central retinal artery, before it pierces the retrobulbar optic nerve, and from branches of the short posterior ciliary arteries more anteriorly. The central retinal artery may supply several small intraneural branches in the retrolaminar region.

The rich capillary beds of each of the 4 regions within the anterior optic nerve are anatomically confluent. Venous drainage of the anterior optic nerve occurs almost exclusively via a single vein, the central retinal vein. In the NFL, blood drains directly into the retinal veins, which then join to form the central retinal vein. In the prelaminar, laminar, and retrolaminar regions, venous drainage also occurs via the central retinal vein or axial tributaries to the central retinal vein.

Mackenzie PJ, Cioffi GA. Vascular anatomy of the optic nerve head. *Can J Ophthalmol.* 2008;43(3):308–312.

Glaucomatous Optic Neuropathy

Characteristic changes in the optic nerve head are the defining feature of glaucoma (Fig 5-4). Histologic examination reveals that early glaucomatous cupping begins with structural damage to the lamina cribrosa. Subsequently, there is apoptotic loss of RGCs and their axons, blood vessels, and glial cells. RGC axonal damage begins at the level of the lamina cribrosa. It is most pronounced at the superior and inferior poles of the ONH. In many cases, although not always, structural optic nerve changes may precede detectable functional loss as measured by standard perimetry.

Glaucomatous optic neuropathy is a progressive degeneration of RGCs and their axons in association with lamina cribrosa damage characterized by rupture of the laminar beams and enlargement of the optic disc cup. Transsynaptic neurodegeneration extends from the optic nerve to the major vision centers in the brain, such as the lateral geniculate nucleus and occipital cortex. Intraocular pressure (IOP) plays a major role in the development of glaucomatous optic neuropathy in most affected individuals and is considered the most significant risk factor. IOP can cause mechanical stress and strain on the posterior structures of the eye, particularly the lamina cribrosa, which is the weakest point in the posterior wall of the eye, and its adjacent tissues. IOP-induced stress and strain may result in compression, deformation, and remodeling of the lamina cribrosa with consequent mechanical axonal damage and disruption of axonal transport. Studies involving cats and monkeys with experimentally induced ocular hypertension have also demonstrated blockade of both orthograde and retrograde axonal transport at the level of the lamina cribrosa. Blockage of axonal transport occurs early in the pathogenesis of glaucoma and interrupts retrograde delivery of essential trophic factors to RGCs from their brainstem target (relay neurons of the lateral geniculate nucleus). Disrupted axonal transport also results in collections of vesicles and disorganization of microtubules and neurofilaments

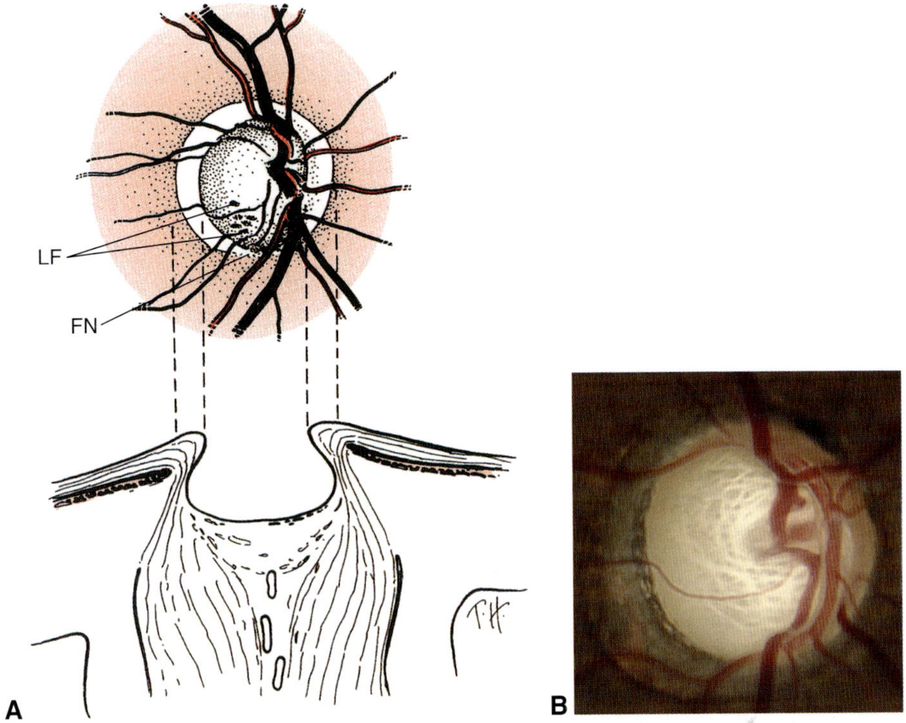

Figure 5-4 Two views of glaucomatous optic nerves. **A,** Glaucomatous optic nerve (anterior ONH and transverse view, right eye). Note thinning, undermining, and focal notching (FN) of inferior neuroretinal rim; enlarged central cup with visible laminar fenestrations (LF); nasal shift of retinal vessels; and peripapillary atrophy. **B,** Clinical view of glaucomatous ONH demonstrating extensive loss of the neuroretinal rim. *(Part A reprinted with permission from Wright KW, ed.* Textbook of Ophthalmology. *Williams & Wilkins; 1997. Part B courtesy of Ronald L. Gross, MD.)*

in the prelaminar and postlaminar regions. Similar ultrastructural changes in optic nerve fibers are observed in postmortem human eyes with glaucoma.

Although the role of IOP as a risk factor for the development and progression of glaucoma has been well established, up to one-third of primary open-angle glaucoma (POAG) patients in North America have IOP levels within statistically normal limits. For reasons that are unclear, an even larger proportion of POAG patients in certain Asian populations, such as Japanese and Korean, have normal IOP. In Japan, for example, 90% of POAG patients have statistically normal IOP. Whether there are any pathophysiological differences between glaucoma at low and high pressures is unknown (see Chapter 7). Impaired microcirculation, altered immunity, excitotoxicity, and oxidative stress may also contribute to the pathogenesis of glaucomatous damage. Current thinking recognizes that glaucoma comprises a heterogeneous family of disorders mediated, most likely, by many factors.

Weinreb RN, Aung T, Medeiros FA. The pathophysiology and treatment of glaucoma: a review. *JAMA*. 2014;311(18):1901–1911.

Clinical Examination of the Optic Nerve Head

Clinical examination of the ONH is preferably performed with a *slit-lamp biomicroscope* combined with a high-magnification posterior pole lens (60, 78, or 90 diopter [D] lens). The slit beam, rather than diffuse illumination, is useful for determining subtle changes in the contour of the nerve head. This system provides high magnification, excellent illumination, and a stereoscopic view. In addition, adjusting the height of the slit beam enables quantitative measurement of the diameter of the ONH. The disc is viewed through the handheld lens and the height of the slit beam is adjusted so that it is the same as the vertical diameter of the disc. The disc diameter can then be calculated, adjusting for the magnification of the lens used as follows:

- with a 60 D lens, the height of the slit equals the disc diameter, in millimeters, read directly from the scale
- with a 78 D lens, multiply the height of the slit by 1.1
- with a 90 D lens, multiply the height of the slit by 1.3

The normal ONH ranges from approximately 1.5 to 2.2 mm in diameter. Note that the patient's refractive error will affect this measurement, resulting in underestimation in patients with myopia and overestimation in those with hyperopia.

The *direct ophthalmoscope* also may be used for clinical examination of the ONH. However, this instrument may not provide sufficient stereoscopic detail to detect subtle changes in ONH topography. The head-mounted *indirect ophthalmoscope* can be used for examination of the ONH in young children and in patients who are unable to cooperate with slit-lamp biomicroscopy. Lower-power lenses (15 D) can also be helpful when slit-lamp biomicroscopy is not possible and a more detailed view of the optic nerve is needed. Although cupping of the optic nerve can be detected with the indirect ophthalmoscope, in general, optic nerve cupping and pallor appear less pronounced than with slit-lamp methods, and the magnification offered by the indirect ophthalmoscope is often inadequate for detecting subtle or localized details important in the evaluation of glaucoma. Thus, the indirect ophthalmoscope is not recommended for routine use in examining the ONH.

The ONH is usually round or slightly oval in shape and contains a central *cup*. The tissue between the cup and the disc margin is called the *neural rim* or *neuroretinal rim*. The size of the physiologic cup is developmentally determined and is related to the size of the disc. For a given number of nerve fibers, the larger the overall disc area is, the larger the cup will be. The cup–disc ratio alone is not an adequate assessment of the ONH for possible glaucomatous damage. For example, a 0.7 cup–disc ratio in a large ONH may be normal, whereas a 0.3 cup–disc ratio in a very small disc is likely pathologic. Thus, assessment of the disc size is important; in healthy subjects, a small disc (vertical disc diameter < 1.5 mm) will have a small cup, whereas a large disc (vertical disc diameter > 2.2 mm) will have a large cup. Individuals of African ancestry, on average, have larger disc areas and larger cup–disc ratios than do White individuals, although substantial overlap exists.

Differentiating a large physiologic or normal cup from acquired *glaucomatous cupping* of the ONH can be difficult. The early changes of glaucomatous optic neuropathy are subtle and include the following (Table 5-1):

- generalized enlargement of the cup
- focal rim thinning
- superficial disc hemorrhage
- retinal nerve fiber layer (RNFL) atrophy
- asymmetry of cupping
- peripapillary atrophy (PPA) of the beta (β) zone

Diffuse neuroretinal rim thinning associated with generalized enlargement of the cup may be an early sign of glaucomatous damage. However, diffuse loss may be difficult to appreciate unless previous objective documentation of the ONH (eg, photographs) is available. Comparing 1 eye with the fellow eye may be helpful, because cup–disc ratio asymmetry greater than 0.2 is unusual in healthy eyes in the absence of disc size asymmetry (Fig 5-5). The vertical cup–disc ratio typically ranges between 0.1 and 0.4, although up to 5% of individuals without glaucoma will have cup–disc ratios larger than 0.6. Asymmetry of the cup–disc ratio of more than 0.2 occurs in fewer than 1% of individuals without glaucoma. This asymmetry may be related to disc size asymmetry. Increased size of the physiologic cup may be a familial trait, and it is also observed with high myopia. An oblique insertion of the optic nerve into the globe of individuals with high myopia may also cause the ONH to appear tilted. Examination of other family members may clarify whether a large cup is inherited or acquired.

Localized loss of the neuroretinal rim usually occurs first at the inferior and superior temporal poles of the optic nerve in early glaucomatous optic neuropathy (Fig 5-6).

Table 5-1 Ophthalmoscopic Signs of Glaucoma

Generalized	Focal	Less Specific
Large optic cup	Notching of the rim	Exposed lamina cribrosa
Asymmetry of the cups	Vertical elongation of the cup	Nasal displacement of vessels
Progressive enlargement of the cup	Cupping to the rim margin	Baring of circumlinear vessels
	Nerve fiber layer hemorrhage	Peripapillary atrophy
	Nerve fiber layer loss	

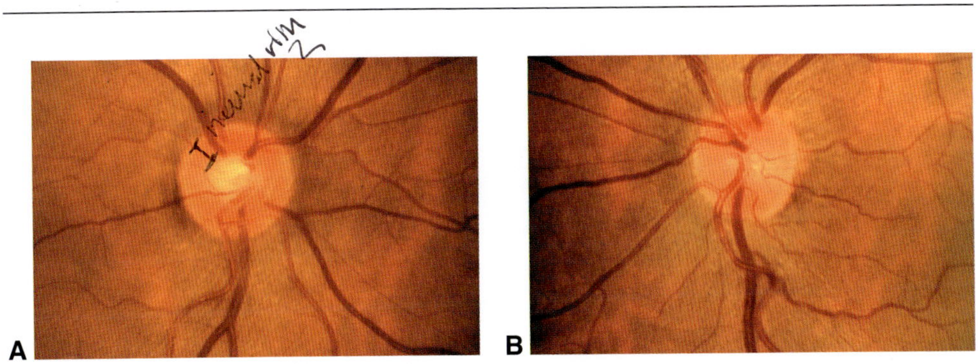

Figure 5-5 ONH photographs showing asymmetry of optic nerve cupping. Note the generalized enlargement of the cup in the right eye **(A)** as compared with the normal left eye **(B).** *(Courtesy of G.A. Cioffi, MD.)*

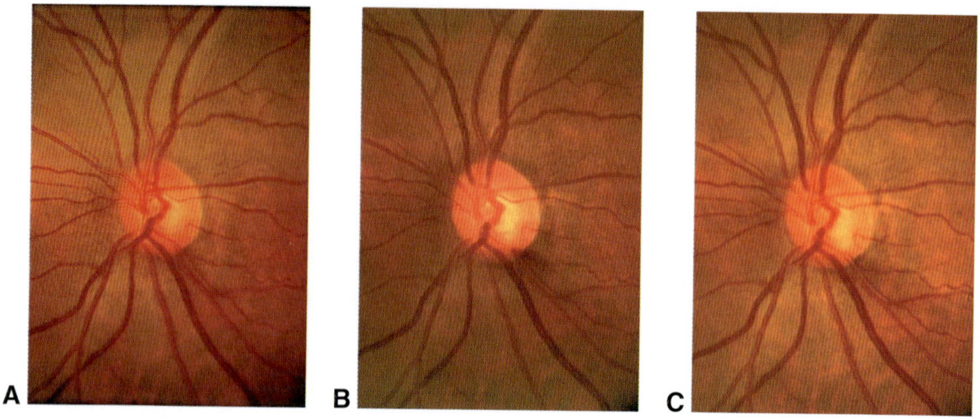

Figure 5-6 Progressive optic disc excavation in a patient with uncontrolled open-angle glaucoma over a 3-year period. The overall size of the optic disc is small. **A,** The inferior overall cup size is larger than expected for a small optic disc and the inferior neuroretinal rim is thinner than the superior rim, suggestive of early glaucomatous optic neuropathy. **B,** There is progressive thinning of the inferior neuroretinal rim at 5 o'clock, and an optic disc hemorrhage is present in the same location. **C,** Further inferior neuroretinal rim loss is evident at the 5-o'clock position, where a notch is developing. *(Courtesy of Angelo P. Tanna, MD.)*

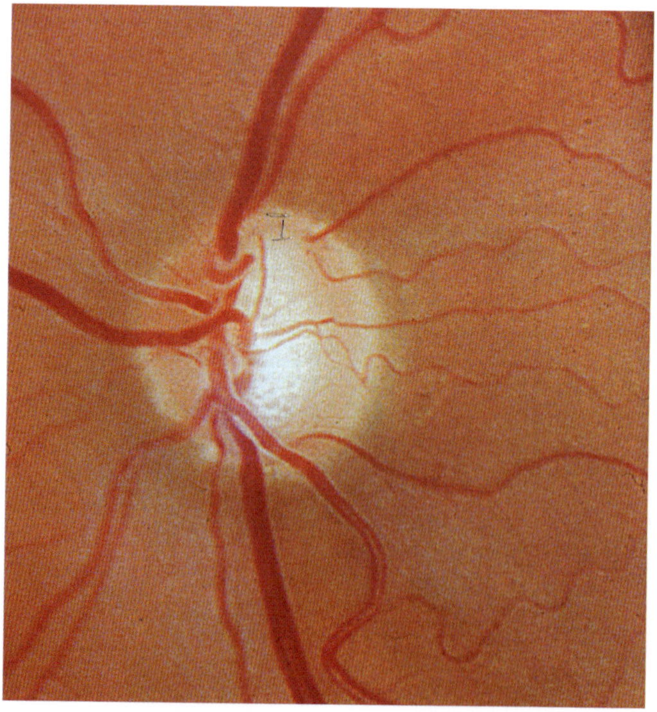

Figure 5-7 ONH photograph showing vertical elongation of the cup with localized thinning of the inferior and superior neuroretinal rim in the left eye of a patient with moderately advanced glaucoma. *(Courtesy of Felipe A. Medeiros, MD, PhD.)*

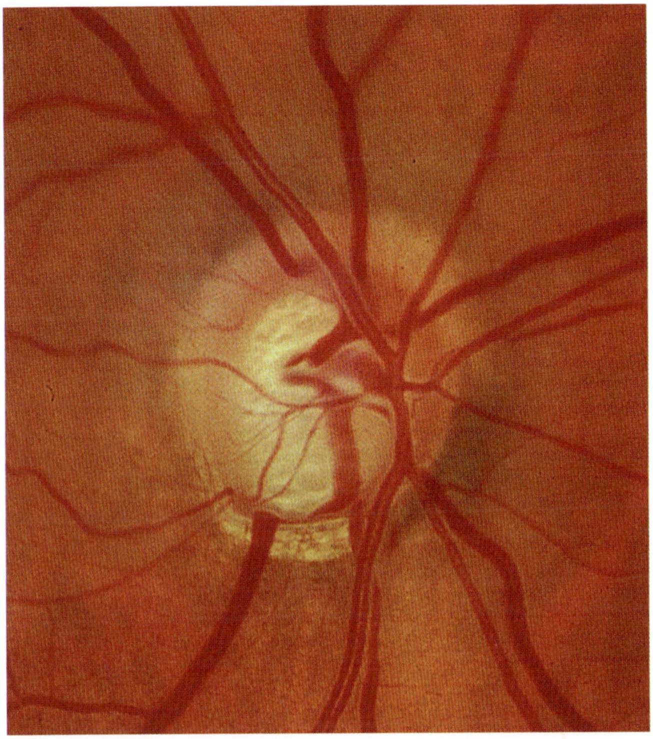

Figure 5-8 Acquired optic disc pit located in the inferior temporal region. Note the absence of rim tissue. *(Courtesy of Felipe A. Medeiros, MD, PhD.)*

The preferential loss of rim tissue in the superior and inferior poles leads to a vertically elongated cup in glaucomatous nerves (Fig 5-7). To help identify subtle thinning of the neuroretinal rim, a convention referred to as the *ISNT rule* may be useful. In healthy eyes, the *I*nferior neuroretinal rim is generally the thickest, followed by the *S*uperior rim, the *N*asal rim, and finally the *T*emporal rim. Therefore, if the rim widths do not follow this pattern, there should be increased concern for focal loss of rim tissue. However, violation of the ISNT rule is not highly specific and may also be observed in healthy eyes. Deep localized notching, in which the lamina cribrosa is visible at the disc margin, is sometimes termed an *acquired optic disc pit* (Fig 5-8). Patients with acquired pits are at especially high risk for progression. Even in the healthy eye, laminar trabeculations or pores may be visible as grayish dots in the base of the physiologic cup. In glaucomatous optic neuropathy, optic disc excavation is characterized by extensive exposure of the underlying lamina cribrosa and its pores or striations in the optic nerve cup (Fig 5-9). The backward bowing, strain, and compression of the lamina cribrosa cause damage to the laminar pores and beams. Glaucomatous damage to the lamina may also cause tearing of the connective tissue bundles between the pores, leading to coalescence of small pores and formation of larger ones. As the cup enlarges, nasal migration of the central retinal artery and central retinal vein is often observed.

Retinal nerve fiber layer hemorrhages can be a sign of glaucoma and usually appear as a linear red streak on or near the disc surface (Fig 5-10). However, their appearance can

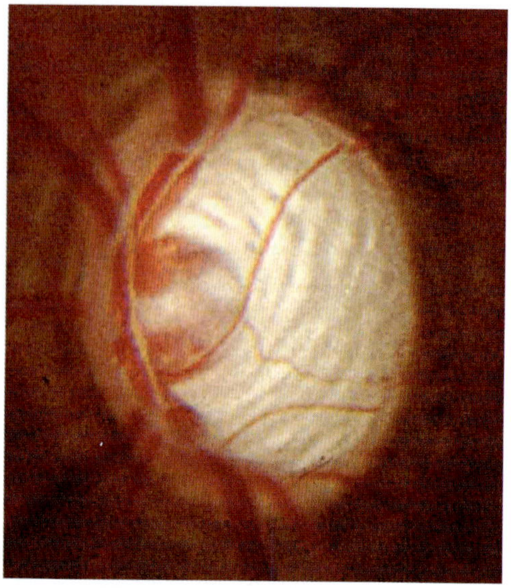

Figure 5-9 Striations of the lamina cribrosa in an optic nerve with severe glaucomatous damage. *(Courtesy of Felipe A. Medeiros, MD, PhD.)*

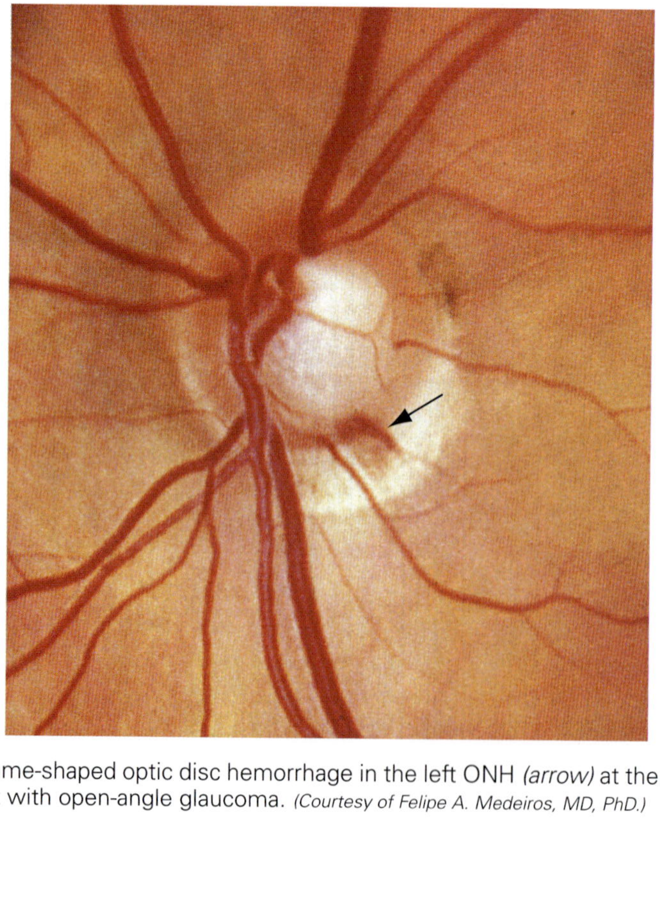

Figure 5-10 Flame-shaped optic disc hemorrhage in the left ONH *(arrow)* at the 5-o'clock position in a patient with open-angle glaucoma. *(Courtesy of Felipe A. Medeiros, MD, PhD.)*

be highly variable, and hemorrhages may be difficult to detect unless the clinician actively searches for them. At some time during the course of their disease, one-third of patients with glaucoma may develop hemorrhages, which typically clear over several weeks to a few months. Some glaucoma patients have repeated episodes of optic disc hemorrhage, whereas others have none. Disc hemorrhages are an important prognostic sign of the development or progression of visual field loss, and the presence of a disc hemorrhage in any patient warrants detailed evaluation and follow-up. In many cases, disc hemorrhages are followed by localized notching of the rim and visual field loss. Disc hemorrhages may also be caused by posterior vitreous detachments, diabetes mellitus, retinal vein occlusions, and anticoagulation therapy.

The RNFL of the healthy eye is best visualized with red-free (green) illumination. As the nerve fibers extend from the peripheral retina to converge at the ONH, they appear as fine striations created by the bundles of axons. In the healthy eye, the brightness and striations of the NFL are more easily visible superiorly and inferiorly. In an eye with progressive glaucomatous optic neuropathy, the NFL thins and becomes less visible. The loss may be diffuse (generalized) or localized (Fig 5-11). With diffuse loss, there is a general decrease in the RNFL brightness, with a reduction of the usual difference between the superior and inferior poles in comparison to the temporal and nasal regions. Localized RNFL loss appears as wedge-shaped dark areas emanating from the ONH in an arcuate pattern. Nonspecific slitlike defects may also be observed in the NFL; however, these do not usually extend to the disc margin. *Diffuse nerve fiber loss* is more common in glaucoma than is focal loss but is also more difficult to observe. The RNFL can be visualized clearly in high-contrast black-and-white photographs, and with good-quality photographs, experienced clinicians can recognize even early disease. However, such photographs are difficult to obtain and have been largely abandoned in clinical practice due to the availability of imaging methods to quantify RNFL thickness, which are discussed later in this chapter.

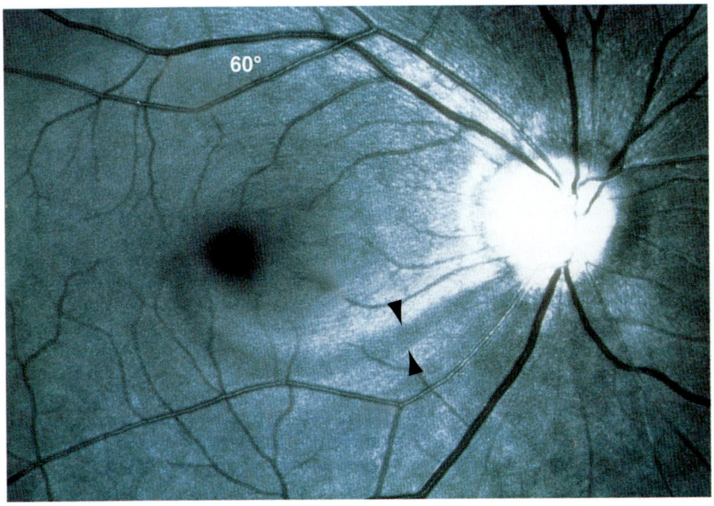

Figure 5-11 Nerve fiber layer photograph shows a nerve fiber bundle defect *(arrowheads)*. *(Courtesy of Louis B. Cantor, MD.)*

Slit-lamp techniques and direct ophthalmoscopy can be successfully employed to observe the RNFL. The combination of a red-free filter, a wide slit beam, and posterior pole lens at the slit lamp affords the best view.

PPA can be classified into 2 general types: alpha (α) zone and beta (β) zone. Alpha zone is present in most nonglaucomatous eyes as well as in eyes with glaucoma and is characterized by a region of irregular hypopigmentation and hyperpigmentation of the retinal pigment epithelium (RPE). The more important type of PPA with respect to glaucoma is β zone, which results from atrophy of the RPE and choriocapillaris, leading to increased visibility of the large choroidal vessels and sclera (Fig 5-12). Beta zone is more common and extensive in eyes with glaucoma than in healthy eyes. The area of PPA is spatially correlated with the area of neuroretinal rim loss; the atrophy is largest in the corresponding area of thinner neuroretinal rim. Therefore, an area of β-zone atrophy signals the need for a search for glaucomatous loss in the adjacent neuroretinal rim.

Other, less specific, signs of glaucomatous damage include nasal displacement of the vessels, narrowing of peripapillary retinal vessels, and baring of the circumlinear vessels. With advanced damage, the cup becomes pale and markedly excavated.

Conditions with associated optic nerve changes that can be confounded with glaucoma include congenital pits of the ONH, coloboma, morning glory disc anomaly, arteritic anterior ischemic neuropathy, and compressive optic neuropathies. Pallor of the neuroretinal rim itself is an indication of a nonglaucomatous optic neuropathy and necessitates further investigation (see BCSC Section 5, *Neuro-Ophthalmology*). With rare exceptions, glaucoma results in increased cupping and pallor within the cup, but not pallor of the remaining rim tissue. However, rim pallor that is out of proportion to the degree of cupping may sometimes occur following previous episodes of very high IOP, such as following an episode of acute angle closure. Optic nerve drusen or coloboma are other possible causes of glaucomatous-appearing visual field loss. Finally, the myopic optic disc represents a challenge in the assessment of possible glaucomatous damage.

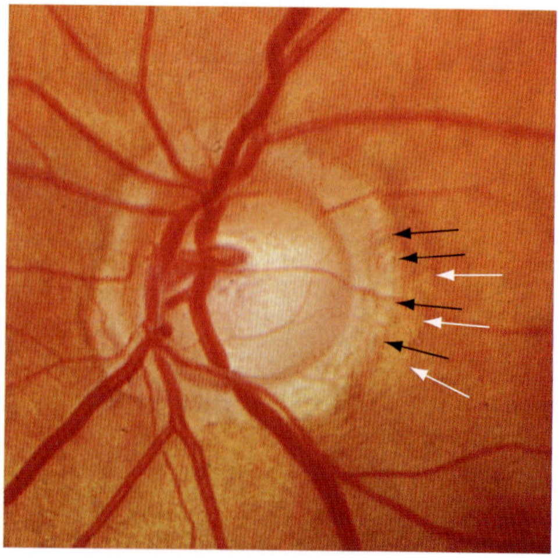

Figure 5-12 In β zone *(black arrows),* there is marked atrophy of the retinal pigment epithelium and the large choroidal vessels can be easily seen. Alpha zone *(white arrows)* is peripheral and adjacent to β zone and is characterized by a region of irregular hypo- and hyperpigmentation. *(Courtesy of Felipe A. Medeiros, MD, PhD.)*

The size, tilting, and associated structural changes often preclude the ability to definitively determine the presence of glaucomatous damage.

Jonas JB, Budde WM, Panda-Jonas S. Ophthalmoscopic evaluation of the optic nerve head. *Surv Ophthalmol.* 1999;43(4):293–320.

Recording of Optic Nerve Findings

Due to the large variability in the appearance of the optic nerve head in healthy subjects, it is frequently not possible to confirm the presence of glaucomatous damage on the basis of a single cross-sectional observation. Therefore, glaucoma diagnosis frequently requires longitudinal monitoring and detection of progressive damage over time. Careful documentation is essential in order to allow adequate comparison of the ONH appearance over time, both for diagnosis of the disease in individuals suspected of having glaucoma and for detection of progression in those with established disease.

It is common practice to grade an ONH by comparing the diameter of the cup with the diameter of the disc. This ratio is usually expressed as a decimal, for example, 0.2; but such a description poorly conveys the appearance of the ONH. A detailed, annotated diagram of the ONH topography is preferable to the recording of a simple cup–disc ratio. However, even very detailed descriptions or drawings of the ONH are generally insufficient to detect the subtle changes that may occur as the result of glaucomatous progression over time. Therefore, for objective documentation, it is preferable to also obtain photographs or other imaging of the ONH whenever possible.

Photography, particularly simultaneous stereophotography, is an excellent method for recording the appearance of the optic nerve for detailed examination and sequential follow-up. This record allows the examiner to compare the present status of the patient with the baseline status without resorting to memory or grading systems. If stereoscopic photographs are not available, even simple monoscopic photographs are preferable to drawings for documenting the appearance of the ONH. However, evaluation of ONH photographs is subjective and does not provide direct quantitative information about the degree of neural loss or rates of disease progression.

Imaging of the Optic Nerve Head, Macula, and Retinal Nerve Fiber Layer

Since the 1850s, the appearance of the optic nerve head has been recognized as critical in assessing glaucoma. However, assessment of the ONH at the slit lamp or with photographs is subjective and shows relatively large interobserver and intraobserver variation. Quantitative imaging devices provide an objective means to obtain reproducible and high-resolution images of ocular structures relevant to glaucoma. In addition, imaging devices contain normative databases that allow the user to determine the probability that observed measurements are within the normal range, assisting in the differentiation of optic nerve damage from normal variation. Imaging assessment is also helpful for detecting progressive structural damage and for assessment of rates of disease progression.

Advancements in ocular imaging technologies over the last 3 decades include OCT, confocal scanning laser ophthalmoscopy (CSLO), and scanning laser polarimetry (SLP). Of these technologies, OCT is now the most widely used because of its versatility as well as its high resolution and the reproducibility of the measurements that can be obtained.

Optical Coherence Tomography for Glaucoma Diagnosis

OCT employs the principles of low-coherence interferometry and is analogous to ultrasound B-mode imaging, but it uses light instead of sound to acquire high-resolution cross-sectional images of ocular structures. The original time-domain OCT (TD-OCT) has been superseded by Fourier- or spectral-domain OCT (SD-OCT), which has improved spatial resolution and image acquisition speed, resulting in enhanced image quality and better reproducibility. OCT is able to provide quantitative measurements of the peripapillary RNFL thickness, ONH topography, and macular thickness, which can discriminate glaucomatous eyes from healthy eyes.

OCT RNFL thickness measurements are usually acquired in the peripapillary area, that is, at a fixed radius around the ONH. Most commercially available OCT devices acquire RNFL thickness measurements in a peripapillary circle located at a certain distance from the ONH, usually 3.45 mm. RNFL thickness measurements are generally lower in glaucomatous eyes compared with those in nonglaucomatous eyes, although considerable interindividual variability exists. Measurement parameters presented in OCT reports include the global average peripapillary RNFL thickness, which corresponds to the average of all thickness measurements in the peripapillary circle, as well as average RNFL thickness in quadrants (superior, inferior, temporal, nasal) or in small clock-hour sectors. Figure 5-13 shows an example of RNFL analysis provided by SD-OCT in a patient with glaucomatous RNFL loss in the right eye and normal RNFL thickness in the left eye. Sensitivities and specificities for detection of glaucomatous damage vary depending on the specific parameter evaluated and the characteristics of the studied population. In general, the parameters with best diagnostic accuracy are the average peripapillary RNFL thickness and thicknesses in the inferior and superior quadrants. This is supported by studies that demonstrated that the superior and inferior areas of the optic nerve are most commonly affected in glaucoma.

Note that, although sectorial RNFL parameters may increase the chance of detecting localized RNFL damage in glaucoma, these parameters may suffer from lower reproducibility, because measurements are averaged over relatively small areas. By contrast, the global average RNFL thickness has generally been shown to be the most reproducible parameter, which is not surprising considering that its calculation involves averaging measurements over a relatively large area. The improved reproducibility may offer gains in the ability to detect progression over time. The gain in reproducibility, however, may come at the expense of discovering localized RNFL defects, which are averaged out in the calculation. However, some commercially available OCT devices are able to acquire and visualize a 3-dimensional map of the RNFL thickness in the peripapillary region; such maps may facilitate identification of localized arcuate RNFL defects that may be missed with summary parameters.

SD-OCT devices are also able to provide topographical measurements of the ONH, including measurements of the optic disc area, neuroretinal rim area, and cup–disc ratio. These parameters and the methods for calculating them differ across platforms. Although

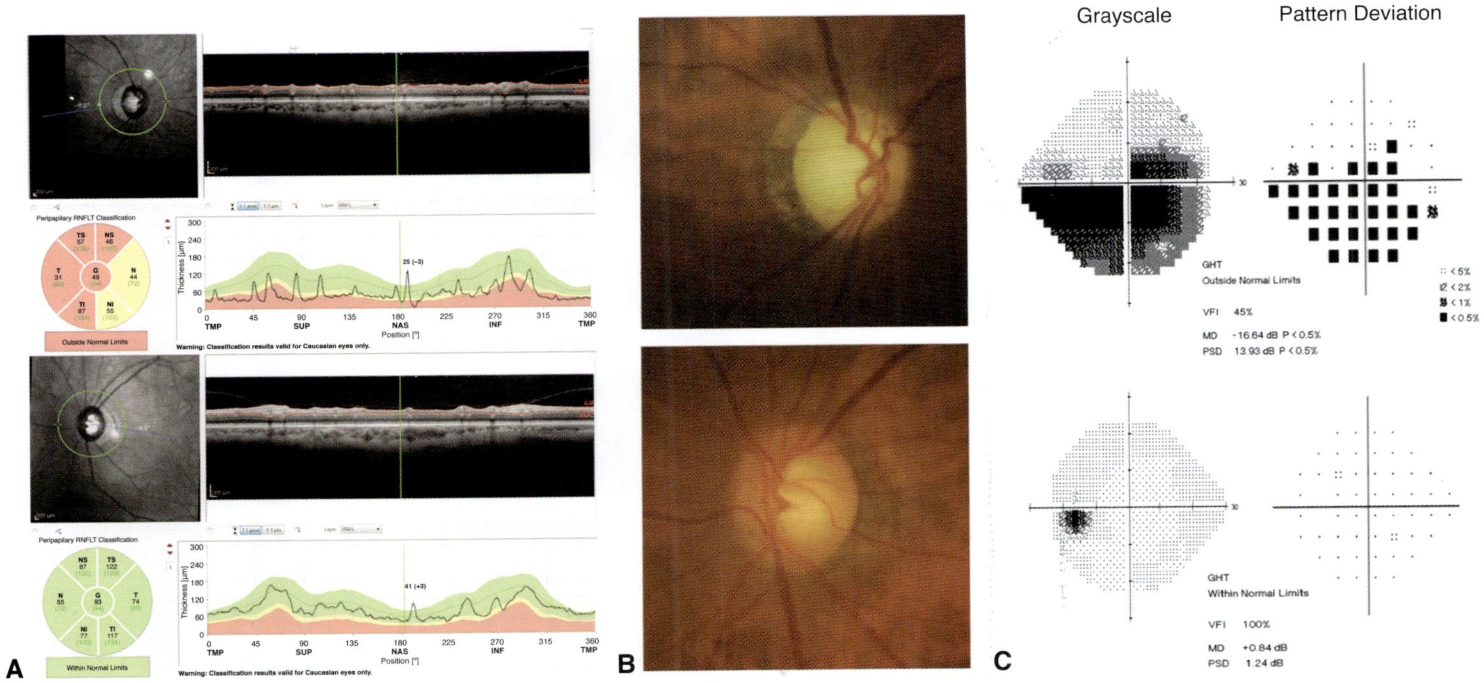

Figure 5-13 Example of RNFL analysis with spectral-domain optical coherence tomography (SD-OCT). *Top:* The right eye shows diffuse RNFL thinning on SD-OCT **(A),** which is consistent with the neuroretinal rim thinning and enlarged cup shown in the photographs of the ONH **(B),** and with the visual field loss that is evident on standard automated perimetry (SAP) **(C).** *Bottom:* The left eye shows normal RNFL thickness on SD-OCT **(A),** normal appearance of the ONH **(B),** and normal visual field **(C).** *(Courtesy of Felipe A. Medeiros, MD, PhD.)*

previous versions of the OCT technology were also able to provide such measurements, considerable data interpolation was required, resulting in poor reproducibility of the measurements. The improved resolution of SD-OCT has greatly reduced the need for interpolation, resulting in much better delineation of the ONH structures.

In general, with OCT, the border of the optic disc is defined by the termination of Bruch membrane, or its "opening." The Bruch membrane opening–minimum rim width (BMO-MRW) is a parameter for measuring the neuroretinal rim thickness at the optic disc border with SD-OCT. BMO-MRW is defined as the minimum distance from the termination of Bruch membrane (BMO) to the inner aspect of the neuroretinal rim averaged around the disc. Studies suggest that BMO-MRW may be more sensitive than other rim-based parameters for diagnosing glaucoma. Figure 5-14 shows an example of an SD-OCT printout with calculations of BMO-MRW measurements.

Increased attention has been directed toward the macular region for evaluation of glaucomatous damage. Because much of the total macular thickness consists of RNFL and ganglion cell bodies, this region is an attractive area for identifying structural glaucoma damage. The macular RGC layer contains more than 50% of the RGCs of the entire retina. Investigations have also suggested that, contrary to previous belief, glaucomatous damage frequently affects the macular region even early in the disease process, leading to central visual field loss that can go undetected with conventional perimetry. SD-OCT enables quantitative assessment of either the entire macular thickness or the thickness of specific layers

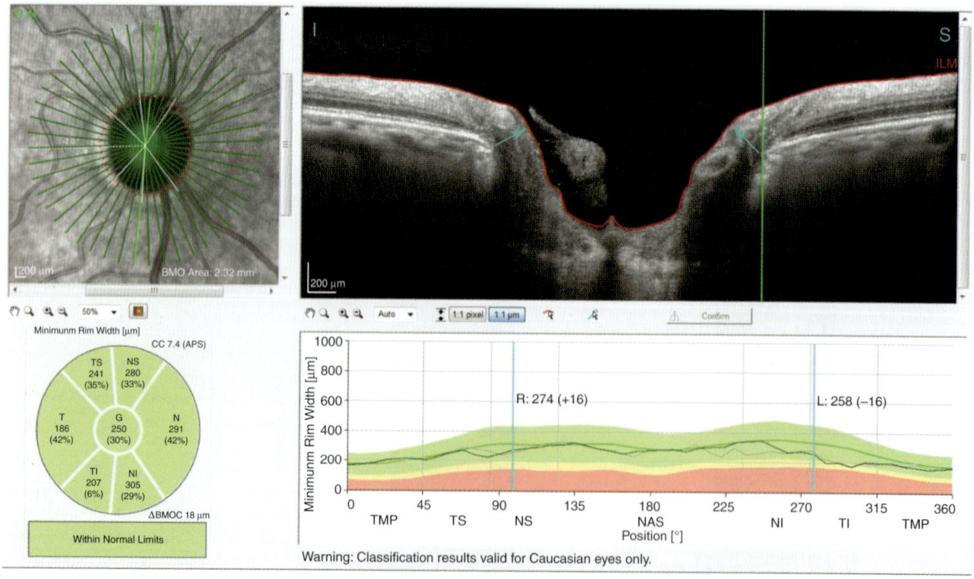

Figure 5-14 SD-OCT scan showing results for the Bruch membrane opening–minimum rim width (BMO-MRW) parameter. The B scan on the right shows how the BMO-MRW measurement is obtained. It corresponds to the minimum distance extending from the border of Bruch membrane to the internal limiting membrane *(arrows)*. The global and sectoral BMO-MRW measurements are then calculated and compared with a normative database. *(Courtesy of Felipe A. Medeiros, MD, PhD.)*

that may be important in glaucoma. The retinal layers that are included in the macular thickness measurements for glaucoma evaluation vary with the different OCT platforms. The thickness of the ganglion cell layer combined with the inner plexiform layer (GCIPL) is a commonly used parameter, as is the *ganglion cell complex (GCC),* which is composed of the RNFL, the ganglion cell layer, and the inner plexiform layer. The diagnostic ability of macular parameters is similar to that of the peripapillary RNFL. In eyes with myopic discs or large areas of PPA, which can present with artifacts on peripapillary RNFL assessment, macular evaluation may provide an enhanced ability to diagnose and monitor glaucomatous damage. Figure 5-15 shows an example of macular damage detected in a glaucomatous eye with SD-OCT, along with corresponding RNFL scans and optic disc photographs.

Several studies have compared the diagnostic ability of different RNFL, ONH, and macular parameters. The results of these studies have not always been consistent; the differences in the results may be related to differences in the criteria used to select the glaucoma and control subjects, as well as the different characteristics of the populations included in the studies. As in any diagnostic accuracy study, a reference standard needs to be employed to select cases and controls. The ability to distinguish cases and controls, as defined by the reference standard, is then determined for the parameters under investigation. In most studies, the reference criteria for glaucoma cases are glaucomatous field losses with "compatible" optic nerve damage. If the reference criteria include clinician assessment of the optic disc, this increases the chance that patients with obvious abnormalities of optic disc features such as rim or cup, as opposed to those with RNFL abnormalities, will be those selected for inclusion as glaucoma cases in the study. Reference criteria for control cases frequently require "normal" optic discs, which clinically equate to a normal-appearing neuroretinal rim and cup. Such selection criteria can bias studies toward favoring the accuracy of topographic optic disc–based parameters. Furthermore, potential controls with anomalous optic disc characteristics such as tilted discs are often excluded from such studies and from normative databases. As a result, the diagnostic performance of OCT-based parameters for distinguishing eyes with glaucoma from nonglaucomatous eyes in clinical practice is not as good as one might expect on the basis of published findings.

Although imaging technologies are generally helpful in the detection of glaucoma, their diagnostic performance decreases for detection of early disease compared with moderate or advanced disease. Most studies evaluating the diagnostic accuracy of SD-OCT have evaluated the instruments' ability to differentiate the eyes of patients with well-defined glaucomatous visual field defects from those of healthy subjects. Such studies are important for providing an initial exploratory evaluation of newly developed methods to detect glaucomatous damage. However, in clinical practice, a diagnostic test is used to diagnose disease in patients suspected of having the disease, not in patients with a confirmed diagnosis. Therefore, from a practical standpoint, it is of little utility to demonstrate that an imaging device is able to diagnose glaucoma in a patient with a confirmed visual field defect, because such a patient would already have a clear diagnosis established. In fact, studies with a case-control design that includes patients with well-established disease and a separate group of control subjects without glaucoma tend to substantially overestimate the performance of the tests. Therefore, if a test succeeds in initial exploratory diagnostic studies, further steps are necessary to evaluate whether it is able to provide clinically relevant information.

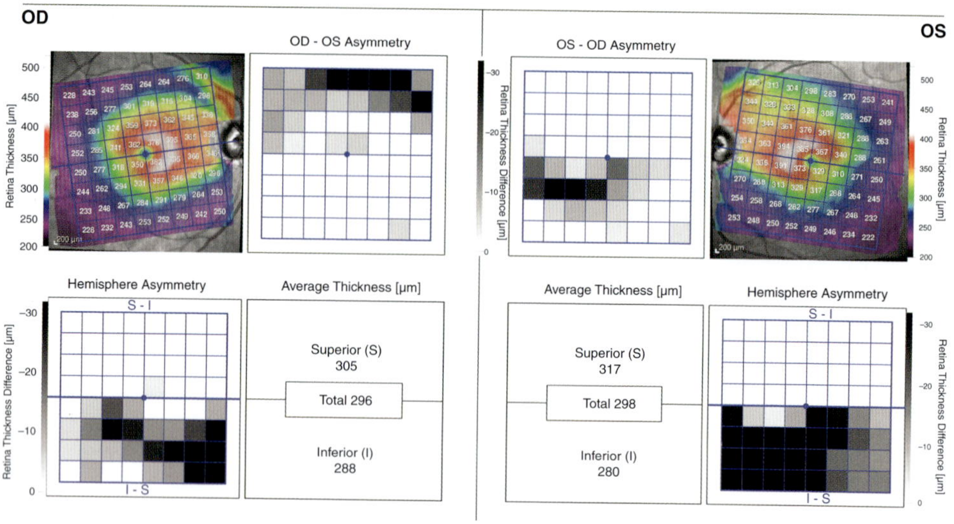

OD
OD - OS Asymmetry
OS - OD Asymmetry
OS
Retina Thickness [µm]
Retina Thickness Difference [µm]
Hemisphere Asymmetry
Average Thickness [µm]
Superior (S) 305
Total 296
Inferior (I) 288
Superior (S) 317
Total 298
Inferior (I) 280
S - I
I - S
A

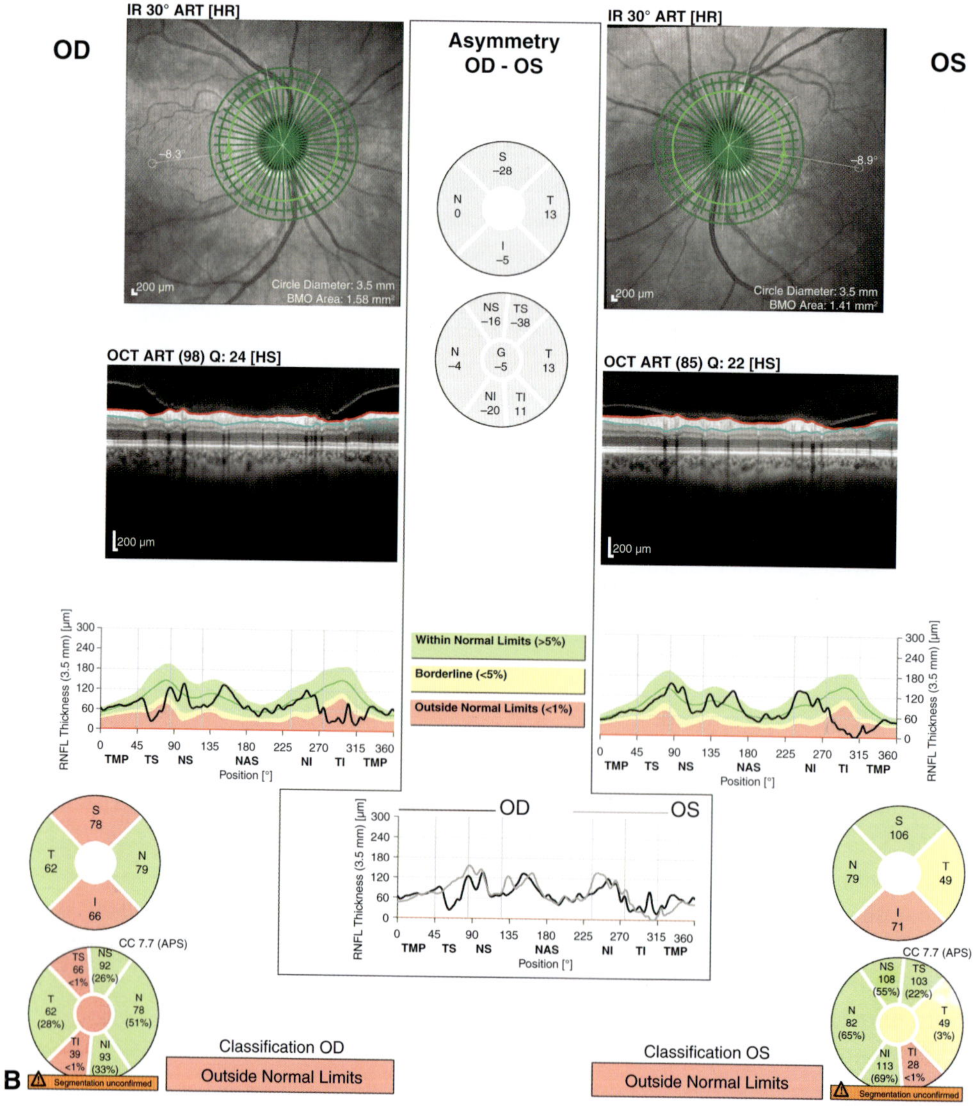

IR 30° ART [HR]
OD
OS
Asymmetry OD - OS
Circle Diameter: 3.5 mm
BMO Area: 1.58 mm²
BMO Area: 1.41 mm²
OCT ART (98) Q: 24 [HS]
OCT ART (85) Q: 22 [HS]
Within Normal Limits (>5%)
Borderline (<5%)
Outside Normal Limits (<1%)
RNFL Thickness (3.5 mm) [µm]
Position [°]
TMP TS NS NAS NI TI TMP
CC 7.7 (APS)
Segmentation unconfirmed
Classification OD
Outside Normal Limits
Classification OS
Outside Normal Limits
B

(Continued)

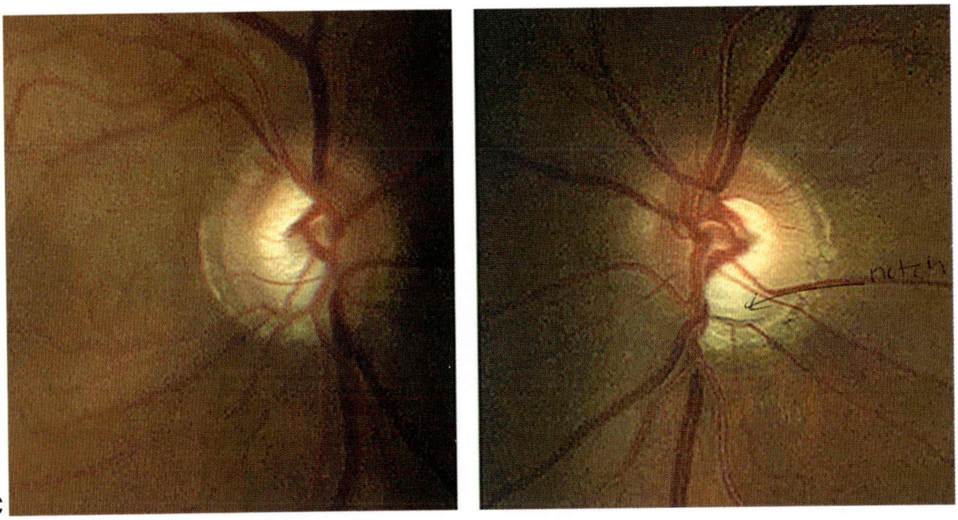

Figure 5-15 *(continued)* Macular (posterior pole) thickness maps of a patient with glaucoma. **A,** The grayscale plots illustrate hemisphere asymmetries for each eye (ie, differences in thickness between the superior and inferior corresponding regions), and the asymmetry map shows differences between the right and left eyes. Note that the right eye shows thinning in the inferior arcuate region, which is easily seen in both the hemisphere asymmetry graph and the color-coded map. The right eye also shows a superior arcuate defect, clearly suggested by the OD–OS asymmetry map. The left eye shows an extensive inferior arcuate defect that clearly involves the paracentral region. The superior region of the left eye seems preserved in the posterior pole analysis. **B,** RNFL scans of the same eyes. The right eye shows localized losses in both the superior and inferior temporal regions, which correspond to the damage shown in the posterior pole scan. The left eye shows damage that seems to be limited to the inferior temporal region, again in agreement with the posterior pole analysis. **C,** Optic disc photographs showing rim thinning and localized RNFL defects in the superior and inferior temporal regions of the right eye. The left eye demonstrates notching and complete loss of the rim in the inferior temporal location, but the superior rim appears well preserved. *(Courtesy of Felipe A. Medeiros, MD, PhD.)*

In fact, the optimal design for assessing a diagnostic test's accuracy is considered to be a prospective, masked comparison of the test and the reference test in a consecutive series of patients from a relevant clinical population—that is, those suspected of having the disease. Some studies have prospectively investigated the ability of SD-OCT to diagnose glaucoma in individuals who were suspected of having the disease by conventional examination at the time of enrollment. In 1 study, assessment of the RNFL with SD-OCT detected abnormalities in one-third of subjects up to 5 years before the first appearance of a visual field defect on standard automated perimetry. Importantly, other studies have shown that RNFL thickness measurements are predictive of development of future visual field losses in glaucoma suspect eyes. Figure 5-16 shows an eye in which the OCT measurements of RNFL thickness were abnormal before the development of visual field defects.

Kuang TM, Zhang C, Zangwill LM, Weinreb RN, Medeiros FA. Estimating lead time gained by optical coherence tomography in detecting glaucoma before development of visual field defects. *Ophthalmology*. 2015;122(10):2002–2009.

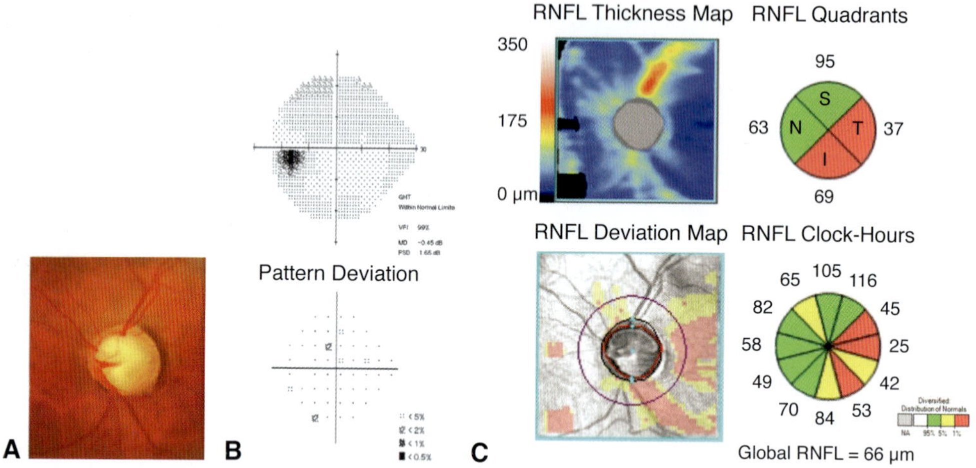

Figure 5-16 Structural damage often precedes detectable visual field damage. **A,** Photograph of the optic nerve head shows marked neuroretinal rim thinning and an enlarged cup. **B,** Standard automated perimetry, by contrast, shows that the visual field is still within normal limits. **C,** Retinal nerve fiber layer (RNFL) analysis with spectral-domain optical coherence tomography shows diffuse loss of the RNFL. *(Courtesy of Felipe A. Medeiros, MD, PhD.)*

Lisboa R, Leite MT, Zangwill LM, Tafreshi A, Weinreb RN, Medeiros FA. Diagnosing preperimetric glaucoma with spectral domain optical coherence tomography. *Ophthalmology.* 2012;119(11):2261–2269.

Optical Coherence Tomography for Detecting Glaucoma Progression

Perhaps the greatest value of optical coherence tomography imaging is in the longitudinal monitoring of structural damage. Several studies have shown that imaging parameters such as RNFL, neural rim, and macular thickness measurements can detect progressive glaucomatous damage. In addition, these parameters can provide quantitative assessment of rates of change in the disease, which are essential for establishing appropriate treatment. Although most glaucoma patients will show some evidence of progression if followed long enough, the rate of deterioration can be highly variable among them. While most patients progress relatively slowly, others have aggressive disease with fast deterioration, which can eventually cause blindness or substantial impairment unless treated appropriately. The use of imaging may assist in detection of patients who are fast progressors in need of more aggressive intervention.

Several studies have used SD-OCT to evaluate the role of RNFL, ONH, and macular measurements in assessing glaucoma progression. However, it is difficult to determine whether 1 parameter is better than another because of the lack of a perfect reference ("gold") standard. Also, although glaucomatous changes reflect loss of RGCs, the temporal relationship between changes to the ONH, RNFL, and macula are still poorly understood. Overall, RNFL, ONH, and macular parameters show faster rates of loss in glaucomatous eyes compared with typical age-related changes observed in control eyes; however, there is considerable variation in reported rates of change. Figure 5-17 shows SD-OCT RNFL scans that were acquired over time in an eye that developed progressive RNFL loss in the inferior temporal region.

Detection of disease progression depends fundamentally on the ability to differentiate true change from the noise of test–retest variability and from changes attributable to a normal aging process. Several studies have shown that measurements of RNFL, ONH, and macular thickness obtained via SD-OCT have excellent short-term reproducibility. These reproducibility studies suggest that a change in global RNFL thickness of 5 µm between tests may indicate progression. However, it is important to exercise caution when interpreting such cutoffs. Most studies examining reproducibility excluded poor-quality scans and analyzed short-term rather than long-term reproducibility. In clinical practice, patients are followed over the course of many years, and long-term variability may be considerably greater than in the short term.

At present, there is no consensus on the best way to detect glaucoma progression using OCT. Although trend-based assessment of RNFL thickness over time has been commonly employed, it is also important to differentiate changes due to glaucoma from age-related changes. Previous longitudinal studies have found mean rates of change of approximately −0.50 µm/year in average RNFL thickness in healthy subjects. Accordingly, high rates of false-positive detection of progression occur when the only criterion required is a statistically significant negative slope of RNFL thickness change as a function of time (ie, a slope that is statistically significantly different from 0 with $P < .05$). For example, after 5 years of annual testing, up to 25% of nonglaucomatous eyes can be falsely identified as having progressed if this criterion is used for change in RNFL thickness. It has been suggested that trend-based analysis of RNFL thickness change should involve at least testing the statistical significance of the change relative to the mean estimate of age-related changes. Doing so would be analogous to evaluating visual field progression using mean deviation instead of mean sensitivity (with the former being an age-adjusted parameter) and could be described as an RNFL mean deviation trend analysis.

Detection of longitudinal changes with OCT is important not only for detecting progression in eyes with existing damage but also for detecting changes in eyes suspected of disease, which would then help confirm the diagnosis of glaucoma. Due to the wide range of normative values, significant changes in RNFL thickness or other parameters may be observed well before the measurements fall into the "outside normal limits" range (Fig 5-18).

Given the relative stability of the BMO as a point of reference for repeat scans, one might suppose that measurements taken relative to BMO would be more helpful than conventional structural measurements for detecting glaucoma progression. However, a recent study has suggested that it may be more difficult to detect changes using measurements of BMO-MRW and BMO–minimum rim area because of a relatively low longitudinal signal-to-noise ratio compared with peripapillary RNFL thickness measurements. This observation may have been the result of changes in the location of the BMO over time, possibly related to fluctuations in IOP or because of connective tissue remodeling as a result of glaucoma progression. One study suggested that BMO is located more posteriorly in older individuals versus younger individuals, suggesting that it may migrate posteriorly with age and is therefore a less stable landmark than previously hoped. Longer-duration studies are needed to determine whether BMO can be used as a long-term stable reference from which to measure glaucomatous changes.

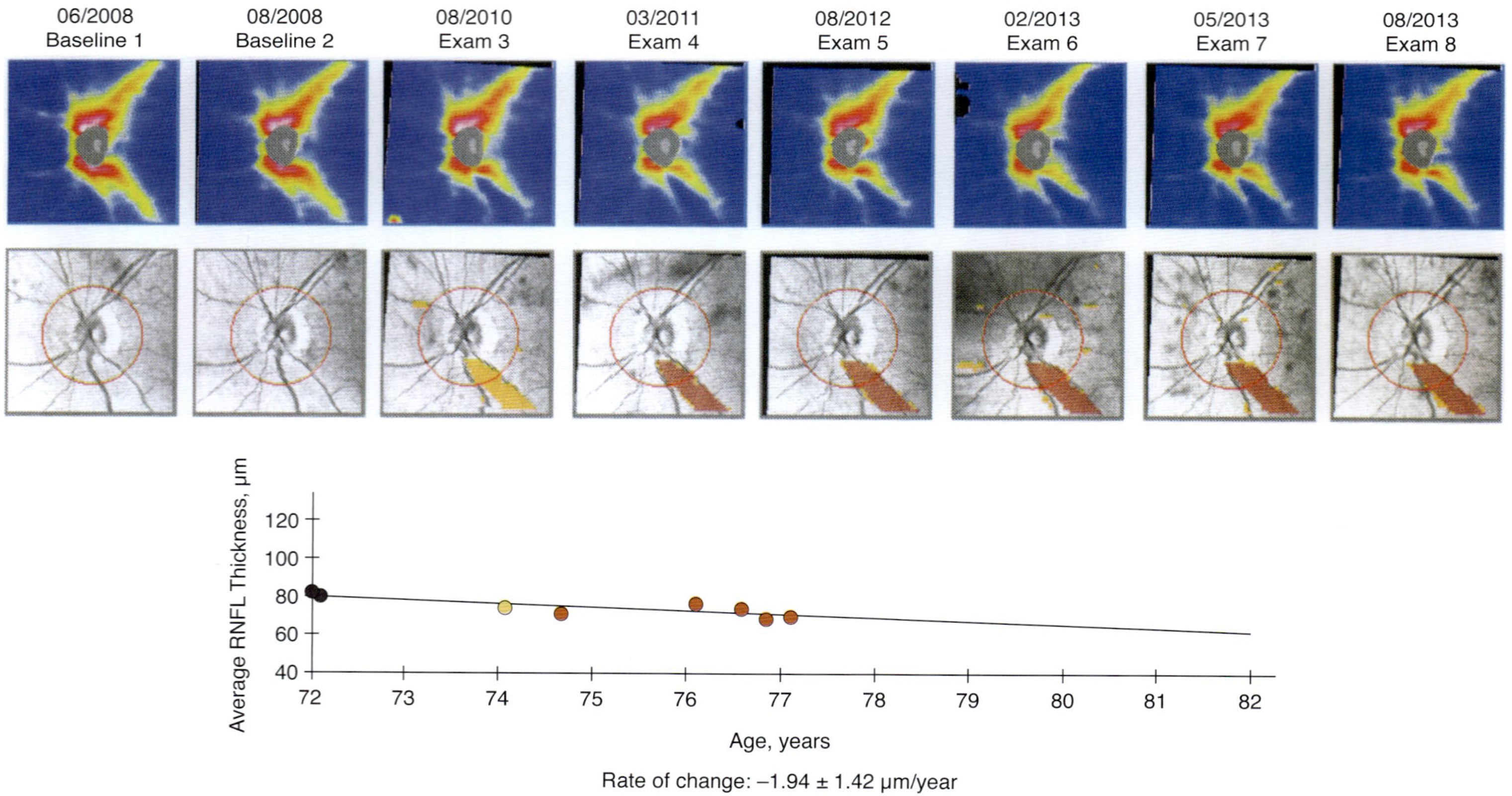

Figure 5-17 SD-OCT images showing progressive RNFL loss. There is progressive loss of the RNFL in the inferotemporal sector. The plot at the bottom of the figure shows the rate of change in the parameter average RNFL thickness. *(Courtesy of Felipe A. Medeiros, MD, PhD.)*

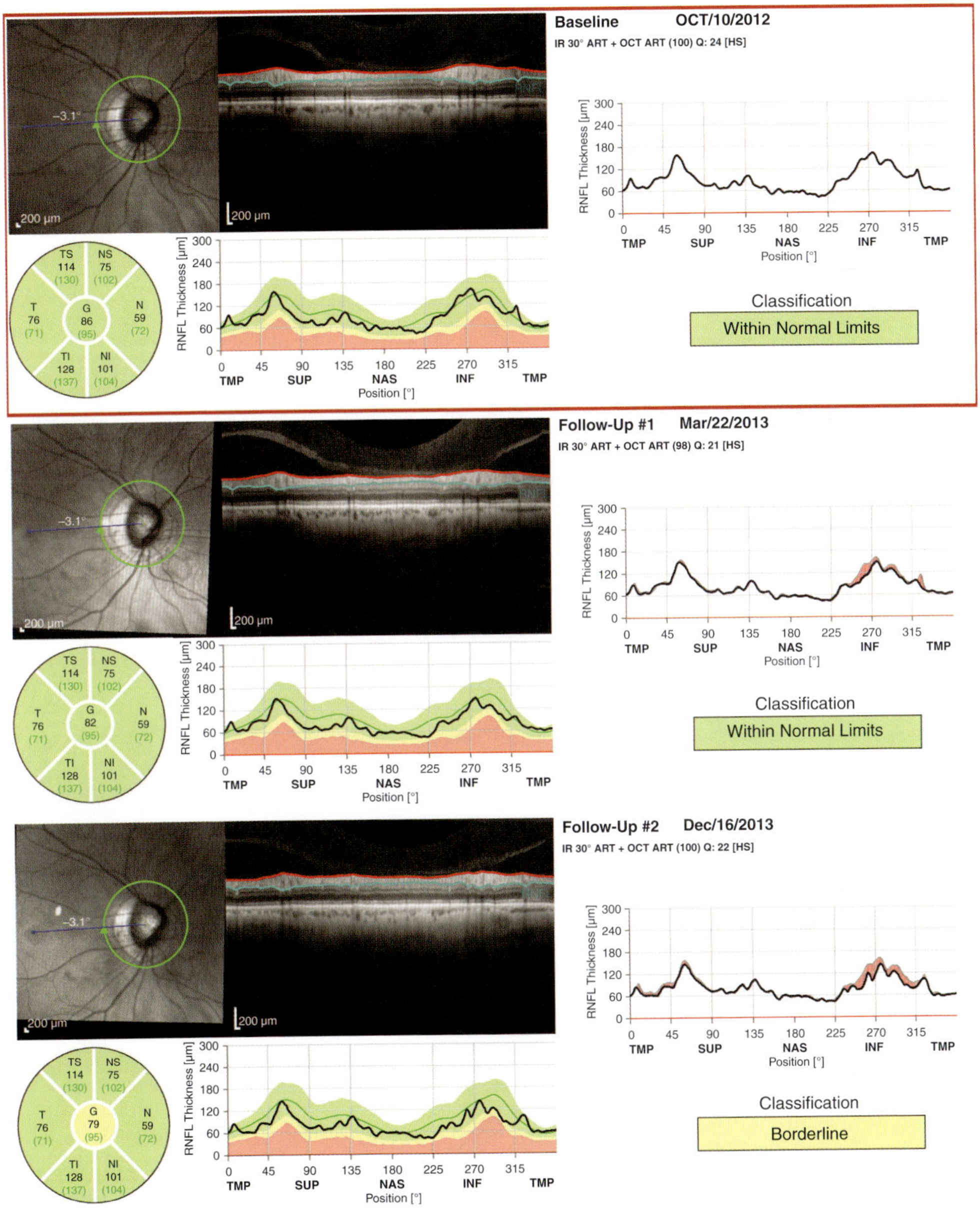

Figure 5-18 Series of SD-OCT RNFL scans of a patient followed from 2012 to 2016. The patient was suspected of having glaucoma at the beginning of follow-up due to the appearance of the optic disc. Note that the initial scan does not show any clear abnormality, and all parameters are within normal limits. There is progressive RNFL loss, initially in the inferior region, but subsequently also affecting the superior region over time. Note that the global and sectoral RNFL thickness parameters become clearly abnormal *(flagged in red)* only after 4 years. *(Courtesy of Felipe A. Medeiros, MD, PhD.)*

(Continued)

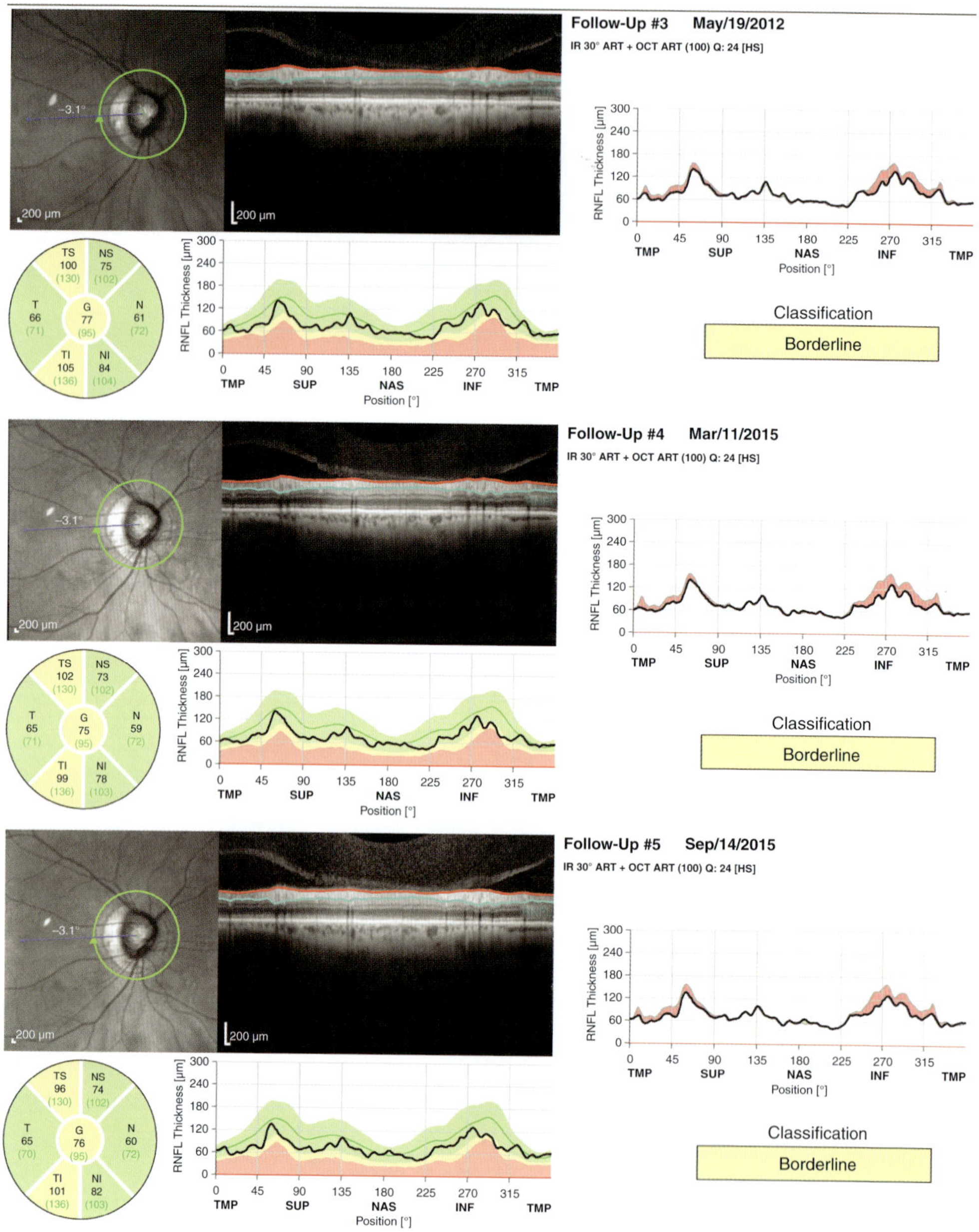

Figure 5-18 *(continued)*

Regardless of which measurement parameter is best, there is now a large body of evidence that progressive changes on OCT are clinically relevant. Faster rates of RNFL loss, visualized by OCT, are also associated with a higher risk for the future development of visual field defects. A study found that each 1-μm/year faster rate of RNFL loss in glaucoma suspects corresponded to a twofold-increased risk for the development of a visual

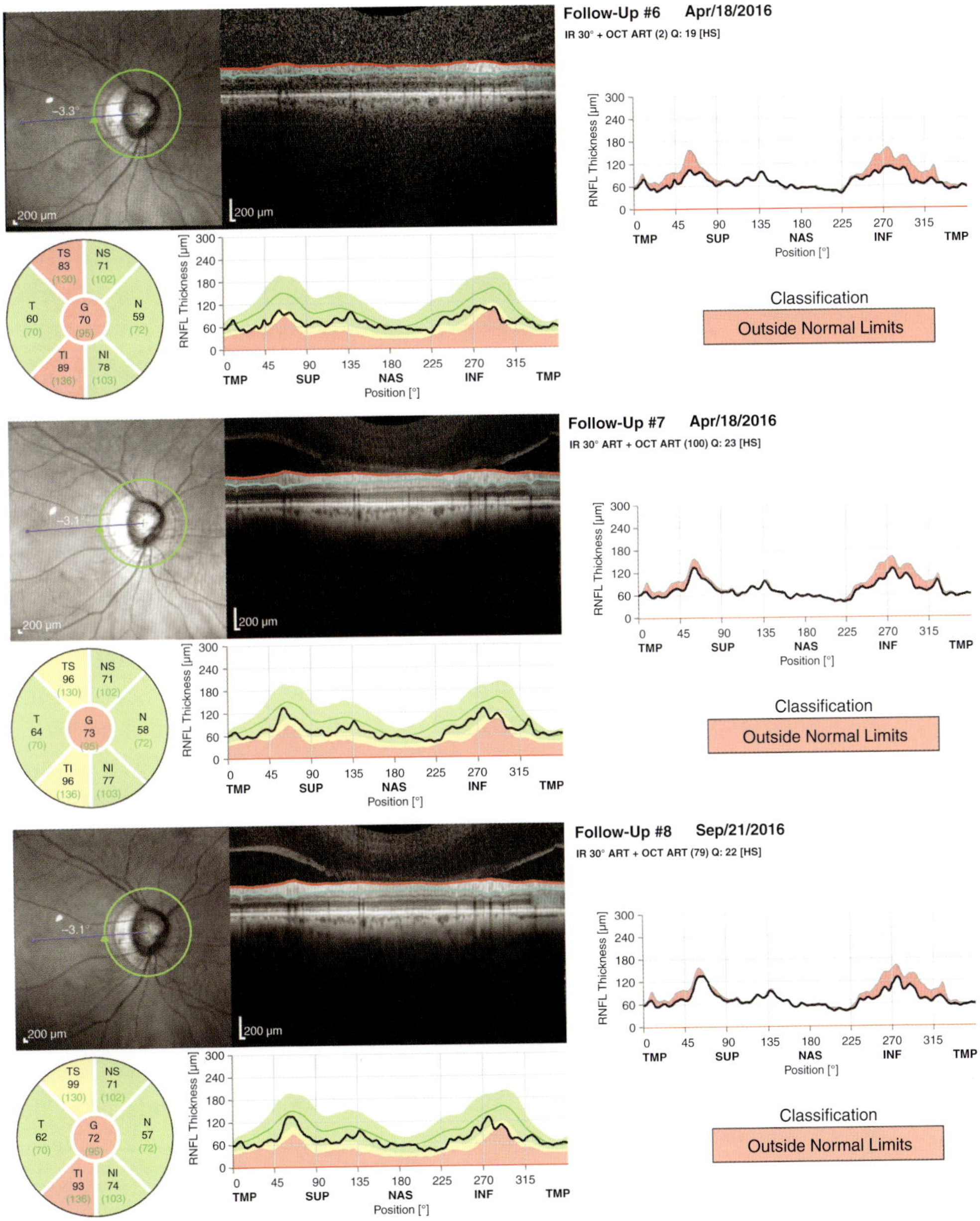

Figure 5-18 *(continued)*

field defect. Similar results have also been described in eyes with established glaucoma, in which progressive RNFL thinning on trend-based progression analysis was strongly predictive of visual field loss. Higher rates of RNFL loss have also been associated with a faster decline in quality of life in patients with glaucoma. Assessment of glaucoma progression on OCT should be combined with an assessment of functional changes in perimetry. The relationship between structural and functional changes in glaucoma is discussed in more detail in Chapter 6.

Since the introduction of OCT more than 25 years ago, our ability to detect and quantify glaucomatous structural changes has improved significantly. OCT provides a means to obtain reproducible measurements of the RNFL, ONH, and macula, each of which is of value in quantifying glaucoma progression. Although visual function is what matters most to patients, progressive structural changes can precede functional loss. In addition, patients who demonstrate a faster rate of change on OCT are at increased risk of worsening vision loss; OCT offers these patients the possibility of escalating treatment at an earlier stage to preserve more vision. The ability to assess glaucoma progression is likely to be improved further by novel approaches that incorporate information from OCT and visual fields, reducing the noise inherent in both tests (for further discussion, see Chapter 6).

Tatham AJ, Medeiros FA. Detecting structural progression in glaucoma with optical coherence tomography. *Ophthalmology*. 2017;124(12 Suppl.):S57–S65.

Imaging of the Lamina Cribrosa

The lamina cribrosa is challenging to image because of its location deep within the ONH. However, advances in OCT, including enhanced depth imaging OCT (EDI-OCT) and swept-source OCT (SS-OCT), have provided a means of imaging deeper ocular structures, including the lamina cribrosa. In EDI-OCT, the OCT source is placed closer to the eye than in typical practice, thereby producing an image in which the most tightly focused illumination is located more posteriorly, at the level of the choroid and inner sclera. The wavelength of light used in an OCT system affects image resolution, and when penetration depth increases, the image resolution and signal strength decrease. Commonly used SD-OCT devices employ wavelengths in the range of 840–880 nm. However, SS-OCT uses wavelengths of 1000 nm, allowing higher penetration with minimum light absorption and dispersion by the vitreous, which provides improved imaging of deeper ONH structures. Figure 5-19 shows imaging with EDI-OCT and SS-OCT of the right eye of a glaucoma patient with a clinically visible lamina cribrosa defect.

Another technology used to evaluate the lamina cribrosa is adaptive optics. This system uses a wave-front sensor to measure ocular aberrations, for example, those induced by the lens and cornea. A deformable mirror or a spatial light modulator is then used to compensate for measured aberrations and improve image quality. Adaptive optics can correct ocular aberrations in real time; its use can be combined with the use of OCT or scanning laser ophthalmoscopy.

Imaging has enabled the identification of general and localized configurational changes in the lamina cribrosa of glaucomatous eyes, including posterior laminar displacement, altered laminar thickness, and focal laminar defects that have spatial association with conventional structural and functional losses. In addition to changes in the depth and thickness of the lamina cribrosa, studies have suggested that focal lamina cribrosa defects may be important structural features in glaucoma and could potentially serve as biomarkers for glaucomatous visual field loss. There is growing evidence of an association

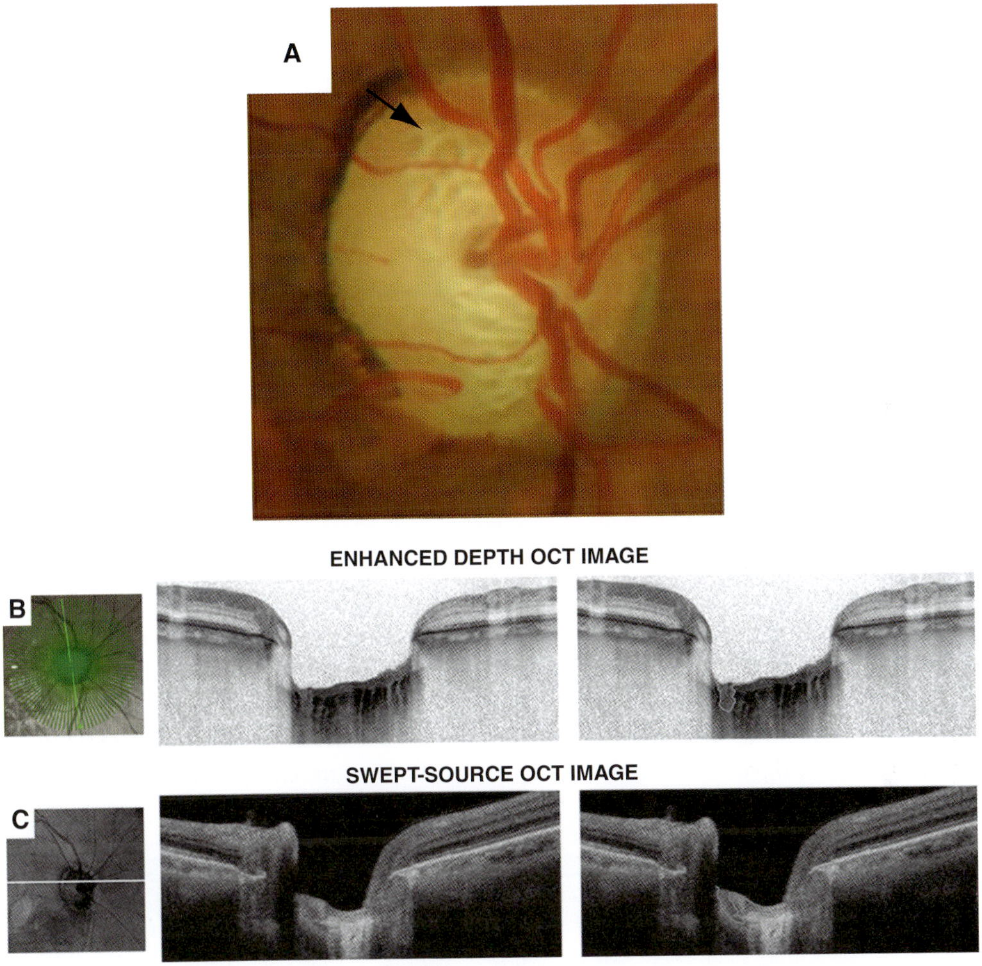

Figure 5-19 Images from the right eye of a patient with glaucoma showing a lamina cribrosa defect. **A,** Optic disc photograph. **B,** Radial scans from an enhanced depth imaging with a SD-OCT device (Spectralis, Heidelberg Engineering) showing an unmarked image and a manually marked focal defect in the superior region of the optic disc. **C,** Axial scans showing the same defect on the superior region of the optic nerve using a swept-source optical coherence tomography device. *(Courtesy of Topcon.)*

between lamina cribrosa structure and other structural and functional measures of glaucoma, suggesting that evaluation of the lamina cribrosa may become a useful addition to clinical imaging options in the detection of glaucoma and in monitoring glaucoma progression. Lamina cribrosa imaging also has the potential to improve understanding of the mechanisms of glaucomatous RGC injury; in addition, although the temporal relationship between lamina cribrosa and neural changes remains uncertain, lamina cribrosa changes may be a useful biomarker of increased risk of neural losses.

Optical Coherence Tomography Angiography

The potential role of the microvasculature and blood flow in the pathophysiology of glaucoma has been extensively investigated and debated. Studies have demonstrated reduced ocular blood flow in the ONH, retina, choroid, and retrobulbar circulations in eyes with glaucoma. These changes may simply be a consequence of glaucomatous damage to the RGCs and may have no predictive value. The lack of a reproducible and relevant in vivo quantitative assessment method has limited the study of both ocular perfusion and microvascular networks as potential predictors of future vision loss. Optical coherence tomography angiography (OCTA) is a new imaging modality that can be used to characterize vasculature in various retinal layers, providing quantitative assessment of the microcirculation in the ONH, peripapillary region, and macula.

The principle of imaging in OCTA is to contrast blood vessels from static tissue by assessing the change in the OCT signal caused by flowing blood cells. OCTA compares the differences in the backscattered OCT signal intensity or amplitude between sequential OCT B scans taken at precisely the same cross section in order to construct a map of blood flow. Axial bulk motion from patient movement is eliminated; sites of motion between repeated OCT B scans are thought to represent erythrocyte movement in retinal blood vessels.

The different OCTA parameters include vessel density, corresponding to the percentage of detected vessel area over the imaged area, and flow index, corresponding to a dimensionless parameter between 0 and 1 representing the average signal. Note that these indices are surrogate measures and that their validity for measurement of blood flow remains to be investigated. Studies have shown significant differences in vessel density and

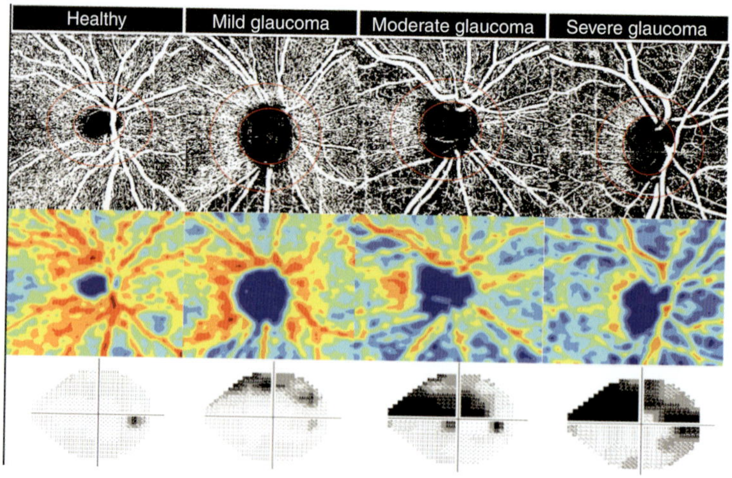

Figure 5-20 Optical coherence tomography angiography (OCTA) scans of a healthy eye and glaucomatous eyes with mild, moderate, and severe damage. The OCTA scans show a dense peripapillary vessel network in the healthy eye, illustrated in red and yellow in the color-coded map. Glaucomatous damage causes a decrease in vessel damage and replacement of the red/yellow areas with blue, indicating either absence of vessels or no flow. *(Courtesy of Yarmohammadi A, Zangwill LM, Diniz-Filho A, et al. Relationship between optical coherence tomography angiography vessel density and severity of visual field loss in glaucoma.* Ophthalmology. *2016;123(12):2498–2508.)*

flow index in the peripapillary and macular regions in eyes of glaucoma patients versus those of healthy subjects. Also, these indices have shown significant association with measures of visual field loss. Figure 5-20 shows OCTA scans of a healthy eye and eyes of glaucoma patients with different levels of damage.

Motion artifacts and projection artifacts are common in OCTA imaging, and a considerable proportion of OCTA images remain suboptimal in quality for interpretation. Poor-quality OCTA scans are more common than poor-quality OCT scans. It remains to be determined whether OCTA will be able to provide additional information that can assist in diagnosis and detection of glaucoma progression beyond what can currently be obtained with OCT.

Jia Y, Wei E, Wang X, et al. Optical coherence tomography angiography of optic disc perfusion in glaucoma. *Ophthalmology*. 2014;121(7):1322–1332.

CHAPTER 6

Perimetry

Highlights

- Standard "white-on-white" automated perimetry remains the gold standard for functional evaluation in glaucoma.
- A high false-positive rate (>15%) is very detrimental to a visual field test and indicates low reliability. Absence of a blind spot is also typically a sign of an unreliable field.
- When assessing the presence of abnormalities in visual field testing, it is important to verify whether the defect is repeatable and present in approximately the same location, and that the abnormalities are not due to artifacts.
- When assessing the visual field for disease progression, it is important to confirm that a new visual field defect or expansion of a preexisting defect is repeatable on subsequent examinations.
- Measuring the rate of visual field change by trend-based analysis is essential for estimating the risk of functional impairment and determining management.

Introduction

For many years, the standard method of measuring the visual dysfunction that occurs with glaucomatous injury has been assessment of the visual field with *perimetry,* which measures differential light sensitivity, or the ability of the subject to detect a stimulus on a uniformly illuminated background.

Perimetry serves 2 major purposes in the management of glaucoma:

1. identification and quantification of abnormalities in the visual field
2. longitudinal assessment to detect glaucomatous progression and measure rates of change

Quantitation of visual sensitivity enables detection of visual field defects by comparison with normative data. Regular visual field testing in known cases of disease provides valuable information for helping to differentiate between stability and progressive loss.

Automated static perimetry is currently the standard method for assessing visual function in glaucoma. With this method, sensitivity measurements are performed at a number of test locations using white stimuli on a white background ("white on white"); this is known as *standard automated perimetry (SAP),* or achromatic automated perimetry. Automated perimetry offers obvious advantages compared with manual perimetry; in automated perimetry, stimulus presentation, as well as the recording of patient responses, can be standardized, which leads to results that are more reproducible. Therefore, manual kinetic perimetry is now rarely performed for visual field assessment in glaucoma. However, kinetic perimetry may be helpful for monitoring visual fields in patients who are unable to perform the automated test. Some perimeters are capable of performing automated kinetic perimetry, although its value for assessing visual field loss in glaucoma is not well established.

Basic Principles of Automated Perimetry

In automated static threshold perimetry, the sensitivity of a patient's central and peripheral vision is quantified using computerized algorithms to accurately ascertain the threshold of sensitivity at each location tested in the patient's field of vision. At each location, stimuli of varying intensities are presented, the patient's responses checked, and the differential light sensitivity measured.

Modern perimeters use the convention introduced with Goldmann perimetry to determine the target sizes for the stimuli. The stimulus sizes are numbered with Roman numerals I through V. Each stimulus covers a 4-fold-greater area, ranging from 0.25 mm^2 for a Size I stimulus to 64 mm^2 for a Size V stimulus. The most commonly used stimulus size for the Humphrey Field Analyzer (HFA; Carl Zeiss Meditec) is stimulus Size III, which corresponds to 4 mm^2. Stimulus Size V may be employed for individuals with severe visual field loss or poor visual acuity.

Threshold strategies start by testing a single location in the field of view. If the stimulus is seen, subsequent stimuli at that location are dimmed a step at a time until no longer seen. If the initial stimulus is not seen, then subsequent presentations are made brighter in steps until the patient responds. This process can be repeated at the same location with reversal of the steps to confirm that the threshold of sensitivity has been accurately ascertained.

The HFA tests light intensities over 5 orders of magnitude, from 10,000 apostilbs (asb) to 0.1 asb. Every log order change in light intensity corresponds to 10 dB; the machine can measure sensitivities over a 50-dB range. Test locations at which a stimulus of 10,000 asb is not detected are assigned a value of 0 dB. It is important to note that this applies to the specific stimulus size that is being used. For example, a 0-dB location when testing with stimulus Size III means that the stimulus with maximum intensity of 10,000 asb and Size III was not seen. However, this does not imply that the location is totally blind. A larger stimulus in the same location, such as stimulus Size V, may be visible and detected by the patient. The threshold values reported for each location reflect the extent to which light can be dimmed (by a series of neutral density filters used in the perimeter) and still detected. For example, a value of 30 dB indicates that the stimulus can be dimmed 1000-fold, from 10,000 to 10 asb, and still be seen.

The state of light adaptation of the eye at the time of the visual field test influences luminance sensitivities. The HFA uses background lighting of 31.5 asb to saturate rod photoreceptors, producing photopic conditions in which cones are primarily tested.

Testing Strategies

The standard method for threshold measurement used by the HFA is currently the Swedish Interactive Threshold Algorithm (SITA). SITA is a Bayesian test strategy that uses information from a database of healthy individuals and persons with disease to generate a probability distribution function (PDF) representing the probabilities that the visual field sensitivity will be of a particular value at a particular visual field location. As the test progresses, the distribution is then adjusted according to how the person being tested responds to prior stimulus presentations. This continues until the PDF distribution is within a small range, at which point the mean of the distribution is selected as the threshold sensitivity estimate. The PDFs are adjusted for the age of the individual, the visual field location tested, the sensitivity values of neighboring test locations, and the results of previous stimulus presentations. Compared with conventional staircase algorithms employed in the older full-threshold strategy, SITA has been demonstrated to have equal or lower test–retest variability, and testing can often be done in half the time.

The SITA strategy is available in the Humphrey perimeters as SITA Standard and SITA Fast. As the name implies, SITA Fast is a faster testing method than SITA Standard and may have similar accuracy and reliability; however, it may be a more difficult test for the patient because the test stimuli tend to be closer to the patient's threshold, thus offering less positive feedback to the patient. Patients who are perceived to have difficulties with SITA Standard should not be shifted to SITA Fast; they should continue with SITA Standard. These patients may benefit from careful instruction by the perimetrist, closer surveillance, and positive feedback.

SITA Faster is a newer strategy; its testing times are approximately 30% shorter than SITA Fast and 50% shorter than SITA Standard. The reduction in testing time is achieved by several modifications, including changes in the starting stimulus intensity and in the number of reversals needed to confirm the threshold, as well as elimination of false-negative and fixation-loss catch trials (see the section Interpretation of a Single Visual Field later in this chapter). Although initial studies indicate that SITA Faster may offer results comparable to SITA Standard, its accuracy for longitudinal monitoring of visual field loss has not been established.

Similar to the SITA testing strategy for the HFA, the *tendency-oriented perimeter (TOP)* algorithm was developed for the Octopus perimeter (Haag-Streit) as an alternative to the lengthy staircase threshold procedures. TOP differs from SITA in that only 1 stimulus is shown at a single location of the visual field. Therefore, in order to estimate the threshold sensitivity at a particular location, TOP supplements this single data point per test location with information obtained at adjoining test locations.

Patterns of Testing Points

The most common patterns used for testing visual function for glaucoma diagnosis and management test the central 24° to 30° of the visual field. The Octopus perimeter implements these in the 32 and G1 patterns, and the Humphrey uses the 24-2 and 30-2 patterns (Fig 6-1). The 24-2 and 30-2 patterns test the central field using a 6° grid. They test points

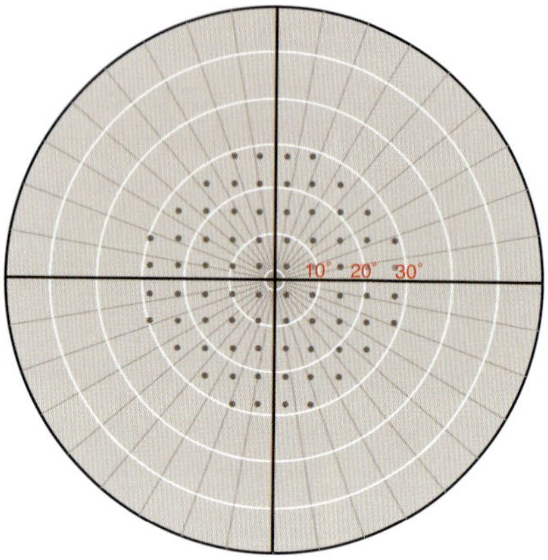

Figure 6-1 Central 30-2 threshold test pattern, right eye. *(Illustration by Mark Miller.)*

3° above and 3° below the horizontal midline, thereby facilitating diagnosis of defects that respect this line. A 24-2 pattern test performed with the SITA Standard strategy for obtaining threshold estimates is then usually referred to as *SITA Standard 24-2.* For patients with advanced visual field loss or with paracentral defects, testing of the central field with the 10-2 or C8 pattern is appropriate (Fig 6-2). These patterns concentrate on the central 8°–10° of the visual field and test points every 1°–2°, enabling the ophthalmologist to follow many more test points within the central island, improving detection of disease progression. Alternatively, a larger stimulus (Size V) can be used in patients with advanced disease or reduced visual acuity.

Although a strategy that tests the visual field between 30° and 60° is available on most static threshold perimeters, it is rarely used because the threshold variability is very high in these more peripheral regions.

Factors Affecting Perimetry Results

Many factors may affect the results obtained from perimetry, including the patient's level of attentiveness, the perimetrist's administration of the test, and other variables, such as refractive correction. The interaction between the perimetrist and the patient is fundamental to enhance the chances of successful perimetric testing.

Patient

Individuals vary in their attentiveness and response time from moment to moment and from day to day. Longer tests are more likely to produce fatigue and diminish the ability of the patient to maintain peak performance.

Perimetrist

Although the influence of the perimetrist on the results of automated perimetry is in general smaller than with manual perimetry, the perimetrist still plays an important role in

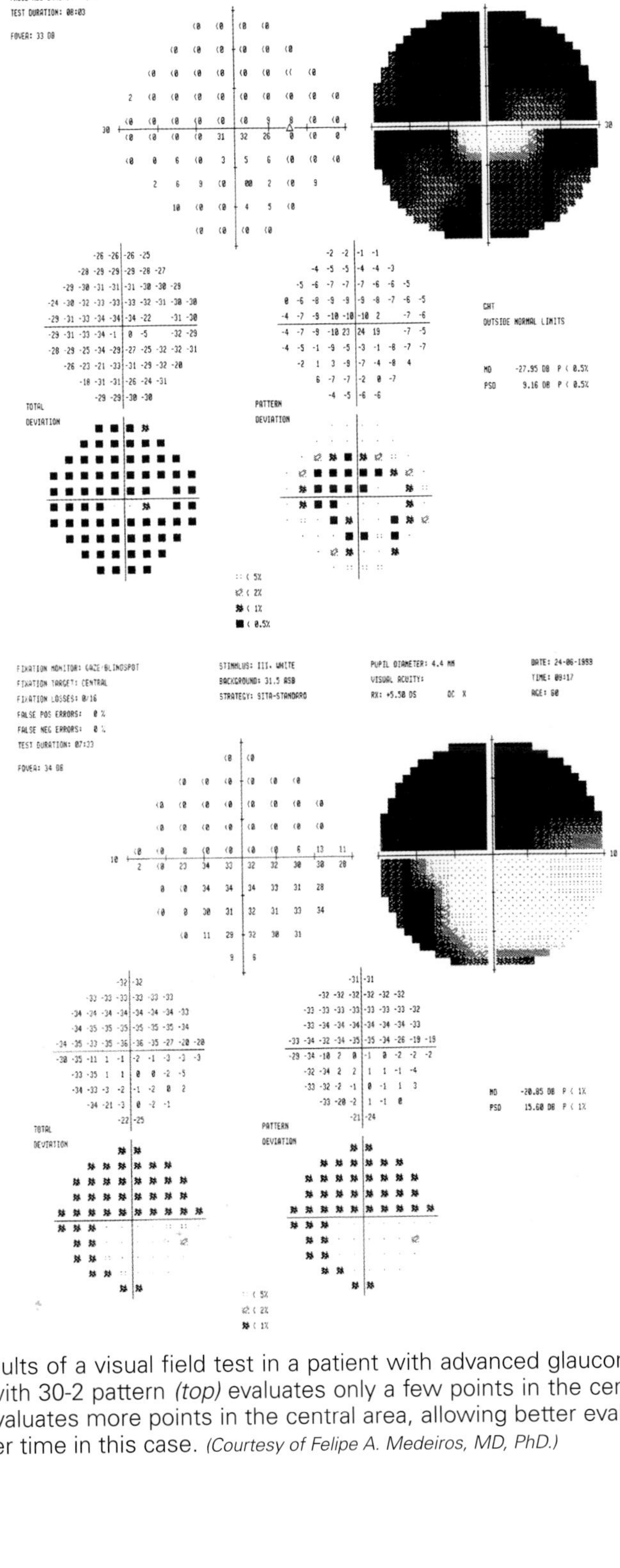

Figure 6-2 Results of a visual field test in a patient with advanced glaucomatous visual field loss. The test with 30-2 pattern *(top)* evaluates only a few points in the central area. The 10-2 test *(bottom)* evaluates more points in the central area, allowing better evaluation of potential progression over time in this case. *(Courtesy of Felipe A. Medeiros, MD, PhD.)*

the outcome of the test. It is important to instruct the patient about what to expect during the test, such as how long the test will take, when to blink, what the stimulus will look like, and where it might appear. Also, it is important to advise patients that the stimuli are likely to be barely visible throughout the test, and that more than half of the stimuli shown may not be visible. This knowledge can decrease a patient's anxiety and improve cooperation during the test. In addition, the perimetrist should explain to the patient how to pause the test if necessary. The patient should be monitored during the test to ensure proper positioning and fixation, and the perimetrist should be available to intervene if necessary to ensure proper testing conditions.

Other Factors

Other factors that may affect perimetry results include patient refraction and pupil size. Uncorrected refractive errors cause blurring on the retina and decrease the visibility of stimuli. Thus, proper neutralization of refractive errors is essential for accurate perimetry. In addition, presbyopic patients must be given a refractive correction that focuses on the perimeter bowl. Care needs to be taken to center the patient close to the correcting lens to avoid a lens rim artifact where the rim blocks peripheral stimuli. A small pupil (<2.5 mm) may produce artifacts on perimetry by reducing the amount of light entering the eye. However, such artifacts are now rare because the use of miotics (eg, pilocarpine) is now less common.

Interpretation of a Single Visual Field

The clinician should exercise caution when interpreting perimetric results. Even with improved strategies, these remain subjective tests. Therefore, confirmation of a new defect or worsening of an existing defect is usually necessary to validate the clinical implication of the visual field in conjunction with all other pertinent data. Evaluation of the visual field involves (1) assessing the quality or reliability of the visual field test, (2) assessing the normality or abnormality, and (3) identifying artifacts.

Test Quality

The first aspect of the visual field test to be evaluated is its quality or reliability. Reliability indices include the percentage of fixation losses, false-positives, and false-negatives. The false-positive response score measures the tendency of the patient to press the response button even when no stimulus has been presented. With the SITA strategy, patient responses that are made at impossible or unlikely times are used to estimate the false-positive response rate. These include responses made before or during the presentation or too soon after presentation, with consideration for the patient's usual reaction times that have been gathered during the test. Of the reliability indices, a high percentage of false-positives is most detrimental to a visual field test. Visual fields with a false-positive rate greater than 15% are likely unreliable and nonrepresentative of the patient's true visual function.

The fixation loss rate measures the patient's gaze stability during the test. A patient who does not maintain correct fixation during the test will produce an unreliable assessment of his or her peripheral vision. Fixation losses are estimated by periodically presenting stimuli at the region of the physiologic blind spot, known as the Heijl-Krakau method. If a patient responds to a stimulus that should have been presented at the blind spot, this is an indication that some eye movement must have occurred. However, this method can sometimes fail in identifying fixation losses when the location of the blind spot has not been appropriately identified at the beginning of the test. Humphrey perimeters also possess a gaze tracker that uses infrared light to check pupil location throughout the test. A record of gaze stability is shown at the bottom of the printout. Lines extending upward indicate gaze error, while lines downward indicate that the tracker was not able to successfully track the gaze direction, for example, during blinks. A high fixation loss rate (>25%) is also indicative of an unreliable field, especially if accompanied by the lack of a well-demarcated blind spot.

Finally, the false-negative error rate was originally devised to assess inattention during the test. This indicates lack of response to stimuli that should have been seen. Although a high false-negative rate could indicate an inattentive patient, damaged areas of the visual field show increased variability, which can lead to a high false-negative rate. Therefore, false-negative response rates can be elevated in abnormal fields regardless of the attentiveness of the patient. Hence, visual field tests should not necessarily be disregarded because of high false-negative rates, and many testing algorithms no longer measure this parameter.

Normality or Abnormality of the Visual Field

The next aspect to be assessed is the normality or abnormality of the visual field. A normal visual field demonstrates the greatest sensitivity centrally, with sensitivity falling steadily toward the periphery. Figure 6-3 shows a single field analysis of a visual field obtained with the HFA. The results are presented as a series of numerical plots and probability maps, including a threshold sensitivity map with the numerical threshold sensitivities for each location and a corresponding grayscale map; a total-deviation plot, showing deviations from age-corrected normal sensitivities; a total-deviation probability map, showing deviations that fall outside the statistical range of normal sensitivity; a pattern-deviation map, showing the localized loss after correcting for overall decreases in sensitivity; and a pattern-deviation probability map.

The Humphrey perimeter also provides a series of summary indices, including the following:

- *Mean deviation (MD).* MD is a weighted average of the total deviation values. Zero equates to no deviation from normal, and more negative values indicate more advanced loss.
- *Pattern standard deviation (PSD).* PSD is a summary index of localized visual field loss.
- *Glaucoma Hemifield Test (GHT).* This index categorizes eyes as within normal limits, borderline, or outside normal limits based on a comparison of visual field sensitivities at corresponding areas of the superior and inferior hemifields. Because glaucoma frequently causes asymmetric damage to the superior and inferior hemifields, the GHT is a powerful tool for identification of glaucomatous visual field defects (Fig 6-4).

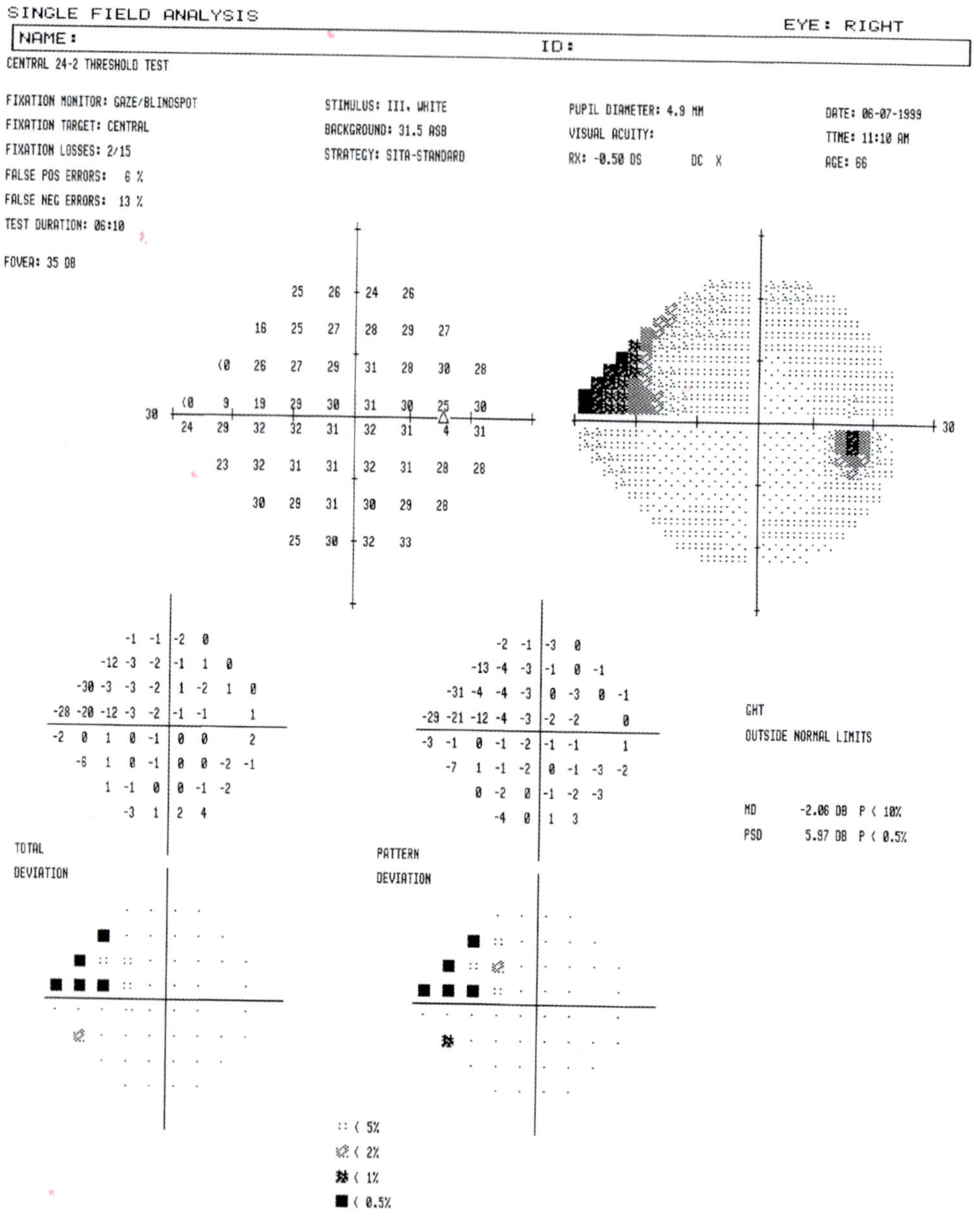

Figure 6-3 Printout of a visual field test obtained with a Humphrey field analyzer using the Swedish Interactive Threshold Algorithm (SITA) Standard 24-2 test.

Several criteria have been proposed for identification of visual field abnormalities. The system employed by the Ocular Hypertension Treatment Study (OHTS) is simple and widely accepted. In the OHTS, an abnormal visual field was defined by the presence of a PSD with $P < 5\%$ or the presence of a GHT with a result outside normal limits. The

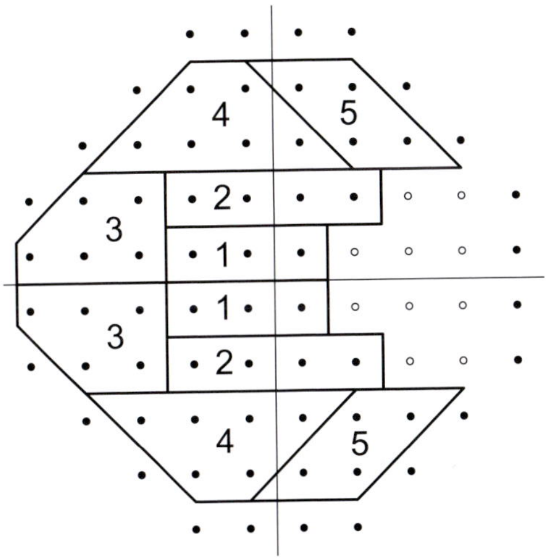

Figure 6-4 The Glaucoma Hemifield Test (GHT) compares pattern-deviation probability values in 5 predetermined zones in the superior hemifield with corresponding zones in the inferior hemifield. *(Courtesy of Michael Boland, MD.)*

abnormality had to be present in 3 consecutive visual field tests. In the analysis of a visual field printout, it is also important to evaluate the probability maps, especially the pattern-deviation probability plot. The presence of a cluster of at least 3 abnormal points ($P<5\%$) on the pattern-deviation plot, with at least 1 of those points with $P<1\%$, is also commonly used to define a visual field as abnormal.

It is important to emphasize that the clinician should examine the visual fields to verify whether the defect is repeatable and present in approximately the same location, and that the abnormalities are not due to the presence of artifacts. Although the points that are abnormal will not be exactly the same in all confirmatory tests, the area of visual field abnormality should be similar among the tests.

Artifacts

Identification of artifacts is the next step in evaluation of visual field test results. Common artifacts seen on automated perimetry include the following:

- *Lens rim.* If the machine's corrective lens is decentered or set too far from the eye, the lens rim may block more peripheral stimuli (Fig 6-5).
- *Inappropriate corrective lens.* If an inappropriate corrective lens is used, the resulting field may show generalized depression. This commonly occurs, for example, when testing young pseudophakic patients or when the patient is wearing a contact lens that is not considered when selecting the corrective lens power.
- *Eyelid artifact.* Partial eyelid ptosis may lead to a superior visual field defect.
- *Cloverleaf visual field.* If a patient stops paying attention and ceases to respond partway through a visual field test, a distinctive visual field pattern may develop. Figure 6-6 shows a cloverleaf visual field, the result of the testing order of the Humphrey 30-2 perimeter, which begins testing with the points circled in this figure and proceeds outward. This pattern may also be seen if a patient is malingering.

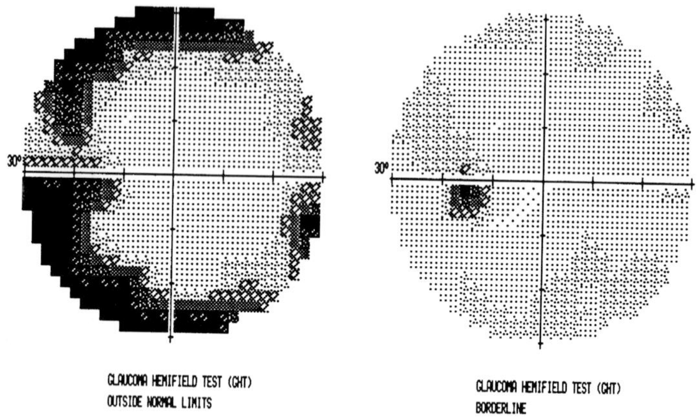

Figure 6-5 Lens rim artifact. The 2 visual fields shown were obtained 9 days apart. The visual field on the left shows a typical lens rim artifact, whereas the corrective lens was positioned appropriately for the visual field on the right (Humphrey 30-2 program).

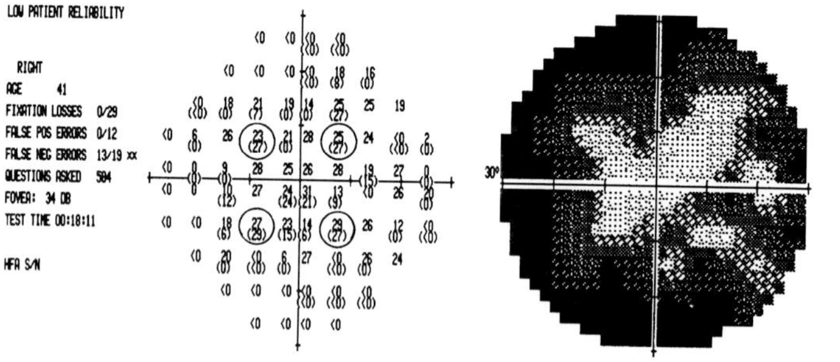

Figure 6-6 Cloverleaf visual field. In the Humphrey visual field perimeter test, 4 circled points are checked initially and the testing in each quadrant proceeds outward from these points. If the patient stops responding after only a few points have been tested, the result is some variation of the cloverleaf visual field shown at right (Humphrey Full Threshold 30-2 program).

- *High false-positive rate.* When a patient responds at a time when no test stimulus is being presented, a false-positive response is recorded. False-positive rates greater than 15% suggest an unreliable test that can mask or minimize an actual scotoma and can, in extreme cases, result in a visual field with impossibly high threshold values (Fig 6-7). Careful instruction of the patient may sometimes resolve this artifact.

Patterns of Visual Field Loss in Glaucoma

The hallmark defect of glaucoma is the nerve fiber bundle defect that results from damage at the optic nerve head. The pattern of nerve fibers in the retinal area served by the damaged nerve fiber bundle will correspond to the specific defect. The common names for the classic visual field defects are derived from their appearance as plotted on a kinetic visual

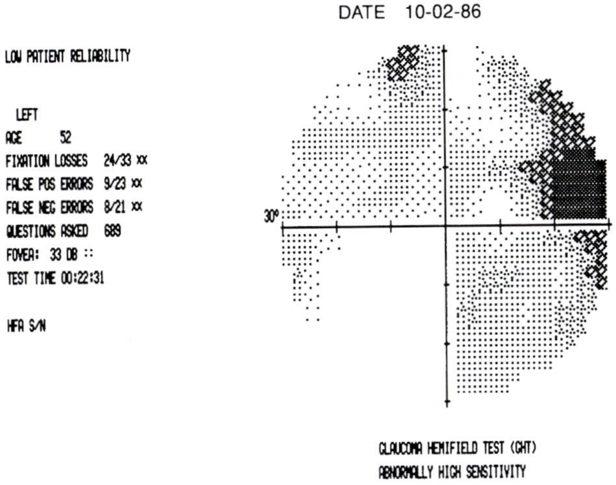

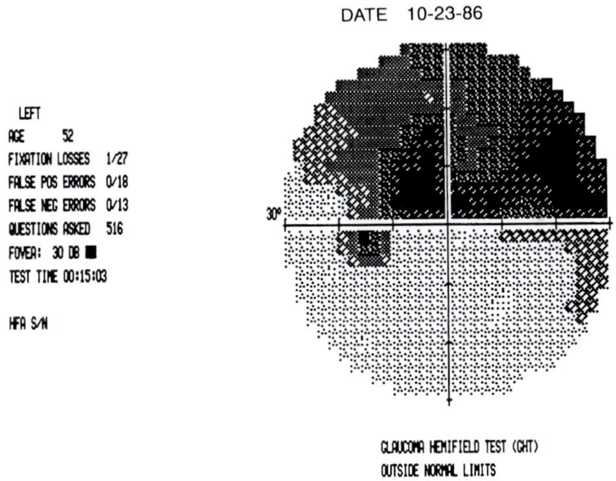

Figure 6-7 High false-positive rate. The top visual field contains characteristic "white scotomas," which represent areas of impossibly high retinal sensitivity. On the return visit 3 weeks later, the patient was carefully instructed to respond only when she saw the light, resulting in the bottom visual field, which shows good reliability and demonstrates the patient's dense superior visual field loss (Humphrey 30-2 program).

field chart. In static perimetry, however, the sample points are in a grid pattern, and the representation of visual field defects on a static perimetry chart generally lacks the smooth contours suggested by such terms as *arcuate.*

Glaucomatous visual field defects include the following:

- arcuate or Bjerrum scotoma (Fig 6-8)
- nasal step (Fig 6-9)
- paracentral scotoma (Fig 6-10)
- altitudinal defect (Fig 6-11)

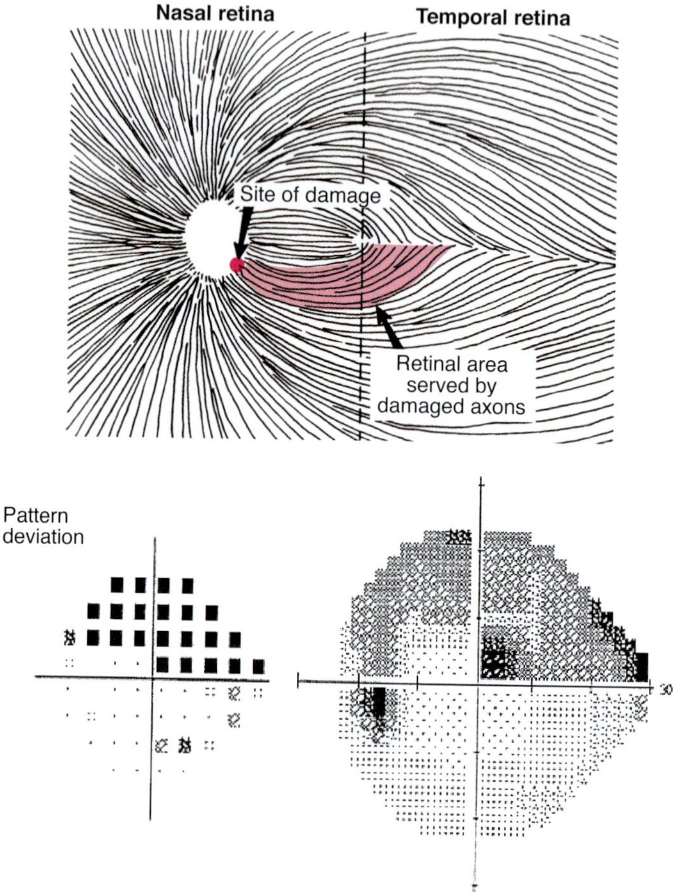

Figure 6-8 An *arcuate scotoma* occurs in the area 10°–20° from fixation. Glaucomatous damage to a nerve fiber bundle containing axons from both the inferonasal and inferotemporal retina resulted in the arcuate defect shown. The scotoma often begins as a single area of relative loss, which then becomes larger, deeper, and multifocal. In its full form, an arcuate scotoma arches from the blind spot and ends at the nasal raphe, becoming wider and closer to fixation on the nasal side (Humphrey 24-2 program). *(Visual field courtesy of G.A. Cioffi, MD.)*

- generalized depression (rare in glaucoma in the absence of localized loss)
- temporal wedge (rare)

The superior and inferior poles of the optic nerve are most susceptible to glaucomatous damage. However, damage to small, scattered bundles of optic nerve axons commonly produces a generalized decrease in sensitivity, which is harder to recognize than focal defects. Combinations of superior and inferior visual field loss, such as double arcuate scotomas, may occur, resulting in profound peripheral vision loss. Typically, the central island of vision and the inferotemporal visual field are retained until late in the course of glaucomatous optic nerve damage (see Fig 6-2).

Heijl A, Bengtsson B, Patella VM. *Effective Perimetry.* 4th ed. Carl Zeiss Meditec AG; 2012.

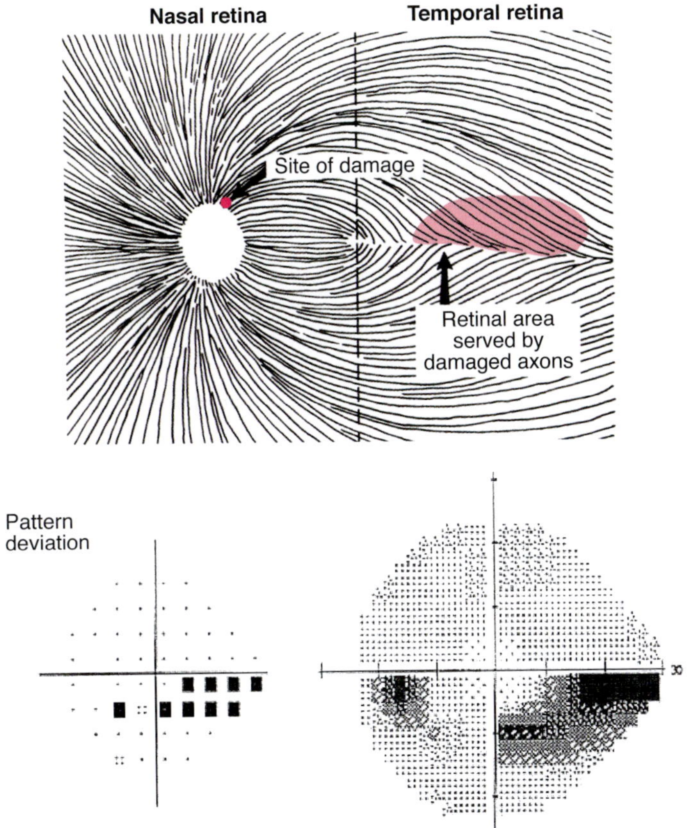

Figure 6-9 A *nasal step* is a relative depression of 1 horizontal hemifield compared with the other. Damage to superior nerve fibers serving the superotemporal retina beyond the paracentral area resulted in this nasal step. In kinetic perimetry, the nasal step is defined as a discontinuity or depression in 1 or more nasal isopters near the horizontal raphe (Humphrey 24-2 program). *(Visual field courtesy of G.A. Cioffi, MD.)*

Interpretation of a Series of Visual Fields and Detection of Visual Field Progression

Interpretation of serial visual fields should meet 2 goals:

1. separating real change from ordinary variation
2. using the information obtained from visual field testing to determine the likelihood that a change is related to glaucomatous progression

Visual field testing is a subjective examination, and different responses may be obtained each time the test is performed or even during the same test. This fluctuation can greatly confound the detection of disease progression. In order to detect true visual field progression, the clinician needs to evaluate whether the observed change exceeds the expected variability for a particular point or area.

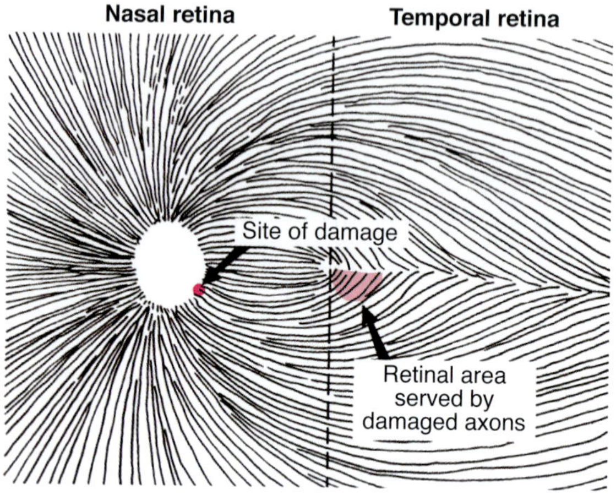

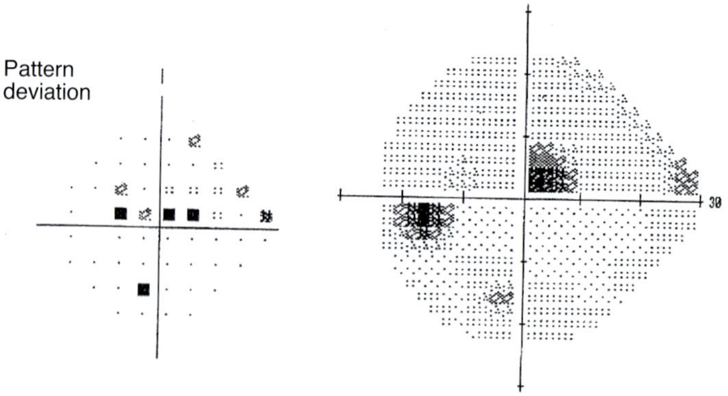

Figure 6-10 A *paracentral scotoma* is an island of relative or absolute vision loss within 10° of fixation. Loss of nerve fibers from the inferior pole, originating from the inferotemporal retina, resulted in the superonasal scotoma shown. Paracentral scotomas may be single, as in this case, or multiple, and they may occur as isolated findings or may be associated with other early defects (Humphrey 24-2 program). *(Visual field courtesy of G.A. Cioffi, MD.)*

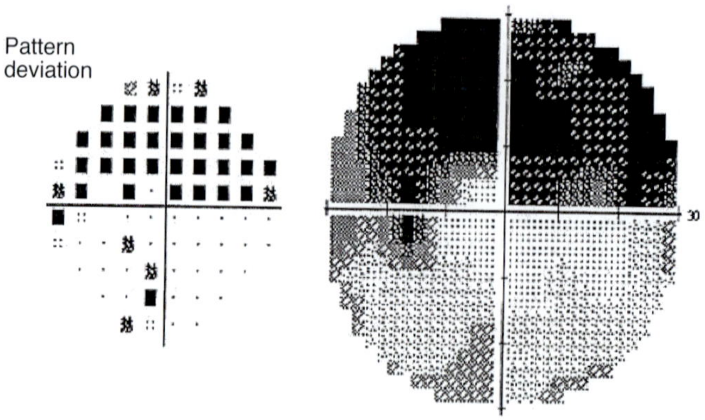

Figure 6-11 Altitudinal defect with nearly complete loss of the superior visual field, characteristic of moderate to advanced glaucomatous optic neuropathy (left eye). *(Visual field courtesy of G.A. Cioffi, MD.)*

There are, in general, 2 main approaches to analyzing visual field progression. The first approach is to compare the results of the current test (or a few recent tests for confirmation) with those obtained at baseline (often a pair of baseline visual field tests). If the results of the follow-up examination(s) are significantly worse than baseline, progression is said to have occurred. This approach, which is called *event-based analysis,* defines progression based on a predefined incremental deterioration compared to baseline.

In the second approach, called *trend-based analysis,* instead of comparing the current test with a baseline test, the clinician looks for progressive change by analyzing changes in visual field points or summary statistics for all tests available in a specific period. Change is observed as a trend in the values plotted over time, and significant deterioration can be assessed by observing the slope of the regression line. In addition to evaluating whether progression has occurred, trend-based analysis allows estimation of the rate of progression. It is well known that some patients decline faster than others; estimating each individual's rate of progression is helpful for predicting the risk of functional impairment and determining how aggressive treatment should be.

There are a variety of tools available to assist clinicians in identifying visual field progression, and there is no consensus about the best method for detecting change. The simplest and most general method uses the MD index plotted against time. A statistically significant decline would indicate progressive deterioration. Deterioration of the MD index may represent glaucomatous progression or progression of cataract or other media opacities. Conversely, in a glaucoma patient who has undergone cataract surgery, true underlying glaucoma progression may be masked by this method.

The Humphrey perimeter provides Guided Progression Analysis (GPA) software to assist in detection of visual field progression (Fig 6-12). This software presents an event-based method that is based on the pattern-deviation plot and, therefore, adjusts for the potential confounding effects of diffuse loss of sensitivity from media opacities. New or worsening visual field defects are identified by comparison to a pair of baseline tests; therefore, it is critical to have reliable baseline examinations. Often, the patient experiences a learning effect, and the second visual field may show substantial improvement over the first. To address this phenomenon, at least 2 visual field tests should be performed as early as possible in the course of a patient's disease. If the results are quite different, a third test should be performed. The software automatically selects the first 2 available examinations as the baseline tests. However, this selection can be easily overridden to a more suitable time point (eg, change in therapy after progression) or to avoid initial learning effects (which could reduce the sensitivity to detect progression). The software then compares each follow-up test to the average of the baseline tests (Fig 6-13). It identifies points that show change greater than the expected variability (at the 95% significance level), as determined by previous studies with stable glaucoma patients. If significant change is detected in at least 3 points and repeated for the same points in 2 consecutive follow-up tests, the software will flag the last examination as *Possible Progression.* If significant change is detected and repeated for the same 3 or more points in 3 consecutive follow-up tests, the GPA software will flag the last examination as *Likely Progression.*

GPA software also provides the Visual Field Index (VFI) and VFI progression plot (Fig 6-14). The VFI is calculated as the percentage of normal visual field, after adjustment

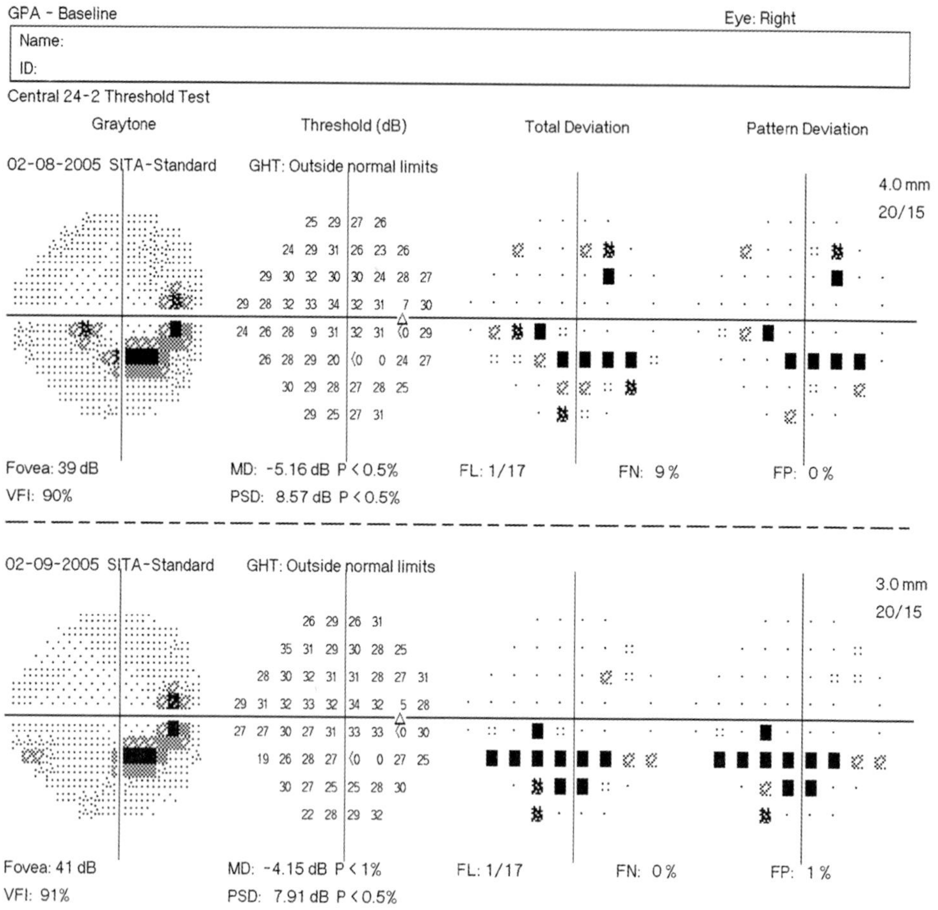

Figure 6-12 Analysis of visual field progression using the Guided Progression Analysis software of the Humphrey perimeter. These visual fields were selected as the baseline. Results of each follow-up visual field test (see Fig 6-13) are compared with the average of the 2 baseline fields. *(Courtesy of Felipe A. Medeiros, MD, PhD.)*

for age. Therefore, a VFI of 100% represents a completely normal visual field, while a VFI of 0% represents a perimetrically blind visual field. The VFI is shown on the GPA printout as a percentage value for each examination. A trend-based analysis of VFI as a function of the patient's age is presented with a future projection that predicts the VFI, assuming the same regression slope, 5 years in the future. Whereas the MD is based only on the total-deviation map, and is thus affected by cataract, the VFI is based both on the pattern-deviation probability map, for the identification of possibly progressing points, and on the total-deviation map, used for the actual calculation of change of the total-deviation value. In addition, the algorithm applies different weights to different locations, giving more weight to more central points, which have greater impact on the patient's quality of vision. The final VFI score is the mean of all weighted scores.

The Octopus perimeter also provides a comprehensive statistical package (EyeSuite) for evaluation of visual field progression. The software calculates rates of progression in

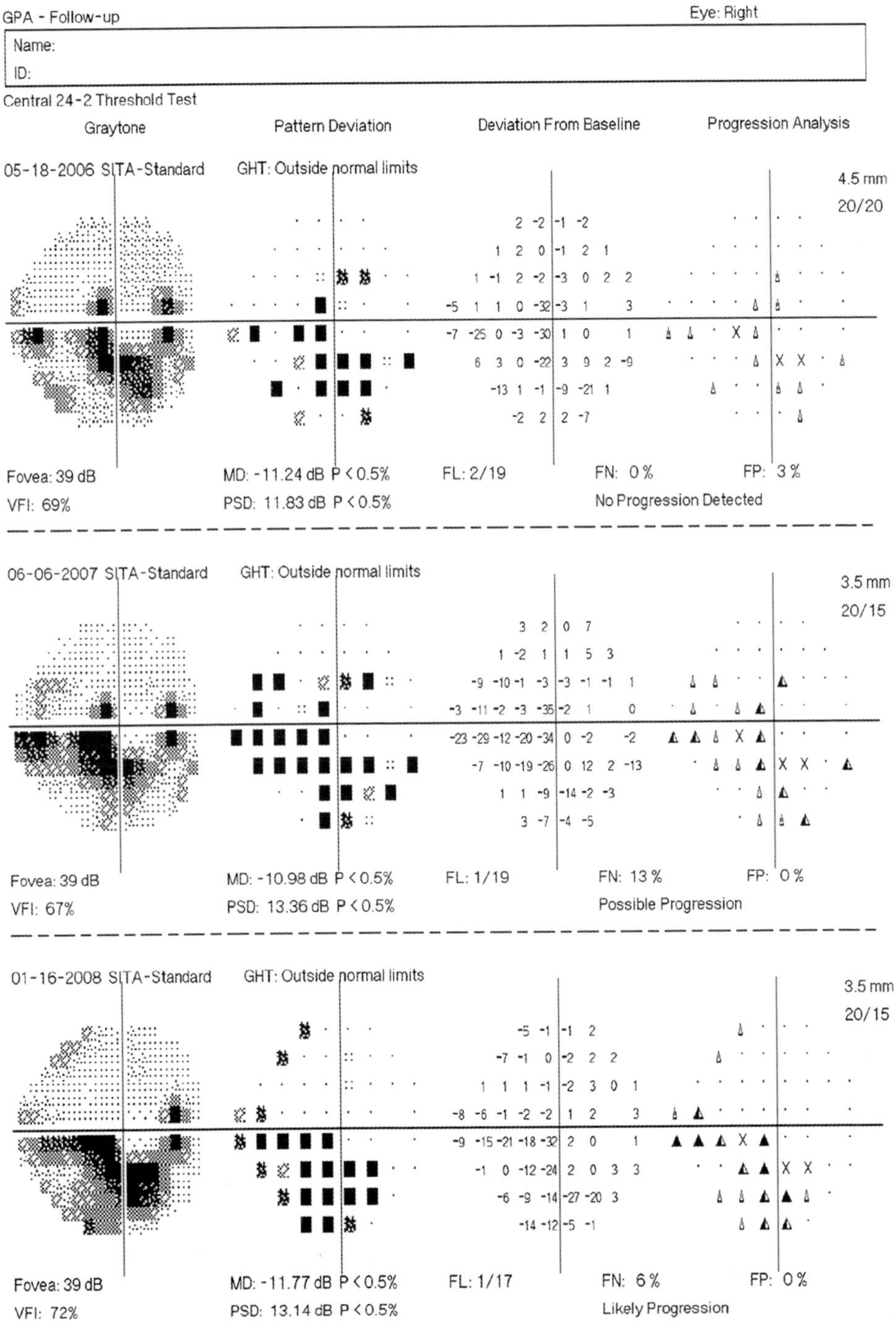

Figure 6-13 Visual fields from consecutive follow-up examinations (see Fig 6-12 for baseline visual field tests for this patient). Several points are flagged as showing significant deterioration. A number of points in the inferonasal region show repeatable significant change *(black-filled triangles)*. The last visual field is then flagged as Likely Progression. *(Courtesy of Felipe A. Medeiros, MD, PhD.)*

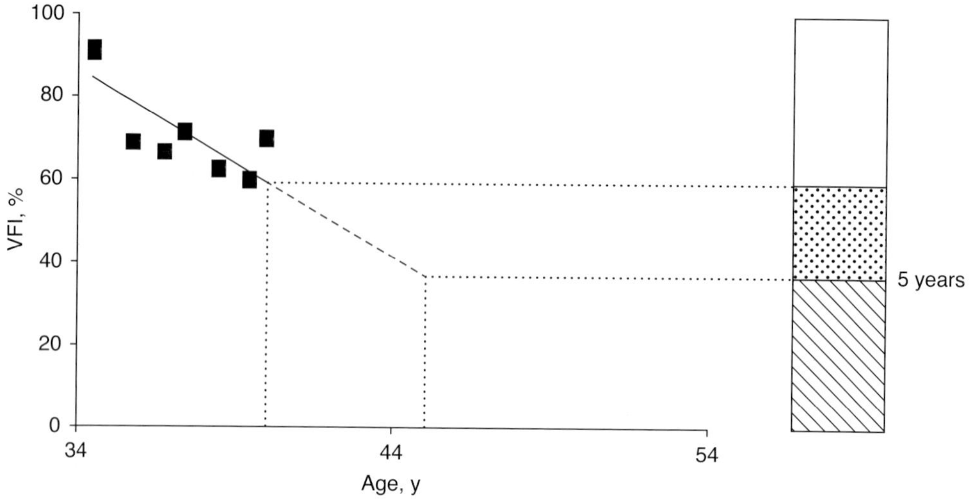

Rate of progression: –4.5 ± 3.3%/year (95% CI)
Slope significant at *P* < 5%

Figure 6-14 Humphrey Visual Field Index (VFI) plot corresponding to the visual fields shown in Figures 6-12 and 6-13. The slope of change was significant and estimated at –4.5% per year. CI = confidence interval. *(Courtesy of Felipe A. Medeiros, MD, PhD.)*

terms of mean defect change per year (in dB/year), similar to the MD index from Humphrey perimetry. In addition, the software provides an analysis of progression by individual test points (pointwise linear regression) and by clusters, where test locations are combined according to nerve fiber bundle patterns.

Frequency of Testing

Accurate and timely detection of progressive changes can be difficult because of the inherent variability of visual field testing. The time required to detect new visual field loss depends on the frequency of testing and follow-up scheme used. The recommended frequency of testing varies depending on patient characteristics such as age, disease severity, presence of risk factors for progression, concomitant clinical findings, and risk for functional impairment. In order to precisely estimate a rate of progression, many tests are needed over time. Studies have shown that the strategy of acquiring only 1 visual field test per year may be insufficient in a large number of cases, resulting in delayed detection of disease progression and imprecise estimation of rates of change. Although the optimal testing strategy will vary, obtaining at least 2 or 3 tests per year during the first 2 years of follow-up is recommended in order to exclude the possibility of fast progression. Thereafter, a testing strategy consisting of 2 tests per year may be sufficient in most cases.

Wu Z, Saunders LJ, Daga FB, Diniz-Filho A, Medeiros FA. Frequency of testing to detect visual field progression derived using a longitudinal cohort of glaucoma patients. *Ophthalmology*. 2017;124(6):786–792.

Structure and Function Relationship

It is important to correlate changes in the visual field (function) with those in the optic nerve (structure). If such correlation is lacking, the ophthalmologist should consider other causes of vision loss, such as ischemic optic neuropathy, demyelinating or other neurologic disease, or pituitary tumor. This consideration is especially important in the following situations:

- The patient's optic nerve head seems less cupped than would be expected for the degree of visual field loss.
- The pallor of the optic nerve head is more impressive than the cupping.
- The rate of visual field loss seems too rapid for a patient with treated glaucoma.
- The pattern of visual field loss is uncharacteristic for glaucoma—for example, it respects the vertical midline.
- The location of the cupping or thinning of the neural rim does not correspond to the location of the visual field defect.

It should be noted, however, that progressive visual field loss may sometimes be seen in the absence of optic nerve head changes and vice versa. In cases of early disease, progressive structural changes of the optic nerve and retinal nerve fiber layer can frequently be seen despite lack of apparent visual field progression. Conversely, in cases of more severe disease, progressive visual field losses tend to occur despite a lack of detectable structural change. This apparent disagreement may be explained by the different characteristics of the tests, including scaling, variability, and presence of floor/ceiling effects. Therefore, follow-up of patients with glaucoma should be performed using both structural and functional assessments.

Recent studies have suggested that early glaucomatous visual field defects may sometimes be seen in the macular area and detected with central 10-2 testing in the absence of defects detected with the 24-2 pattern. This has led to the suggestion that central tests be incorporated into the regular management scheme of patients with glaucoma or in those suspected of disease. However, the benefit of adding more 10-2 pattern tests in these cases needs to be weighed against the increased patient burden and the missed opportunity of obtaining another regular 24-2 pattern test. The Humphrey perimeter offers a combined perimetric strategy that tests the 24-2 pattern along with 10 additional locations in the central 10°, the 24-2C pattern; its utility is under investigation.

Medeiros FA, Zangwill LM, Bowd C, Mansouri K, Weinreb RN. The structure and function relationship in glaucoma: implications for detection of progression and measurement of rates of change. *Invest Ophthalmol Vis Sci.* 2012;53(11):6939–6946.

Other Perimetric Tests

Other psychophysical tests of visual function include frequency-doubling technology (FDT), short-wavelength automated perimetry (SWAP), and flicker-defined form (FDF) perimetry (Fig 6-15). These tests aim to target subpopulations of retinal ganglion cells (RGCs) by evaluating specific aspects of visual function (eg, motion perception, contrast

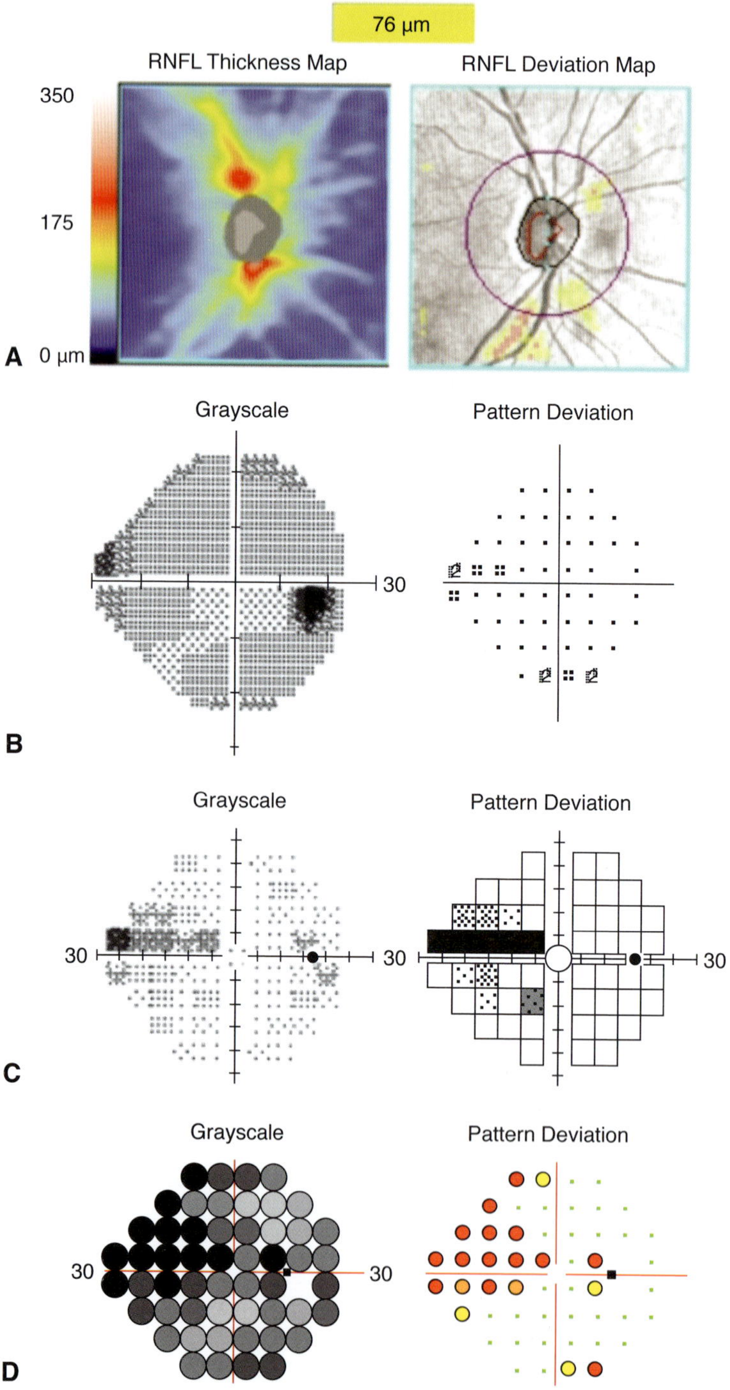

Figure 6-15 Findings from a right eye with glaucoma. **A,** Inferior retinal nerve fiber layer (RNFL) thinning is visible on optical coherence tomography (OCT). **B,** Standard automated perimetry (SAP) shows a small corresponding superonasal visual field defect that is more pronounced on frequency-doubling technology perimetry **(C)** and Heidelberg Edge Perimetry **(D).** *(Courtesy of Felipe A. Medeiros, MD, PhD.)*

sensitivity, color vision) and thereby reduce the ability of the visual system to use other pathways to compensate. It has been hypothesized that in its early stages, glaucoma may damage predominantly magnocellular RGCs projecting to the magnocellular layers of the lateral geniculate nucleus (ie, the magnocellular [M] pathway), although whether such preferential loss indeed occurs is still unclear.

FDT perimetry, which tests the patient's ability to detect a flickering stimulus at a high temporal frequency, was designed to selectively evaluate the M pathway, but evidence shows that the response to motion, including the flicker of FDT, may be generated by many ganglion cell types and is cortically mediated. Nevertheless, FDT has shown promise for glaucoma detection, and longitudinal studies have shown that abnormalities on FDT may precede detectable SAP changes in many patients. The FDT Matrix (Carl Zeiss Meditec) is a commercially available perimeter that features FDT stimuli. It uses sinusoidal grating targets smaller than the original FDT perimeter to enable 24-2 and 30-2 patterns like those used in SAP. Although the first-generation FDT perimeter was able to evaluate visual field sensitivity in only 17 or 19 locations, the FDT Matrix is capable of testing 54 (24-2 pattern) or 69 (30-2 pattern) locations. This technology potentially improves the ability of monitoring progression over time; however, it is not widely used and is limited by the absence of analytic tools for detecting progression.

SWAP is designed to stimulate the small bistratified ganglion cells, which project their axons to the koniocellular layers of the lateral geniculate nucleus. It uses a blue-violet stimulus (440-nm wavelength) against a bright yellow background. SWAP generally does not have better diagnostic ability than SAP and is now performed in clinical practice only in rare cases.

The FDF stimulus has been proposed as an alternative method for detecting glaucomatous vision loss. FDF perimetry is believed to stimulate the M pathway, and there is emerging evidence that it may be useful for early glaucoma diagnosis.

Although psychophysical tests such as FDT, SWAP, and FDF perimetry attempt to minimize potential input from other pathways, it is unlikely any stimulus can be 100% specific for a single visual pathway or a single subset of RGCs. Furthermore, it is unlikely a single ganglion cell type is always affected first in glaucoma. Perimetric tests are also subjective examinations, and therefore responses may vary on repeat testing, or during the same test, reducing the ability to confidently detect genuine early abnormalities.

Other tests that measure the integrity of the visual field include contrast sensitivity perimetry, flicker sensitivity, microperimetry, visual evoked potential, and multifocal electroretinography. These tests are not commonly employed in the evaluation of patients with glaucoma. Several of these tests are discussed in greater detail in BCSC Section 12, *Retina and Vitreous*, and in Section 5, *Neuro-Ophthalmology*.

Meira-Freitas D, Tatham AJ, Lisboa R, et al. Predicting progression of glaucoma from rates of frequency doubling technology perimetry change. *Ophthalmology.* 2014;121(2):498–507.

CHAPTER 7

Primary Open-Angle Glaucoma

Highlights

- Important risk factors for primary open-angle glaucoma include age, race, family history, central corneal thickness, myopia, and intraocular pressure (IOP).
- The relationship between blood pressure and open-angle glaucoma is complex; however, lower ocular perfusion pressure (difference between blood pressure and IOP) is a risk factor.
- Open-angle glaucoma can develop across a wide range of IOPs.
- Lowering IOP with medication, laser surgery, or incisional surgery is currently the only means of treating open-angle glaucoma.
- Treatment of ocular hypertension reduces the risk of progression to glaucoma.

Primary Open-Angle Glaucoma

Primary open-angle glaucoma (POAG) is typically a chronic, slowly progressive optic neuropathy with characteristic patterns of optic nerve damage and visual field loss. Numerous clinical factors affect an individual's susceptibility to POAG, which is a multifactorial disease process. These factors include intraocular pressure (IOP), age, race, central corneal thickness, myopia, and a family history of glaucoma. Other factors that may contribute to disease susceptibility include low corneal hysteresis, low ocular perfusion pressure, low cerebrospinal fluid pressure, abnormalities of axonal or ganglion cell metabolism, and disorders of the extracellular matrix of the lamina cribrosa. Unfortunately, we do not yet fully understand the interplay of the multiple factors involved in the development of POAG. Secondary open-angle glaucoma (OAG) differs from POAG in that identifiable factors contribute to its development, such as the dispersed pigment in pigmentary glaucoma and the pseudoexfoliative material of pseudoexfoliation syndrome. (For more on secondary OAG, see Chapter 8.)

Clinical Features

POAG is typically insidious in onset, slowly progressive, and painless. It is usually bilateral but can be asymmetric. Patients may seem relatively asymptomatic until the later stages of the disease, when central vision is affected. POAG is diagnosed with findings from the assessment of the optic nerve and nerve fiber layer and the results of visual field testing.

Gonioscopic findings

The diagnosis of POAG requires verification that the anterior chamber angle is open. Gonioscopy (discussed in Chapter 4) is indicated for all patients evaluated for glaucoma. In patients with established OAG, gonioscopy should be repeated periodically to monitor for progressive angle closure caused by lens-induced changes, particularly in patients with hyperopia. Repeated gonioscopy is also indicated when the anterior chamber becomes shallow, when strong miotics are prescribed, after argon laser trabeculoplasty* (ALT) or laser peripheral iridotomy has been performed, and when IOP increases.

Optic nerve head appearance and visual fields

Although elevated IOP is an important risk factor for OAG, diagnosis of this disease is based primarily on the appearance of the optic nerve head, or optic disc, and on the results of visual field testing. See Chapters 5 and 6 for a detailed discussion of the optic nerve and visual fields. Careful periodic evaluation of the optic nerve and visual field testing are essential in the management of glaucoma. Stereophotographic documentation of the optic nerve or computerized imaging of the optic nerve, retinal nerve fiber layer, and macula aids the detection of subtle changes over time. Visual field loss typically correlates with the appearance of the optic nerve, and significant discrepancies between the pattern of visual field loss and optic nerve appearance warrant additional investigation.

American Academy of Ophthalmology Glaucoma Panel, Hoskins Center for Quality Eye Care. Preferred Practice Pattern® Guidelines. *Primary Open-Angle Glaucoma—2015.* American Academy of Ophthalmology; 2015. www.aao.org/ppp

Jonas JB, Budde WM, Panda-Jonas S. Ophthalmoscopic evaluation of the optic nerve head. *Surv Ophthalmol.* 1999;43(4):293–320.

Atypical Findings

In patients who present with atypical findings that cannot be explained by the clinical circumstances—for example, unilateral disease, decreased central vision, dyschromatopsia, young age, presence of a relative afferent pupillary defect, neuroretinal rim pallor, or visual field loss inconsistent with optic nerve appearance—additional medical and neurologic evaluation should be considered. This evaluation may include assessment for a compressive etiology, carotid artery insufficiency, anemia, syphilis, certain vitamin deficiencies, giant cell arteritis or other causes of systemic vasculitis, and exposure to a toxic substance. Noninvasive tests of carotid circulation (eg, carotid Doppler ultrasonography) may be helpful. In cases of optic nerve pallor or visual field loss suggestive of a neurologic defect, evaluation of the anterior visual pathway, including the optic chiasm, with magnetic resonance imaging or computed tomography may be warranted. See also BCSC Section 5, *Neuro-Ophthalmology.*

Risk Factors

Intraocular pressure

Elevated IOP is an important risk factor for glaucoma but is not required for a POAG diagnosis. Large population-based studies suggest a mean IOP of 15.5 mm Hg (standard

*Note: This term is based on the historical use of argon laser technology; most green lasers currently used in ophthalmology are diode-pumped solid state (eg, frequency-doubled Nd:YAG or Nd:YLF) lasers.

deviation ± 2.6) in European-derived populations, but the normal distribution of IOP varies across racial and ethnic groups. This finding led to the definition of "normal" IOP as 2 standard deviations above and below the mean IOP or a range between 10 and 21 mm Hg. IOP greater than 21 mm Hg was thus traditionally defined as "abnormal," but this definition has shortcomings.

It is known that IOP in the general population is not represented by a Gaussian distribution but rather is skewed toward higher pressures (see Chapter 2, Fig 2-4). Thus, IOPs of 22 mm Hg and above may not necessarily be abnormal from a statistical standpoint. More importantly, IOP distribution curves for glaucomatous and nonglaucomatous eyes show a great deal of overlap. Several studies indicate that as many as 30%–50% of individuals in the general population with glaucomatous optic neuropathy and/or visual field loss have initial IOP measurements below 22 mm Hg. Higher IOP, across its entire range observed in a population, is a continuous risk factor for POAG.

IOP may vary considerably over a 24-hour period, and elevations of IOP may occur only intermittently in some glaucomatous eyes (see Chapter 2). Thus, a single IOP measurement taken during office hours does not provide an accurate assessment of IOP variability over time. Table 7-1 lists some of the reasons that elevated IOP may be undetected in patients. Large diurnal fluctuation in IOP has been identified as an independent risk factor for progression of glaucoma in some studies, but not in others. Regardless, elevation of IOP is a strong risk factor for glaucoma progression.

As discussed in Chapter 2, central corneal thickness (CCT) affects the measurement of IOP. Thicker corneas resist the deformation inherent in most methods of tonometry, resulting in an overestimation of IOP. In contrast, tonometry in eyes with thin corneas underestimates the IOP. The average CCT in adult eyes, determined by ultrasonic pachymetry, ranges between about 525 and 550 µm and varies with race and ethnicity. For example, in persons of African ancestry, mean CCT is lower than in those of European ancestry.

Bengtsson B, Leske MC, Hyman L, Heijl A; Early Manifest Glaucoma Trial Group. Fluctuation of intraocular pressure and glaucoma progression in the early manifest glaucoma trial. *Ophthalmology.* 2007;114(2):205–209.

Bhan A, Browning AC, Shah S, Hamilton R, Dave D, Dua HS. Effect of corneal thickness on intraocular pressure measurements with the pneumotonometer, Goldmann applanation tonometer, and Tono-Pen. *Invest Ophthalmol Vis Sci.* 2002;43(5):1389–1392.

Table 7-1 Potential Reasons for Undetected High-Tension Glaucoma

Primary open-angle glaucoma with diurnal IOP fluctuation
Intermittent IOP elevation
Asymptomatic angle closure
Glaucomatocyclitic crisis
Secondary glaucoma (eg, pigmentary, pseudoexfoliation, uveitic)
Normalized IOP in an eye with previously elevated IOP (eg, corticosteroid-induced, uveitic, pigmentary, hyphema)
Use of medications that may lower IOP (eg, systemic β-blocker)
Inaccurate IOP measurement (due to thin central cornea, reduced scleral rigidity, uncalibrated device, poor examiner technique)

IOP = intraocular pressure.

Brandt JD, Beiser JA, Kass MA, Gordon MO. Central corneal thickness in the Ocular Hypertension Treatment Study (OHTS). *Ophthalmology.* 2001;108(10):1779–1788.
Liu JH, Kripke DF, Twa MD, et al. Twenty-four-hour pattern of intraocular pressure in the aging population. *Invest Ophthalmol Vis Sci.* 1999;40(12):2912–2917.

Older age

The Baltimore Eye Survey found that the prevalence of glaucoma increases dramatically with age, particularly among individuals of African descent, in whom prevalence exceeded 11% among those older than 80 years. In the Collaborative Initial Glaucoma Treatment Study (CIGTS; see Clinical Trial 7-1 at the end of this chapter), visual field defects were 7 times more likely to progress in patients 60 years or older than in those younger than 40 years. The Ocular Hypertension Treatment Study (OHTS; see Clinical Trial 7-2 at the end of this chapter) found an increased risk of progression to OAG with age (per decade): 43% in the univariate analysis and 22% in the multivariate analysis. Older age is an independent risk factor for both the development and the progression of glaucoma.

Race

The prevalence of POAG in the United States is 3–4 times greater in individuals of African descent or Hispanic ethnicity than in primarily European-derived populations. Blindness from glaucoma is at least 4 times more common in Black individuals than in White individuals. In addition, glaucoma is more likely to be diagnosed in Black patients at a younger age and at a more advanced stage than it is in White patients. In a univariable analysis, the OHTS found that glaucoma was 59% more likely to develop in Black patients with ocular hypertension (defined in this study as IOP ≥24 mm Hg in the absence of optic nerve or visual field abnormalities) than in White patients with ocular hypertension. However, this relationship was not present after controlling for corneal thickness and baseline vertical cup–disc ratio in a multivariable analysis (on average, Black patients had thinner CCT and larger baseline vertical cup–disc ratios).

Thin central cornea and low corneal hysteresis

A thinner cornea is an important risk factor for disease progression in individuals with POAG (who have higher baseline IOPs) and for the development of glaucoma in individuals with ocular hypertension. This risk may not be entirely due to the underestimation of IOP measured by Goldmann tonometry in patients with thin corneas; therefore, attempting to correct IOP according to CCT is not supported by evidence. Thin corneas may be a biomarker for disease susceptibility. As mentioned previously, Black patients have thinner corneas on average than White patients. Studies of corneal biomechanics, particularly hysteresis, have shown a relationship between these measurements and glaucoma progression (see Chapter 2).

Brandt JD, Gordon MO, Gao F, Besider JA, Miller JP, Kass MA; Ocular Hypertension Treatment Study. Adjusting intraocular pressure for central corneal thickness does not improve prediction models for primary open-angle glaucoma. *Ophthalmology.* 2012;119(3):437–442.

Family history

In the Baltimore Eye Survey, the relative risk of POAG increased approximately 3.7-fold for individuals who had a sibling with POAG. Increased risk of glaucoma within families is likely based on genetics, although simple mendelian inheritance of glaucoma is not common (see Chapter 1).

Myopia

Population-based data support an association between POAG and myopia. In the Beaver Dam Eye Study (United States), myopia of greater than 1 diopter (D) spherical equivalent was significantly associated with a diagnosis of glaucoma. In the Rotterdam (Netherlands) follow-up study, high myopia of greater than 4 D was associated with a hazard ratio of 2.3 for developing glaucoma over 10 years. Myopia was also shown to be a risk factor in the Beijing Eye Study, in which high myopia (greater than 6 D spherical equivalent) conferred an odds ratio of 8 for having glaucoma compared to emmetropic eyes. The Blue Mountains Eye Study (Australia) found an odds ratio of 3.3 for participants with myopia of greater than 3 D. However, in the OHTS, no association between myopia and progression to glaucoma was observed.

The concurrence of POAG and myopia may complicate diagnosis and management in several ways. Evaluation of the optic nerve head is particularly challenging in highly myopic eyes that have tilted discs or posterior staphylomas. Also, the myopic refractive error may cause optical minification of the optic nerve, further complicating accurate optic nerve assessment. Myopia-related retinal degeneration or anomalies can cause visual field abnormalities that are difficult to distinguish from those caused by glaucoma (see Chapter 10, Myopia and Pathologic Myopia, in BCSC Section 12, *Retina and Vitreous*). In addition, patients who are highly myopic may have difficulty performing visual field tests, making interpretation of visual field abnormalities more challenging.

Mitchell P, Hourihan F, Sandbach J, Wang JJ. The relationship between glaucoma and myopia: the Blue Mountains Eye Study. *Ophthalmology.* 1999;106(10):2010–2015.

Varma R, Ying-Lai M, Francis BA, et al; Los Angeles Latino Eye Study Group. Prevalence of open-angle glaucoma and ocular hypertension in Latinos: the Los Angeles Latino Eye Study. *Ophthalmology.* 2004;111(8):1439–1448.

Wong TY, Klein BE, Klein R, Knudtson M, Lee KE. Refractive errors, intraocular pressure, and glaucoma in a white population. *Ophthalmology.* 2003;110(1):211–217.

Xu L, Wang Y, Wang S, Wang Y, Jonas JB. High myopia and glaucoma susceptibility: the Beijing Eye Study. *Ophthalmology*. 2007;114(2):216–220.

Association with Systemic Conditions

Diabetes mellitus

The evidence related to diabetes mellitus as a risk factor for glaucoma is difficult to interpret. The Beaver Dam Eye Study, the Blue Mountains Eye Study, and the Los Angeles Latino Eye Study found an increased risk of OAG in participants with diabetes. However, the Framingham Study, the Baltimore Eye Survey, the Barbados Eye Study, and a revised analysis of the Rotterdam Study did not find an association. Furthermore, the Rotterdam Study and the Barbados Eye Study, which were large longitudinal population-based studies, did not identify diabetes as a risk factor for the incident development of glaucoma. In the OHTS, depending on how the analysis was performed, diabetes was either associated with a reduced risk of developing glaucoma or it was not associated with glaucoma. One possible explanation for these results is that the cohort of diabetic patients was skewed in this study because the presence of retinopathy was an exclusion criterion for participants in the OHTS.

de Voogd S, Ikram MK, Wolfs RC, et al. Is diabetes mellitus a risk factor for open-angle glaucoma? The Rotterdam Study. *Ophthalmology.* 2006;113(10):1827–1831.

Hypertension

The Baltimore Eye Survey found that systemic hypertension was associated with a lower risk of glaucoma in younger (<65 years) patients and a higher risk of glaucoma in older patients. The hypothesis is that younger individuals with high blood pressure may have better perfusion of the optic nerve, but as these patients age, their chronic hypertension may have adverse effects on the microcirculation of the optic nerve and increase its susceptibility to glaucomatous optic neuropathy. Conversely, in the Barbados Eye Study, the relative risk of developing glaucoma among study participants with systemic hypertension was less than 1 in all age groups, including those aged 70 years and older.

Lower ocular perfusion pressure

There is compelling evidence that lower ocular perfusion pressure (OPP; defined as diastolic blood pressure + 1/3 systolic blood pressure − IOP) is a risk factor for the development of glaucoma. The Baltimore Eye Survey found a sixfold increase in the prevalence of glaucoma in those patients with the lowest levels of OPP. Low systolic perfusion pressure was also a risk factor for glaucoma progression in the Early Manifest Glaucoma Trial (hazard ratio 1.42 for systolic perfusion pressure ≤160 mm Hg). Although the concept of OPP oversimplifies actual ocular blood flow, several factors, including autoregulatory mechanisms in central nervous system perfusion, make the association between OPP and glaucoma intriguing. The overtreatment of systemic hypertension may contribute to glaucoma progression and should be considered in some cases (eg, worsening of seemingly well-treated glaucoma).

Costa VP, Harris A, Anderson D, et al. Ocular perfusion pressure in glaucoma. *Acta Ophthalmol.* 2014;92(4):e252–e266.

Other associated conditions

Sleep apnea, thyroid disorders, hypercholesterolemia, migraine headaches, low cerebrospinal fluid pressure, and Raynaud phenomenon have been identified in 1 or more studies as potential risk factors for the development of glaucoma. Further research is required in order to clarify the significance of these conditions in patients with POAG and their relationship to glaucoma, if any.

Prognosis and Therapy

Most patients with POAG retain useful vision for their entire lives. The patients at greatest risk of blindness are those who present with visual field loss at the time of diagnosis. In a single-institution study, the cumulative risk of unilateral and bilateral blindness in patients with OAG was 7.4% and 3.4%, respectively, within 10 years of diagnosis, and 13.5% and 4.3%, respectively, within 20 years of diagnosis.

Treatment with topical medication, laser surgery, and incisional surgery to lower IOP has been shown to significantly reduce the risk of glaucomatous progression (see the Clinical

Trials at the end of this chapter). Patients with symptomatically decreased visual function (eg, visual acuity worse than 20/40, severe visual field damage, decreased contrast sensitivity) can be referred to a vision rehabilitation specialist. These specialists can help improve visual function by optimizing lighting, enhancing contrast, reducing glare, and providing adaptations to enhance activities of … be consulted and vision substitution … ove daily function and quality of life f… nal-mology's Initiative in Vision Rehab… ow -vision-and-vision-rehab) provides … ent handouts and information about … nd those provided by the ophthalmolo… *ion Rehabilitation*, for in-depth discussi…

> glaucoma suspect: one of the below things:
>
> ☐ suspicious ON – but no VF changes
>
> ☐ VF changes but no optic nerve abnormalities
>
> ☐ FHx (first-degree relatve)
>
> ☐ elevated IOP w/o ON changes

American Academy of Ophthalmol… for Quality Eye Care. Preferred P… American Academy of Ophthalm…

Boland MV, Ervin AM, Friedman D… angle glaucoma: a systematic revi… *Med*. 2013;158(4):271–279.

Malihi M, Moura Filho ER, Hodge … blindness in Olmsted County, Mi…

The Glaucoma Suspect

A glaucoma suspect is defined as an individual who has 1 or more of the following characteristics:

- a suspicious optic nerve or nerve fiber layer appearance in the absence of a visual field defect
- a visual field defect suggestive of glaucoma in the absence of a corresponding glaucomatous optic nerve abnormality
- a family history of glaucoma in a first-degree relative
- elevated IOP without evidence of optic nerve damage (see the following section Ocular Hypertension)

Patients with such findings are typically monitored for the development of glaucoma with periodic evaluation of the optic nerve, retinal nerve fiber layer, and visual field. In patients with an absence of visual field defects on standard perimetry (see Chapter 6), the use of frequency-doubling technology perimetry, short-wavelength perimetry, and pattern electroretinography have all been proposed, although the role of each is not well supported by available evidence. If signs of optic nerve damage are present, the diagnosis of early POAG and initiation of treatment should be considered. In uncertain cases, however, close monitoring of the patient without treatment is reasonable in order to better establish a diagnosis (ie, confirm initial findings or detect progressive changes) before initiation of therapy. Glaucoma suspects who have elevated IOP and structural or functional findings that are not clearly due to glaucoma may be difficult to diagnose.

Ocular Hypertension

In this book, *ocular hypertension* is defined as a condition in which IOP is elevated above an arbitrary cutoff value, typically 21 mm Hg, in the absence of optic nerve, retinal nerve fiber layer, or visual field abnormalities. This condition is discussed in its own section given the availability of high-quality clinical trial data that are not available for other categories of glaucoma suspects. Estimates of the prevalence of ocular hypertension in the United States vary considerably and may be as high as 8 times that of diagnosed POAG. Studies of individuals with elevated IOP for various lengths of time suggest that a higher baseline IOP is associated with a greater risk of developing glaucoma. However, for most persons with elevated IOP, the risk of developing glaucoma is low.

Distinguishing between ocular hypertension and early POAG is often difficult. The ophthalmologist must look [illegible] mage to the optic nerve, such as focal notching, asymmetry [illegible] nage, nerve fiber layer defects, or subtle visual field defects.

There is no clear consensus about whether elevated IOP should be treated in the absence of signs of early damage. Some clinicians, after assessing all risk factors, select and treat those individuals thought to be at greatest risk of developing glaucoma. In the OHTS, patients 40–80 years of age with IOP between 24 and 32 mm Hg were randomized to either observation or treatment with topical ocular hypotensive medications (see Clinical Trial 7-2 at the end of this chapter). During a 5-year period, 4.4% of participants in the treatment group versus 9.5% of participants in the observation group progressed to glaucoma as determined by optic nerve or visual field changes. Thus, topical medications reduce the risk of progression to glaucoma in patients with ocular hypertension. It should be noted, however, that most untreated participants did not progress over a 5-year period. In the OHTS, the risk of developing glaucoma was increased by 10% for every increase in mm Hg of the IOP over the mean study IOP; the risk was increased by 32% for each 0.1 increment in vertical cup–disc ratio.

Results from the OHTS suggest that older age, higher IOP, thinner corneas, a larger baseline cup–disc ratio, and higher pattern standard deviation on standard automated perimetry are important risk factors for the development of POAG. The increased risk of glaucoma progression attributed to thinner corneas in this study, however, was not fully explained by the estimated artifactual error in measured IOP. Thinner corneas may therefore be a biomarker for glaucoma susceptibility based on factors other than IOP. The increased risk of glaucoma progression in Black participants (in univariate but not multivariate analyses) may be attributed to thinner corneas and greater cup–disc ratios. Interestingly, a family history of glaucoma was not identified as a significant risk factor in the OHTS, possibly because of inadequate assessment from self-reporting. Clinicians should consider family history when evaluating a patient's risk of glaucoma. Other potential risk factors, such as myopia, diabetes mellitus, migraine, and high or low blood pressure, were not confirmed in the OHTS as significant risk factors for glaucomatous progression.

Initial reports from the OHTS clearly demonstrate that lowering IOP in individuals with ocular hypertension reduces the risk of progression to glaucoma. It is important to recognize, however, that the incremental structural or functional change that constituted a progression endpoint in the OHTS would likely not manifest as symptomatic vision loss. Therefore, the question remains whether delaying treatment is associated with poorer outcomes than early initiation of IOP-lowering therapy. The results from the OHTS suggest that clinicians may safely consider delaying the treatment of ocular hypertension, particularly among patients with a lower risk of conversion to glaucoma (see Clinical Trial 7-2). This suggestion is supported by the longer-term follow-up of the OHTS participants in which it was found that delayed initiation of treatment still resulted in a decrease in the rate of developing glaucoma, just as it did earlier in the course. After 13 years, 71% of the original participants were still in the study; 22% of those originally assigned to observation (and offered treatment after the first phase of the study) developed glaucoma, compared to 16% in the group assigned to medication.

The decision of whether to treat a patient with ocular hypertension may be based on a combination of the results from the OHTS, findings from the clinical examination, and discussions with the patient. The clinician and patient should consider whether the risk of developing glaucoma outweighs the inconvenience, cost, and potential side effects of therapy for the patient. Additional factors to consider include the patient's age and likely life span; for patients with no damage and a relatively short life expectancy, it may be reasonable to observe rather than treat. Data from the OHTS and the European Glaucoma Prevention Study were combined to create a risk calculation model (https://ohts.wustl.edu/risk) to help clinicians predict the 5-year risk of conversion from ocular hypertension to glaucoma, based on risk factors in the 2 studies (ie, older age, higher IOP, thinner corneas, a larger baseline cup–disc ratio, higher pattern standard deviation on standard automated perimetry).

Gordon MO, Beiser JA, Brandt JD, et al. The Ocular Hypertension Treatment Study: baseline factors that predict the onset of primary open-angle glaucoma. *Arch Ophthalmol.* 2002; 120(6):714–720; discussion 829–830.

Kass MA, Gordon MO, Gao F, et al. Delaying treatment of ocular hypertension: The Ocular Hypertension Treatment Study. *Arch Ophthalmol.* 2010;128(3):276–287.

Kass MA, Heuer DK, Higginbotham EJ, et al. The Ocular Hypertension Treatment Study: a randomized trial determines that topical ocular hypotensive medication delays or prevents the onset of primary open-angle glaucoma. *Arch Ophthalmol.* 2002;120(6):701–713; discussion 829–830.

Retinal vein occlusion

Glaucoma and ocular hypertension are risk factors for the development of central retinal vein occlusion (CRVO). Consideration may be given to treating elevated IOP in patients with a history of hemicentral retinal vein occlusion or CRVO in order to reduce the risk of a vein occlusion in the fellow eye.

Open-Angle Glaucoma Without Elevated IOP (Normal-Tension Glaucoma, Low-Tension Glaucoma)

Controversy remains as to whether normal-tension glaucoma (NTG) represents a distinct disease entity or whether it is simply POAG developing in individuals with IOP within the statistically normal range. Glaucoma can develop at any level of IOP within the range observed in the general population. Thus, IOP is a continuous risk factor for glaucoma, and any cutoff between "normal" and "abnormal" IOP is arbitrary. Accordingly, many authorities believe the terms *normal-tension glaucoma* and *low-tension glaucoma* should be abandoned.

Risk Factors and Clinical Features

As previously emphasized, glaucoma is a multifactorial disease process for which elevated IOP is just 1 of several risk factors. Studies of Japanese populations have found that the proportion of OAG patients with IOPs in the average range is particularly high. Other risk factors may play a greater role in individuals with NTG than in those with POAG with higher IOPs. One hypothesis is that local vascular factors may have a significant role in the development of NTG in these persons. Some studies suggest that patients with NTG have a higher incidence of vasospastic disorders (eg, migraine and Raynaud phenomenon), ischemic vascular disease, autoimmune disease, sleep apnea, systemic hypotension, and coagulopathies than patients with high-tension POAG. However, these findings have not been consistent.

As in POAG, NTG is characteristically bilateral but often asymmetric. In glaucomatous eyes with IOPs that are within the statistically normal range but asymmetric, worse damage typically occurs in the eye with the higher IOP. Optic disc hemorrhage (Fig 7-1) may be more common among patients with NTG than among those with high-tension POAG.

The visual field defects in NTG tend to be more focal, deeper, and closer to fixation, especially with early disease, than those commonly seen with high-tension POAG. Also, a dense paracentral scotoma encroaching near fixation is not an unusual initial finding on the visual field tests of NTG patients. However, these differences may be due to detection

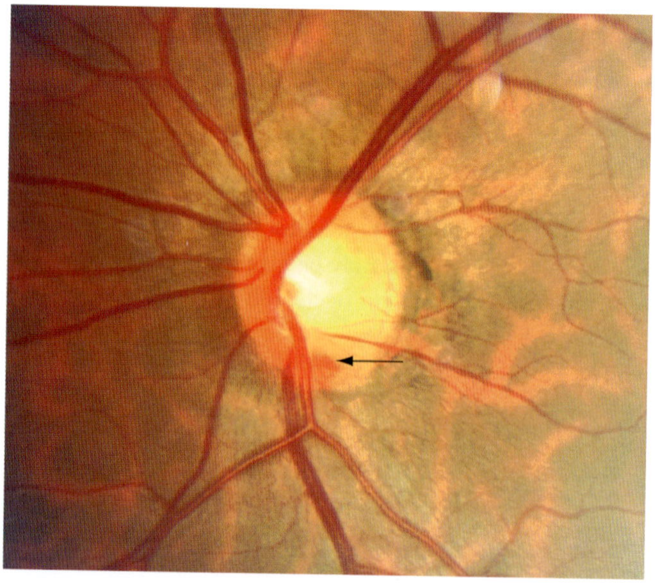

Figure 7-1 Subtle optic disc hemorrhage *(arrow)* in a patient with normal-tension glaucoma. *(Courtesy of Wallace L.M. Alward, MD. ©The University of Iowa.)*

bias, given that patients experiencing visual disturbance are more likely to seek care. Further, differences in optic nerve appearance and visual field defects between patients with NTG and those with high-tension POAG have not been uniformly confirmed in studies. Therefore, for any individual patient, there is no characteristic abnormality of the optic nerve or visual field that distinguishes NTG from high-tension POAG.

Cartwright MJ, Anderson DR. Correlation of asymmetric damage with asymmetric intraocular pressure in normal-tension glaucoma (low-tension glaucoma). *Arch Ophthalmol.* 1988;106(7):898–900.

Sommer A. Ocular hypertension and normal-tension glaucoma: time for banishment and burial. *Arch Ophthalmol.* 2011;129(6):785–787.

Differential Diagnosis

NTG can be mimicked by conditions other than glaucoma. It is therefore essential to distinguish glaucoma from other optic neuropathies (eg, optic nerve drusen, ischemic optic neuropathy) because appropriate therapy will differ (Table 7-2). Visual field defects in some of these conditions may appear similar to those seen with NTG and can even be progressive.

Patients with "normal" IOP in clinic may experience higher pressures outside clinic hours. Diurnal IOP measurement may therefore help in the determination of target IOPs by identifying peak IOPs and IOP fluctuation, but it does not capture nocturnal patterns of IOP. Also, elevated IOP can be obscured in patients taking systemic medication, particularly systemic β-blockers. In addition, some patients with apparent NTG may have artifactually low tonometry readings because of altered corneoscleral biomechanics, 1 marker of which may be a thin central cornea. Similarly, decreased corneal thickness in patients who have undergone refractive surgery may result in underestimation of true IOP.

Diagnostic Evaluation

The clinical assessment in patients with NTG should mirror that of any other open-angle glaucoma (see Chapter 3). In addition, the clinician must carefully review the patient's medical history for conditions that cause an optic nerve appearance and/or visual field defects similar to those seen in NTG: these conditions include significant systemic hemorrhage associated with low blood pressure, myocardial infarction, or shock.

Table 7-2 Differential Diagnosis for Glaucomatous Optic Neuropathy

Congenital anomalies (eg, coloboma, optic nerve pit, myopic optic discs)
Physiologic cupping due to a large scleral canal
Optic nerve drusen
Compressive lesions of the optic nerve and chiasm
Anterior ischemic optic neuropathy
Posterior ischemic optic neuropathy
Toxic or nutritional optic neuropathy (eg, methanol, vitamin B_{12} deficiency)

Prognosis and Therapy

The initial goal of therapy is often to achieve a near 30% IOP reduction from a carefully determined baseline IOP. Once this is established, routine evaluations with appropriate individualized adjustments for target pressure are recommended. These adjustments should take into account relevant factors, including baseline severity of optic nerve damage and visual field loss, potential risks of therapy, comorbid conditions, and life expectancy of the patient. Target pressure may be reassessed and adjusted as needed during follow-up visits in order to maintain visual function.

In a secondary analysis of the Collaborative Normal-Tension Glaucoma Study (CNTGS; see Clinical Trial 7-3 at the end of the chapter), IOP lowering by at least 30% reduced the 5-year risk of visual field progression from 35% to 12%, supporting the role of IOP in NTG. It should be noted that the protective effect of IOP reduction was evident only after adjusting for the effect of cataracts, which were more frequent in the treated group. Considering the findings of the CNTGS, treatment of NTG is generally recommended unless the optic neuropathy is determined to be stable. Interestingly, about half of the patients who did not receive treatment in this study did not progress over the study duration, whereas 12% of patients progressed in that they had worsening glaucomatous visual field damage despite a 30% reduction of IOP. Factors in addition to IOP are likely important in patients with this disease. In those who worsened, the rate of visual field progression was highly variable yet slow in most but not all patients. In addition, this study showed a lower treatment benefit among patients with a baseline history of a disc hemorrhage.

Treatment of NTG differs little from that of other OAGs. Some glaucoma specialists are wary of treating NTG with topical β-blocker medications because of their association with low OPP (see the subsection "Lower ocular perfusion pressure"). The Low-Pressure Glaucoma Treatment Study showed a high rate of glaucomatous progression in patients treated with timolol. However, there was a significant loss of follow-up in this study, and its results must be interpreted with that in mind. In the Early Manifest Glaucoma Trial (EMGT; see Clinical Trial 7-4), IOP lowering with the combination of betaxolol and ALT was minimal in eyes with baseline IOPs of 15 mm Hg or lower. This finding suggests that patients with a lower baseline IOP who are progressing may need incisional surgery or medications other than β-blockers to stabilize their disease. Such tailoring of treatment to each patient is relevant to all forms of glaucoma. See Chapter 13 for further discussion of indications for surgery.

Bhandari A, Crabb DP, Poinoosawmy D, Fitzke FW, Hitchings RA, Noureddin BN. Effect of surgery on visual field progression in normal-tension glaucoma. *Ophthalmology.* 1997;104(7):1131–1137.

Collaborative Normal-Tension Glaucoma Study Group. Comparison of glaucomatous progression between untreated patients with normal-tension glaucoma and patients with therapeutically reduced intraocular pressures. *Am J Ophthalmol.* 1998;126(4):487–497.

Collaborative Normal-Tension Glaucoma Study Group. The effectiveness of intraocular pressure reduction in the treatment of normal-tension glaucoma. *Am J Ophthalmol.* 1998;126(4):498–505.

CLINICAL TRIAL 7-1

Collaborative Initial Glaucoma Treatment Study (CIGTS) Essentials

Purpose: To determine whether patients with newly diagnosed open-angle glaucoma (OAG) are better treated by initial treatment with medications or by immediate filtering surgery.

Participants: A total of 607 patients with OAG (primary, pigmentary, or pseudoexfoliation) recruited between 1993 and 1997.

Study design: Multicenter randomized controlled clinical trial comparing initial medical therapy with initial surgical therapy for OAG.

Results: Although intraocular pressure (IOP) was lower in the surgery group, initial medical and initial surgical therapy resulted in similar visual field outcomes after up to 9 years of follow-up. Early visual acuity loss was greater in the surgery group, but the differences between groups converged over time. Also, cataracts were more common in the surgery group. At the 8-year follow-up examination, substantial worsening (≥3 dB) of visual field mean deviation from baseline was found in 21.3% of the initial surgery group and 25.5% of the initial medical group. Patients with worse baseline visual fields were less likely to progress if treated with trabeculectomy first. Patients with diabetes mellitus were more likely to progress if treated initially with surgery.

The quality of life (QOL) reported by the 2 treatment groups was similar. The most persistent QOL finding was a greater number of symptoms reported at a higher frequency by the surgery group.

The overall rate of progression of OAG was lower in CIGTS than in many clinical trials, possibly because of more aggressive IOP-lowering goals and the stage of the disease. Individualized target IOPs were determined according to a formula that accounted for baseline IOP and visual field loss. Over the course of follow-up, IOP in the medical therapy group averaged 17–18 mm Hg (IOP reduction of approximately 38%), whereas IOP in the surgery group averaged 14–15 mm Hg (IOP reduction of approximately 46%). IOP fluctuation was a risk factor for progression in the medically treated group but not the surgically treated group. The rate of cataract removal was greater in the surgically treated group.

CLINICAL TRIAL 7-2

Ocular Hypertension Treatment Study (OHTS) Essentials

Purpose: To evaluate the safety and efficacy of topical ocular hypotensive medications in preventing or delaying the onset of visual field loss and/or optic nerve damage in participants with ocular hypertension.

Participants: A total of 1637 patients with ocular hypertension recruited between 1994 and 1996.

(Continued on next page)

(continued)

Study design: Multicenter randomized controlled clinical trial comparing observation and medical therapy for ocular hypertension.

Results 2002: Topical ocular hypotensive medication was effective in delaying or preventing the onset of primary open-angle glaucoma (POAG). The incidence of glaucoma was lower in the medication group than in the observation group (4.4% vs 9.5%, respectively) at 60 months' follow-up. No increase in adverse events was detected in the medication group.

The 5-year risk of developing POAG was associated with the following baseline factors: older age (22% increase in relative risk per decade), larger vertical and horizontal cup–disc ratios (32% and 27% increases in relative risk per 0.1 increase, respectively), higher pattern standard deviation (22% increase in relative risk per 0.2 dB increase), and higher baseline IOP (10% increase in relative risk per 1 mm Hg increase). Central corneal thickness (CCT) was found to be a powerful predictor for the development of POAG (81% increase in relative risk for every 40 µm thinner). The corneas in OHTS participants were thicker than those in the general population, and African American participants had thinner corneas than others in the study.

Results 2007: The OHTS prediction model for the development of POAG was independently validated in the European Glaucoma Prevention Study.

Results 2010: Topical ocular hypotensive medication was initiated in the original observation group after 7.5 years (median) without medication, and medication was continued for 5.5 years thereafter. Participants in the original medication group continued topical ocular hypotensive medications for a median of 13 years. The proportion of participants who developed POAG was 0.22 in the original observation group and 0.16 in the original medication group. The primary purpose of the follow-up study was to determine whether delaying treatment resulted in a persistently increased risk of conversion to glaucoma, even after the initiation of therapy. It was found that delayed initiation of treatment still resulted in a decrease in the rate of developing glaucoma, just as it did earlier in the course.

CLINICAL TRIAL 7-3

Collaborative Normal Tension Glaucoma Study (CNTGS) Essentials

Purpose: To determine whether the optic nerve damage seen in eyes without statistically elevated IOP was IOP dependent or IOP independent.

Participants: From 24 centers, a total of 230 eyes of 230 participants were enrolled. Inclusion criteria were as follows:

- the presence of glaucoma in 1 or both eyes (as judged by the investigators)
- age between 20 and 90 years
- had never had a recorded IOP above 24 mm Hg

To determine baseline IOP, each participant was required to undergo 10 IOP readings after medication washout, 6 of which were distributed on a single day. The median of the IOP measurements had to be 20 mm Hg or less, and none could be above 24 mm Hg. Finally, each participant was also required to complete 3 reliable baseline visual fields within 1 month. Exclusion criteria were: systemic β-blockers or clonidine, the presence of other ocular disease that might affect the visual field, previous intraocular surgery, narrow angles, visual acuity worse than 20/30, and severe visual field loss.

Study design: Multicenter randomized controlled clinical trial comparing observation and treatment for normal tension glaucoma (NTG). Randomization to treatment (30% reduction in IOP after treatment with medications, laser trabeculoplasty, or incisional surgery) or observation occurred at enrollment only if there was clear evidence of glaucoma worsening in the time before enrollment. Otherwise, eyes were observed and then randomized after they demonstrated worsening of glaucoma, which was primarily determined using a study-specific analysis of visual fields. Determination of worsening could also be made by observation of optic disc changes.

Results: At the end of the study, 79 eyes had been randomized to observation, 66 to treatment (of which 5 dropped out), and the remaining 85 never showed evidence of worsening. In the intent-to-treat analysis, visual field worsening occurred in 31 eyes (39%) in the observation group and 22 (33%) in the treated group; this difference was not statistically significant. When the data were reevaluated by censoring results obtained after the development of visually significant cataract in a given eye, visual field worsening was determined to be more likely in the observation group (27%) than in the treatment group (12%). The difference in the 2 analyses was attributed to the higher rate of cataract in the sub-group that underwent filtration surgery.

In a secondary analysis of those who met the treatment target, 28 (35%) of the observation eyes and 7 (12%) of the treated eyes worsened after randomization. Visually significant cataract developed in 11 eyes (14%) in the observation group and 23 (38%) in the treated group. Another secondary analysis of the 160 participants in the untreated group showed that after 7 years, only half demonstrated a detectable change in visual field.

CLINICAL TRIAL 7-4

Early Manifest Glaucoma Trial (EMGT) Essentials

Purpose: To evaluate the effectiveness of lowering IOP in patients with early, newly detected OAG.

Participants: Patients 50 to 80 years of age with newly diagnosed OAG and early glaucomatous visual field loss were identified mainly through a

(Continued on next page)

(continued)

population-based screening of more than 44,000 residents of Malmö and Helsingborg, Sweden. Exclusion criteria were thus: advanced visual field loss; mean IOP greater than 30 mm Hg or any IOP greater than 35 mm Hg; and visual acuity less than 0.5 (20/40). Between 1993 and 1997, 255 patients were randomized.

Study design: Multicenter randomized controlled clinical trial comparing observation and treatment with betaxolol and argon laser trabeculoplasty for OAG.

Results: At 6 years, 62% of untreated patients showed progression, whereas 45% of treated patients progressed. On average, treatment reduced IOP by 25%. In a univariate analysis, risk factors for progression included no IOP-lowering treatment, older age, higher IOP, pseudoexfoliation syndrome, more advanced visual field loss, and bilateral glaucoma. In multivariate analyses, the risk of progression with IOP-lowering treatment was reduced by half (HR = 0.50; 95% confidence interval, 0.35–0.71). Each mm Hg of IOP lowering decreased the risk of glaucomatous progression by 10%. Risk factors for progression included higher baseline IOP, older age, pseudoexfoliation syndrome, bilateral disease, worse mean deviation, and frequent disc hemorrhages. IOP fluctuation was not found to be a significant risk factor.

In the observation group, the rate of visual field progression was most rapid in the subgroup of patients with pseudoexfoliation syndrome and slowest in those with baseline IOPs within the normal range.

CLINICAL TRIAL 7-5

Advanced Glaucoma Intervention Study (AGIS) Essentials

Purpose: To compare the clinical outcomes of 2 treatment sequences: argon laser trabeculoplasty–trabeculectomy–trabeculectomy (ATT) and trabeculectomy–argon laser trabeculoplasty–trabeculectomy (TAT).

Participants: A total of 789 eyes of 591 patients with medically uncontrolled OAG recruited from 1988 to 1992.

Study design: Multicenter randomized controlled clinical trial comparing 2 treatment sequences (ATT and TAT) for patients with OAG uncontrolled with medical therapy.

Results:

AGIS 4 and AGIS 13: Black patients treated with the ATT sequence had a lower combined visual acuity and visual field loss than those treated with the TAT sequence. White patients had a lower combined visual acuity and visual field loss at 7 years if initially treated with the TAT sequence. In the initial follow-up period, White patients in the TAT group had greater visual acuity loss than those in the ATT group; by 7 years, this loss was similar.

AGIS 5: The mean IOP at the 4-week postoperative visit was higher in eyes with encapsulated blebs than in those without; with resumption of medical therapy, eyes with and without encapsulated blebs had similar IOPs after 1 year.

AGIS 6: Visual function scores improved after cataract surgery. Adjustment for cataract did not alter the findings of previous AGIS studies.

AGIS 7: Lower IOP was associated with less visual field progression. Less visual field progression was noted for eyes with an average IOP of 14 mm Hg or less during the first 18 months after the first surgical intervention, and for eyes with IOP of 18 mm Hg or less for all study visits.

AGIS 8: Approximately half of the study patients developed cataract in the first 5 years of follow-up. Trabeculectomy increased the relative risk of cataract formation by 78%.

AGIS 9: The treatment protocol with initial trabeculectomy slows the progression of glaucoma more effectively in White patients than in Black patients. The treatment protocol with initial ALT was slightly more effective in Black participants than in White participants.

AGIS 10: Assessment of optic nerve findings showed good intraobserver but poor interobserver agreement.

AGIS 11: Reduced effectiveness of ALT was associated with younger age and higher IOP. The ineffectiveness of trabeculectomy was associated with younger age, higher IOP, diabetes mellitus, and postoperative complications (markedly elevated IOP and inflammation).

AGIS 12: Risk factors for sustained decrease of the visual field included better baseline visual fields, male sex, worse baseline visual acuity, and diabetes mellitus. Risk factors for sustained decrease in visual acuity included better baseline visual acuity, older age, and less formal education.

AGIS 14: In patients with visual field progression, a single 6-month confirmatory visual field test had a 72% probability of verifying a persistent defect. When the number of confirmatory visual field tests was increased from 1 to 2, the percentage of eyes that showed a persistent defect increased to 84%.

2009 AGIS Report: IOP fluctuation was an independent predictor of progression of OAG in eyes with lower baseline IOPs but not in those with higher baseline IOPs.

Most of the relevant findings from AGIS that reflect clinical practice are from post hoc analysis; thus, they may not fully take into account unmeasurable confounding factors and enrollment bias.

CLINICAL TRIAL 7-6

The United Kingdom Glaucoma Treatment Study (UKGTS)

Purpose: To determine the change in the frequency of visual field deterioration in treatment-naïve patients treated with latanoprost compared to those treated with placebo.

Participants: From 10 centers, 516 patients with newly diagnosed mild-to-moderate open-angle glaucoma were enrolled. Potential study participants were excluded for the following reasons:

- mean deviation worse than −10 dB in the better eye or −16 dB in the worse eye
- IOP above 35 mm Hg on 2 visits or IOP that averaged more than 30 mm Hg on 2 visits
- unreliable performance on visual field tests
- poor-quality optic nerve imaging with scanning laser ophthalmoscopy
- the presence of significant cataract
- previous intraocular surgery other than cataract extraction
- diabetic retinopathy

Study design: Enrolled patients were randomized 1:1 to either treatment with latanoprost 0.005% or to placebo and then monitored with frequent visual field tests and optic nerve imaging during 11 visits within 2 years. Visual field worsening was determined with the guided progression analysis (GPA) available on the Humphrey Field Analyzer. The optic nerve was imaged with confocal scanning laser ophthalmoscopy, scanning laser polarimetry, time-domain optical coherence tomography, and monoscopic disc photography. IOP was measured with Goldmann tonometry, dynamic contour tonometry, and the ocular response analyzer. Study endpoints were visual field worsening determined by GPA, IOP greater than 35 mm Hg on 2 visits, and decline of best-corrected visual acuity to worse than 20/60. The UKGTS was designed with the shortest observation period of any of the major therapeutic trials of open-angle glaucoma. This shortened period was achieved by a novel arrangement of the visual field tests in which they were clustered at the beginning and end of the periods of interest, rather than being spaced evenly.

Results: The UKGTS is important because it is the first randomized, placebo-controlled study of the effect of topical glaucoma medications and because of its novel design of testing intervals and clustering, which allowed the investigators to identify differences in visual field worsening in a relatively short time. Over 24 months, 59 participants in the placebo group had worsening of their visual field compared to 35 in the latanoprost group. The mean change in visual field mean deviation in those who worsened was −1.6 dB.

CHAPTER 8

Secondary Open-Angle Glaucoma

Highlights

- Pseudoexfoliation syndrome is the most common cause of secondary open-angle glaucoma (OAG).
- The lens can initiate secondary OAG through a variety of inflammatory mechanisms.
- Ocular inflammatory syndromes may be linked to OAG through both inflammation and the eye's physiological response to steroids.
- Trauma, whether accidental or surgical, is an important cause of secondary OAG.
- Repeated intravitreal injections of anti–vascular endothelial growth factor agents may be associated with increased intraocular pressure.

Secondary Open-Angle Glaucoma

Pseudoexfoliation Syndrome

Pseudoexfoliation syndrome (exfoliation syndrome) is the most common cause of secondary open-angle glaucoma (OAG). It is characterized by the extracellular deposition of distinctive fibrillar material in the anterior segment of the eye. On histologic examination, this material has been found in and on the lens epithelium and capsule, pupillary margin, ciliary epithelium, iris pigment epithelium, iris stroma, iris blood vessels, and subconjunctival tissue. The material has also been identified in other parts of the body, including the skin, lungs, heart, and liver. Mutations in a single gene, *LOXL1*, are present in nearly all cases of pseudoexfoliation syndrome and pseudoexfoliation glaucoma; however, these disease-associated mutations are also common in populations without pseudoexfoliation syndrome, and other genes have also been implicated in genome-wide association studies, suggesting a multifactorial etiology for this disease. The exact relationship between genetic and environmental factors in pseudoexfoliation syndrome remains unclear.

Pseudoexfoliation syndrome is typically asymmetric and often presents unilaterally, although the uninvolved eye may manifest signs of the disease at a later time. This syndrome is strongly age related: it is rarely seen in persons younger than 50 years and occurs most commonly in individuals older than 70 years.

The classic characteristic of pseudoexfoliation syndrome is the deposition of fibrillar deposits in a "bull's-eye" pattern on the anterior lens capsule, which is best viewed after pupillary dilation. This pattern is presumably caused by iris movement that scrapes the pseudoexfoliative material from the lens, causing a clear intermediate area in between a central and a peripheral zone of the material (Fig 8-1). Clinically, this fibrillar extracellular material can be seen on the pupillary margin, zonular fibers of the lens, ciliary processes, inferior anterior chamber angle, corneal endothelium, and anterior vitreous (Figs 8-2, 8-3).

Individuals with pseudoexfoliation syndrome may also have peripupillary atrophy with transillumination defects. In these patients, the pupil often dilates poorly, likely because of

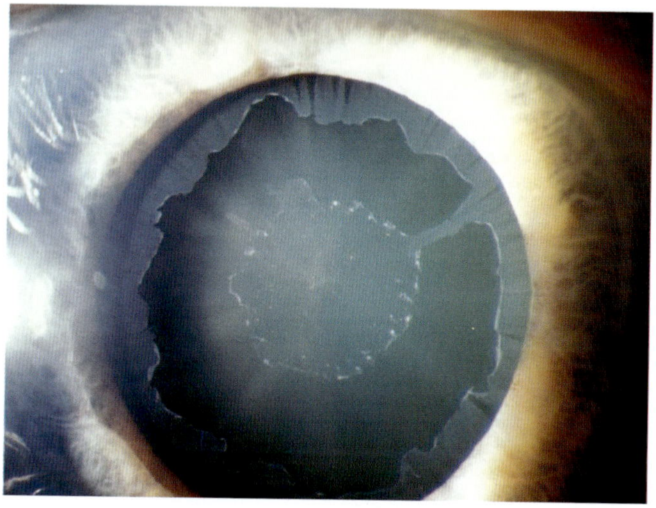

Figure 8-1 Pseudoexfoliation syndrome. Pseudoexfoliative material deposited on the anterior lens capsule in a classic "bull's-eye" pattern in a dilated eye. *(Courtesy of Wallace L.M. Alward, MD. From the* Iowa Glaucoma Curriculum *[curriculum.iowaglaucoma.org]. © The University of Iowa.)*

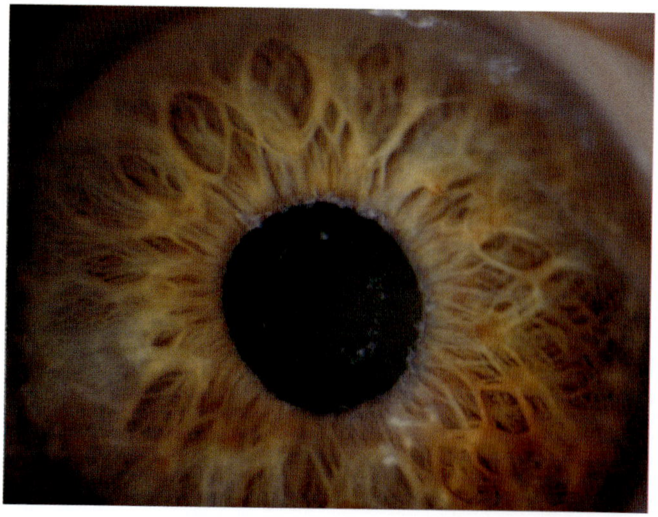

Figure 8-2 Pseudoexfoliative material deposited on the pupillary margin and anterior lens capsule in an undilated eye. *(Courtesy of Wallace L.M. Alward, MD. From the* Iowa Glaucoma Curriculum *[curriculum.iowaglaucoma.org]. © The University of Iowa.)*

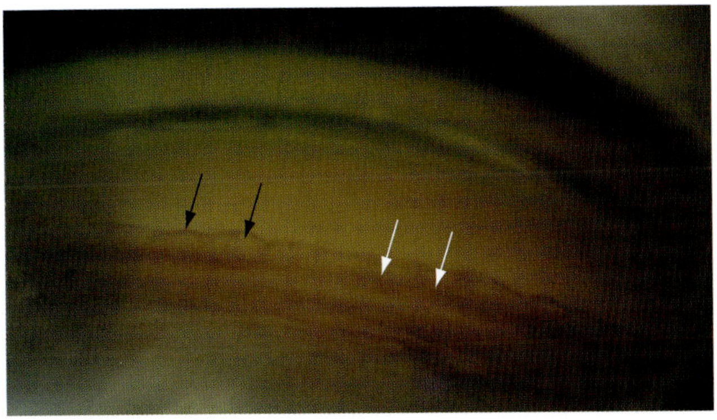

Figure 8-3 Goniophotograph of the anterior chamber angle in an eye with pseudoexfoliation syndrome. Note the Sampaolesi line *(black arrows). White arrows* indicate the anterior border of the pigmented trabecular meshwork. *(Courtesy of Angelo P. Tanna, MD.)*

infiltration of fibrillar material into the iris stroma. Phacodonesis results from the weak zonular fibers. Thus, great care must be taken during cataract surgery to reduce the risk of zonular dehiscence, vitreous loss, lens dislocation, and other complications (see also BCSC Section 11, *Lens and Cataract*). Iris angiography has shown abnormalities of the iris vessels with leakage of fluorescein.

On gonioscopy, the trabecular meshwork is typically heavily pigmented, sometimes in a variegated fashion. Pigment deposition anterior to the Schwalbe line is commonly seen and referred to as the *Sampaolesi line* (see Fig 8-3). Anterior migration of the lens caused by zonular laxity may lead to secondary angle closure.

The intraocular pressure (IOP) elevation associated with pseudoexfoliation syndrome is likely attributable to deposits of fibrillar material in the conventional and uveoscleral outflow pathways that impede the outflow of aqueous humor. In addition, because elastin is an important component of the lamina cribrosa, pseudoexfoliation syndrome may increase the susceptibility of the optic nerve to injury. This increased susceptibility may, in turn, contribute to the increased risk of development and progression of glaucoma in these patients, as was found in the Early Manifest Glaucoma Trial (see Clinical Trial 7-4 at the end of Chapter 7).

Individuals with pseudoexfoliation syndrome with elevated IOP that results in optic nerve damage or visual field loss are described as having *pseudoexfoliation glaucoma.* Pseudoexfoliation syndrome is associated with OAG in all populations, but the prevalence varies considerably. In Scandinavian countries, pseudoexfoliation syndrome accounts for more than 50% of cases of OAG. The risk of progression to glaucoma also varies widely and can be as high as 40% of patients in a 10-year period. Patients with pseudoexfoliation syndrome often have higher IOP, with greater diurnal IOP fluctuations, than do patients with primary open-angle glaucoma (POAG). The overall prognosis for glaucoma is worse for patients with pseudoexfoliation glaucoma than for those with POAG. Laser trabeculoplasty can be very effective, but the duration of the response may be shorter in pseudoexfoliation glaucoma than in POAG.

Aboobakar IF, Johnson WM, Stamer WD, Hauser MA, Allingham RR. Major review: Exfoliation syndrome; advances in disease genetics, molecular biology, and epidemiology. *Exp Eye Res.* 2017;154:88–103.

Thorleifsson G, Magnusson KP, Sulem P, et al. Common sequence variants in the *LOXL1* gene confer susceptibility to exfoliation glaucoma. *Science.* 2007;317(5843):1397–1400.

Pigment Dispersion Syndrome

In pigment dispersion syndrome, the zonular fibers rub the posterior iris pigment epithelium, resulting in the release of pigment granules throughout the anterior segment. Posterior bowing of the iris caused by the so-called "reverse pupillary block" configuration is present in many eyes with pigment dispersion syndrome. This concave iris configuration results in greater contact with the zonular fibers, causing increased release of pigment granules.

Pigment dispersion syndrome classically presents with pigment deposits on the corneal endothelium, trabecular meshwork, and lens periphery, as well as with midperipheral iris transillumination defects in a spokelike pattern. The pigment is typically deposited on the corneal endothelium in a vertical spindle pattern, referred to as a *Krukenberg spindle* (Fig 8-4); the pattern of corneal pigment deposition is the result of aqueous convection currents and subsequent phagocytosis of pigment by the corneal endothelium. The presence of a Krukenberg spindle is not necessary for a diagnosis of pigment dispersion syndrome. Moreover, this sign may be present in other diseases, such as pseudoexfoliation syndrome. The midperipheral iris transillumination defects are a result of contact between the zonular fibers and the posterior iris pigment epithelium (Fig 8-5). On gonioscopy, the trabecular meshwork commonly appears as homogeneous and densely pigmented, with speckled pigment at or anterior to the Schwalbe line (Fig 8-6), often forming a Sampaolesi line. When the eye is dilated, pigment deposits may be seen on the zonular fibers, on the anterior hyaloid, and in the equatorial region of the lens capsule (Zentmayer line/ring or Scheie stripe; Fig 8-7).

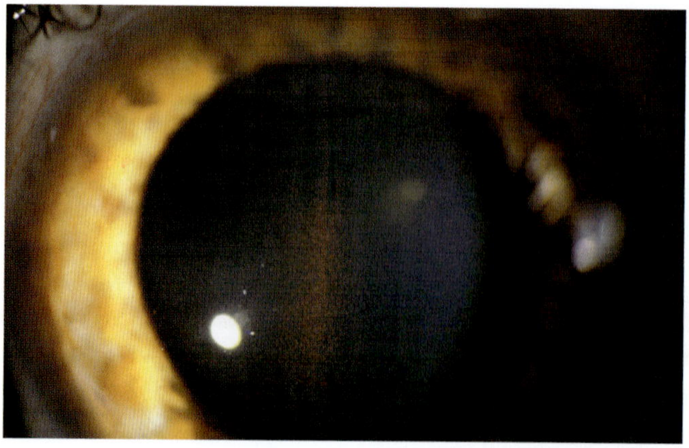

Figure 8-4 Krukenberg spindle in a patient with pigmentary glaucoma. *(Reproduced from Alward WLM, Longmuir RA.* Color Atlas of Gonioscopy. *2nd ed. American Academy of Ophthalmology; 2008:75. Fig 9-1.)*

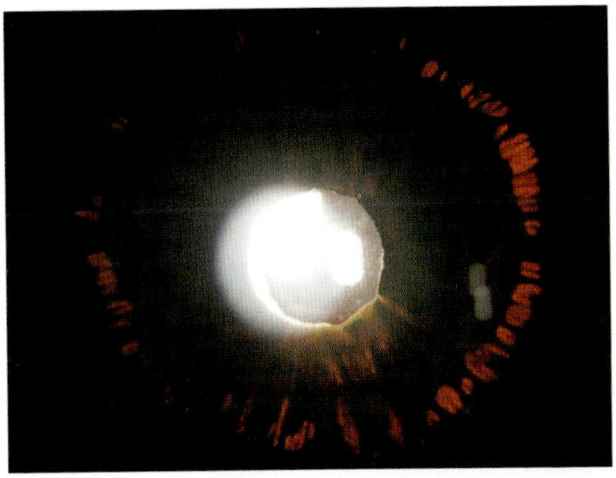

Figure 8-5 Photograph of the classic spokelike iris transillumination defects of pigment dispersion syndrome. *(Courtesy of Angelo P. Tanna, MD.)*

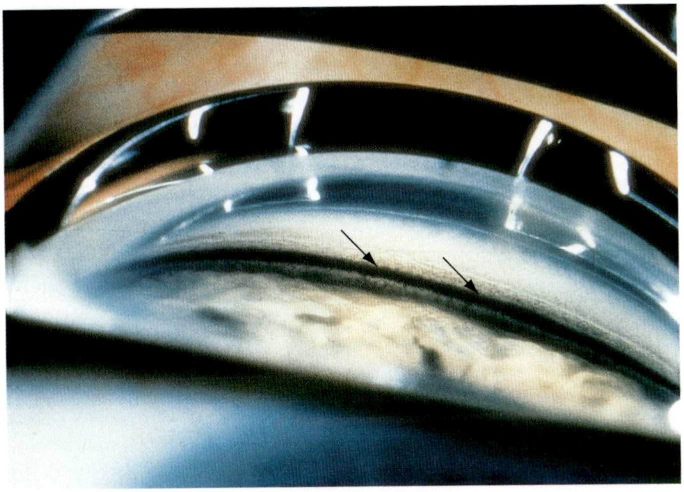

Figure 8-6 Characteristic heavy, uniform pigmentation of the trabecular meshwork *(arrows)* occurring in pigment dispersion syndrome and pigmentary glaucoma. *(Courtesy of M. Roy Wilson, MD.)*

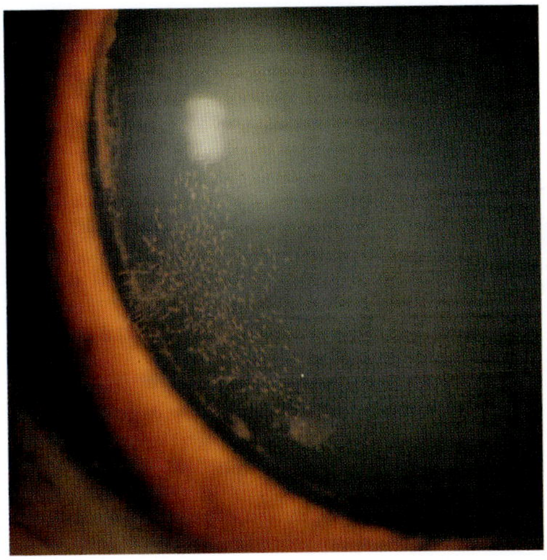

Figure 8-7 In pigment dispersion syndrome, pigment deposits are visible in the equatorial region of the lens capsule (Zentmayer ring or Scheie stripe) and on the zonular fibers. *(Courtesy of Angelo P. Tanna, MD.)*

With increasing age, the signs of pigment dispersion may decrease as a result of normal growth of the lens, inducing a physiologic pupillary block and anterior movement of the iris. Loss of accommodation may also occur. As pigment dispersion is reduced, the deposited pigment may fade from the corneal endothelium, trabecular meshwork, or anterior surface of the iris.

Approximately 15% of cases of pigment dispersion syndrome progress to glaucoma or elevated IOP that requires treatment. Pigmentary glaucoma is 3 times more common in men than in women, particularly men who are young or middle-aged (20–50 years) and myopic. The presumed mechanism of elevated IOP is obstruction of the trabecular meshwork by pigment granules. *Pigmentary glaucoma* is characterized by wide fluctuations in IOP, which can exceed 50 mm Hg in untreated eyes. Affected patients may have extreme elevations in IOP following exercise or pupillary dilation because of an excessive liberation of pigment. Symptoms associated with such elevated IOPs may include halos, intermittent blurry vision, and ocular pain.

Medical treatment is often successful in reducing elevated IOP. Most patients respond reasonably well to laser trabeculoplasty, although its effect may be short-lived. Studies have shown paradoxical elevations of IOP after laser trabeculoplasty in eyes with heavy trabecular meshwork pigmentation including pigmentary glaucoma; thus, it may be advisable to use lower laser energy in this condition. Filtering surgery is usually successful; however, extra care is warranted in young myopic male patients, who are at increased risk for hypotony maculopathy. Laser peripheral iridotomy has been proposed as a means of minimizing posterior bowing of the iris by alleviating the pressure differential between the anterior chamber and the posterior chamber (Fig 8-8). However, multiple studies, including randomized trials, have failed to show a benefit of laser iridotomy for treatment of this condition.

Niyadurupola N, Broadway DC. Pigment dispersion syndrome and pigmentary glaucoma—a major review. *Clin Exp Ophthalmol.* 2008;36(9):868–882.

Reistad CE, Shields MB, Campbell DG, et al; American Glaucoma Society Pigmentary Glaucoma Iridotomy Study Group. The influence of peripheral iridotomy on the

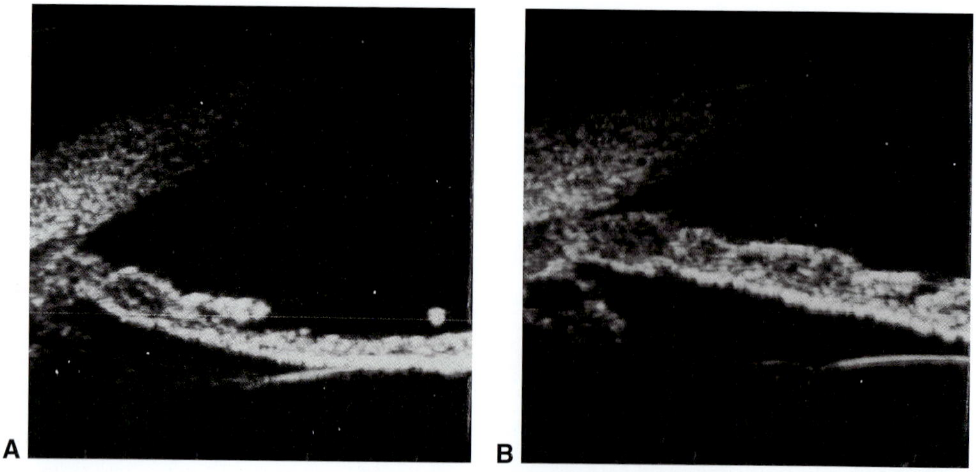

Figure 8-8 Pigment dispersion syndrome. **A,** Ultrasound biomicroscopy image of concave iris configuration in pigmentary glaucoma, before laser peripheral iridotomy (LPI). **B,** Same eye, after LPI, with resolution of the posterior bowing of the iris. *(Courtesy of Charles J. Pavlin, MD.)*

intraocular pressure course in patients with pigmentary glaucoma. *J Glaucoma.* 2005;14(4):255–259.
Siddiqui Y, Ten Hulzen RD, Cameron JD, Hodge DO, Johnson DH. What is the risk of developing pigmentary glaucoma from pigment dispersion syndrome? *Am J Ophthalmol.* 2003;135(6):794–799.

Lens-Induced Glaucoma

The lens can play a role in the development of open-angle and angle-closure glaucoma. Lens-induced OAGs are divided into 3 clinical entities:

- phacolytic glaucoma
- lens particle glaucoma
- phacoantigenic glaucoma

Lens-induced angle-closure glaucomas include phacomorphic glaucoma and ectopia lentis and are discussed in Chapter 10. See also BCSC Section 9, *Uveitis and Ocular Inflammation,* and Section 11, *Lens and Cataract.*

Phacolytic glaucoma

Phacolytic glaucoma is an inflammatory glaucoma caused by the leakage of high-molecular-weight lens protein through microscopic openings in the lens capsule of a mature or hypermature cataract (Fig 8-9) that subsequently obstructs the trabecular meshwork. As the lens ages, its protein composition changes, with an increased concentration of high-molecular-weight lens proteins. Elevated IOP occurs as a result of obstruction of the trabecular meshwork by these high-molecular-weight proteins, lens-laden macrophages, and other inflammatory debris.

Individuals with phacolytic glaucoma are usually older patients with a history of poor vision. They have a sudden onset of pain, conjunctival hyperemia, and worsening vision. Examination reveals markedly elevated IOP, microcystic corneal edema, prominent cell and flare reaction without keratic precipitates (KPs), an open anterior chamber angle, and a mature or hypermature cataract (Fig 8-10). The lack of KPs helps distinguish phacolytic glaucoma from phacoantigenic glaucoma. Cellular debris may be seen layered in the anterior chamber angle, and a pseudohypopyon may be present. Large white particles (clumps of lens protein) may also be present in the anterior chamber. The anterior lens capsule of the

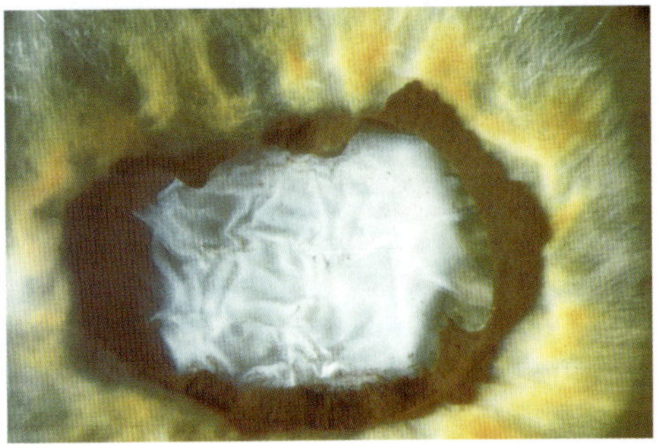

Figure 8-9 Characteristic appearance of hypermature cataract with wrinkling of the anterior lens capsule, which results from loss of cortical volume. Extensive posterior synechiae are present, which suggests previous inflammation. *(Courtesy of Steven T. Simmons, MD.)*

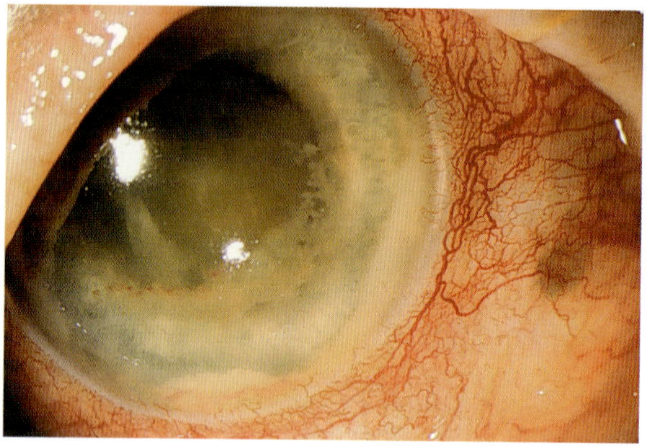

Figure 8-10 Phacolytic glaucoma. The typical presentation of phacolytic glaucoma is conjunctival hyperemia, microcystic corneal edema, mature cataract, and prominent anterior chamber reaction, as shown in this photograph. Note the lens protein deposits on the endothelium and layering in the angle, creating a pseudohypopyon. *(Courtesy of G.A. Cioffi, MD.)*

mature or hypermature (morgagnian) cataract may exhibit wrinkling, which represents loss of volume and the release of lens material (see Fig 8-9). Ocular hypotensive medications may be necessary to reduce the IOP; however, definitive therapy requires cataract extraction.

Lens particle glaucoma

In lens particle glaucoma, retention of lens material in the eye after cataract extraction, capsulotomy, or ocular trauma results in obstruction of the trabecular meshwork. The severity of IOP elevation depends on the quantity of lens material released, the degree of inflammation, the ability of the trabecular meshwork to clear the lens material, and the functional status of the ciliary body, which is often altered after surgery or trauma.

Lens particle glaucoma usually occurs within weeks of the initial surgery or trauma, but it may occur months or years later. Clinical findings include cortical material in the anterior chamber, elevated IOP, moderate anterior chamber reaction, microcystic corneal edema, and, with time, posterior synechiae and peripheral anterior synechiae (PAS).

Medical therapy may be needed to reduce the IOP while the residual lens material resorbs. Appropriate therapy includes medications to decrease aqueous formation, mydriatics to inhibit posterior synechiae formation, and topical corticosteroids to reduce inflammation. If the IOP cannot be controlled, surgical removal of the lens material may be necessary.

Phacoantigenic glaucoma

Phacoantigenic glaucoma (previously known as *phacoanaphylaxis*) is a rare condition in which patients become sensitized to their own lens protein after surgery or penetrating trauma, resulting in a granulomatous inflammation. The clinical picture is quite varied, but most patients present with a moderate anterior chamber reaction with KPs on both the corneal endothelium and the anterior lens surface. In addition, a low-grade vitritis, posterior synechiae, PAS, and residual lens material in the anterior chamber may be present. Glaucomatous optic neuropathy may occur, but it is not common in eyes with phacoantigenic glaucoma. Initiation of topical corticosteroids and aqueous suppressants are recommended to reduce the inflammation and IOP. The residual lens material will likely need to be removed once the inflammation is controlled.

Intraocular Tumors

A variety of tumors can cause unilateral glaucoma. Many of the tumors described in this section are also discussed in BCSC Section 4, *Ophthalmic Pathology and Intraocular Tumors.* Depending on the size, type, and location of the tumor, IOP elevation can result from several different mechanisms, including

- direct tumor invasion of the anterior chamber angle
- angle closure resulting from rotation of the ciliary body or from anterior displacement of the lens–iris interface (see Chapter 10)
- intraocular hemorrhage
- neovascularization of the angle
- deposition of tumor cells, inflammatory cells, and cellular debris within the trabecular meshwork

Choroidal and retinal tumors typically cause a secondary angle-closure glaucoma by the anterior displacement of the lens–iris diaphragm, which results in closure of the anterior chamber angle. Posterior synechiae may develop as a result of inflammation of necrotic tumors; they exacerbate angle closure through a pupillary block mechanism. Choroidal melanomas, medulloepitheliomas, and retinoblastomas may also cause neovascularization of the angle, which can result in angle closure. Neovascularization of the angle may also occur after radiation therapy for intraocular tumors.

The most common cause of IOP elevation associated with primary or metastatic tumors of the ciliary body is direct invasion of the anterior chamber angle. This can be exacerbated by anterior segment hemorrhage and inflammation, which further obstruct aqueous outflow. Necrotic tumor and tumor-laden macrophages may cause obstruction of the trabecular meshwork and result in a secondary OAG. Tumors causing a secondary glaucoma in adults include uveal melanoma and melanocytoma (Figs 8-11, 8-12), metastatic carcinoma, lymphoma, and leukemia. In children, tumors associated with glaucoma include retinoblastoma, juvenile xanthogranuloma, and medulloepithelioma.

Camp DA, Yadav P, Dalvin LA, Shields CL. Glaucoma secondary to intraocular tumors: mechanisms and management. *Curr Opin Ophthalmol.* 2019;30(2):71–81.

Shields CL, Materin MA, Shields JA, Gershenbaum E, Singh AD, Smith A. Factors associated with elevated intraocular pressure in eyes with iris melanoma. *Br J Ophthalmol.* 2001;85(6):666–669.

Ocular Inflammation and Secondary Glaucoma

Inflammatory, or uveitic, glaucoma is a secondary glaucoma that often combines components of open-angle and angle-closure disease. In individuals with uveitis, elevated IOP may be caused by a variety of mechanisms, and appropriate therapy depends on the etiology:

- edema of the trabecular meshwork
- endothelial cell dysfunction of the trabecular meshwork

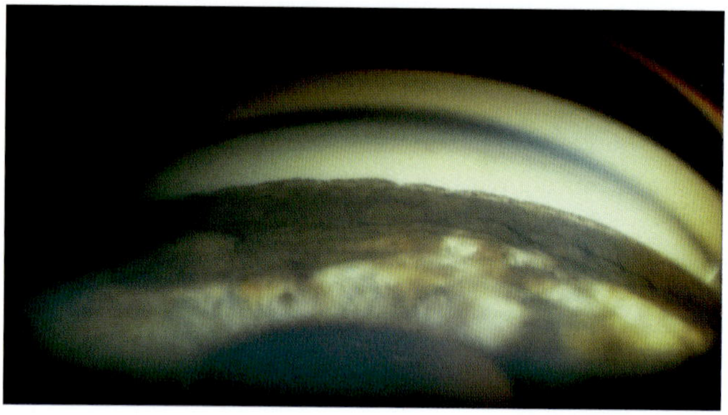

Figure 8-11 Goniophotograph of a ciliary body melanoma in the anterior chamber angle. *(Courtesy of Wallace L.M. Alward, MD. From the* Iowa Glaucoma Curriculum *[curriculum.iowaglaucoma.org]. © The University of Iowa.)*

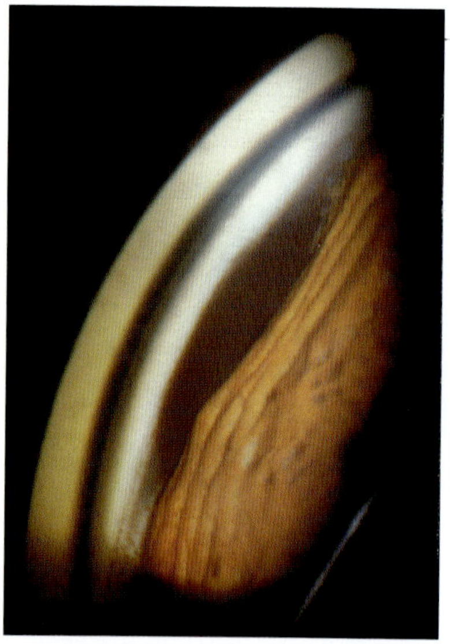

Figure 8-12 Goniophotograph of a ciliary body melanocytoma in the anterior chamber angle. *(Courtesy of Wallace L.M. Alward, MD. From the* Iowa Glaucoma Curriculum *[curriculum.iowaglaucoma.org]. © The University of Iowa.)*

- fibrin and inflammatory cells blocking outflow through the trabecular meshwork or Schlemm canal
- corticosteroid-induced reduction in outflow through the trabecular meshwork
- Peripheral anterior synechiae blocking outflow
- prostaglandin-mediated breakdown of the blood–aqueous barrier

Most cases of anterior uveitis are idiopathic, but uveitides commonly associated with open-angle inflammatory glaucoma include Fuchs uveitis syndrome, herpes zoster iridocyclitis, herpes simplex keratouveitis, toxoplasmosis, juvenile idiopathic arthritis, and pars planitis. See also BCSC Section 9, *Uveitis and Ocular Inflammation.*

The presence of KPs suggests anterior uveitis may be the cause of IOP elevation. Gonioscopic evaluation may reveal subtle trabecular meshwork precipitates. Occasionally, PAS or posterior synechiae with iris bombé may develop, resulting in angle closure.

The treatment of inflammatory glaucoma is complicated by the fact that corticosteroid therapy may increase IOP, likely by increasing outflow resistance, but also possibly by improving aqueous production, which can be decreased in eyes with intraocular inflammation. Miotic agents are not recommended in patients with anterior uveitis because they may exacerbate the inflammation and result in formation of more central posterior synechiae. Prostaglandin analogues may exacerbate inflammation in some eyes with uveitis and herpetic keratitis; however, this relationship is not clear, and some patients may benefit from their IOP-lowering effects without increased inflammation.

Some uveitis patients may have low IOP. The etiology is unclear but may be related to a prostaglandin-mediated increase in uveoscleral outflow. Hyposecretion of aqueous humor (particularly if ciliary body detachment is present) has often been assumed to be the etiology for low IOP but has not been confirmed, because aqueous flow currently cannot be measured in the presence of uveitis.

Glaucomatocyclitic crisis

First described by Posner and Schlossman in 1948, glaucomatocyclitic crisis (also known as *Posner-Schlossman syndrome*) is an uncommon form of open-angle inflammatory glaucoma characterized by acute, unilateral episodes of markedly elevated IOP accompanied by low-grade anterior chamber inflammation. This condition most frequently affects middle-aged persons, who usually present with unilateral blurred vision and mild ocular pain. The anterior uveitis is mild, with few KPs, which are small, discrete, and round and which usually resolve spontaneously within a few weeks. On gonioscopy, KPs may be seen on the trabecular meshwork, suggesting a "trabeculitis." The elevated IOP may range between 40 and 50 mm Hg, and corneal edema may be present. In between episodes, the IOP usually returns to normal, but with increasing numbers of episodes, chronic secondary glaucoma may develop.

The etiology of this condition is unknown; theories include infections (eg, herpes simplex virus, cytomegalovirus [CMV], *Helicobacter pylori*) and autoimmune disease. Recurrent attacks of acute primary angle closure have been mistaken for this condition. In some cases in which glaucomatocyclitic crisis was initially diagnosed, CMV DNA was subsequently detected in the aqueous humor by polymerase chain reaction (see BCSC Section 9, *Uveitis and Ocular Inflammation,* for more on CMV). Distinguishing glaucomatocyclitic crisis from CMV is important, as specific antiviral therapy for CMV is available.

During a glaucomatocyclitic crisis, treatment should be initiated to control IOP and may be considered to reduce inflammation. Topical and often oral ocular hypotensive medications are used to reduce IOP. Prostaglandin analogues may exacerbate the condition but can be used in some patients. Topical corticosteroids and topical and/or oral nonsteroidal anti-inflammatory drugs (NSAIDs; eg, indomethacin) may be of benefit. There is no evidence that long-term suppressive therapy with topical NSAIDs or corticosteroids is effective in preventing attacks. In some cases, filtering surgery is performed to prevent IOP spikes in eyes with advanced optic nerve damage or in those undergoing frequent attacks.

Fuchs uveitis syndrome

Fuchs uveitis syndrome (formerly *Fuchs heterochromic iridocyclitis*) is a relatively rare, insidious, and chronic form of uveitis that is typically unilateral. There is no race or sex predilection,

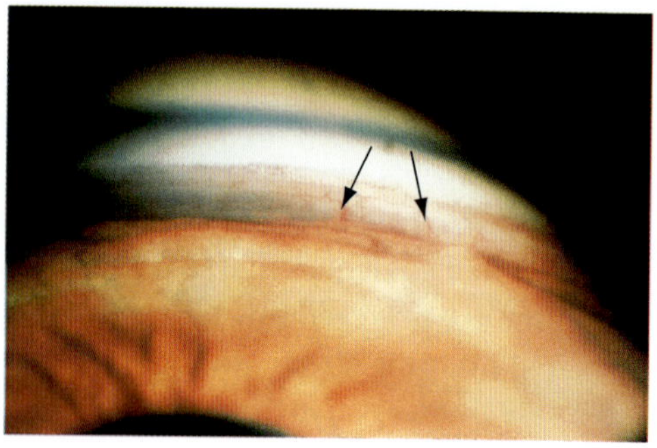

Figure 8-13 Fuchs uveitis syndrome. The goniophotograph shows fine vessels *(arrows)* crossing the trabecular meshwork. This neovascularization is not accompanied by a fibrovascular membrane and does not result in peripheral anterior synechiae formation or secondary angle closure. *(Courtesy of Steven T. Simmons, MD.)*

and it often manifests in young to middle adulthood. It is characterized by iris heterochromia, low-grade anterior chamber inflammation, posterior subcapsular cataracts, and IOP elevation. The heterochromia is caused by loss of iris pigment in the affected eye, which is usually hypochromic in dark irides and hyperchromic in light irides. The low-grade inflammation is often accompanied by small, stellate, pancorneal KPs. Despite the low-grade inflammation, these patients are classically asymptomatic and present with a nonhyperemic eye. Fuchs uveitis syndrome has variously been associated with toxoplasmosis, CMV, herpes simplex, and rubella, although these links are difficult to prove given the frequency of those infectious agents in the population.

Secondary OAG occurs in approximately 15% of patients with this disease. Gonioscopic examination reveals multiple fine vessels that cross the trabecular meshwork (Fig 8-13). These vessels are usually not accompanied by a fibrous membrane and typically do not result in PAS formation and secondary angle closure, although in rare cases the neovascularization may be progressive. The vessels are fragile and may cause an anterior chamber hemorrhage, either spontaneously or resulting from trauma. A classic finding is anterior chamber hemorrhage after a paracentesis during intraocular surgery (Amsler sign).

Treatment of Fuchs uveitis syndrome is directed at controlling the IOP with topical ocular hypotensive medications. IOP control may be difficult, and the IOP does not necessarily correlate with the degree of inflammation. Corticosteroids are generally not effective in treating the low-grade chronic inflammation, and their use can elevate the IOP.

Birnbaum AD, Tessler HH, Schultz KL, et al. Epidemiologic relationship between Fuchs heterochromic iridocyclitis and the United States rubella vaccination program. *Am J Ophthalmol.* 2007;144(3):424–428.

Elevated Episcleral Venous Pressure

Episcleral venous pressure (EVP) is an important factor in the determination of IOP. Normal EVP ranges between 6 and 9 mm Hg, depending on the measurement technique used. Elevated EVP may be caused by conditions that either obstruct venous outflow or involve arteriovenous malformations (Table 8-1).

Patients may note a chronic red eye without ocular discomfort, itching, or discharge. Occasionally, a distant history of a significant head trauma may suggest the cause of a

Table 8-1 Causes of Elevated Episcleral Venous Pressure

Vascular malformations
Arteriovenous fistula
Dural
Carotid-cavernous sinus
Orbital varix
Sturge-Weber syndrome
Venous obstruction
Retrobulbar tumor
Thyroid eye disease
Superior vena cava syndrome
Idiopathic (may be familial)

carotid-cavernous sinus (high-flow) fistula or a dural (low-flow) fistula. However, most cases are idiopathic, and some may be familial. Clinically, patients with elevated EVP present with tortuous, dilated episcleral veins (Fig 8-14). These vascular abnormalities may be unilateral or bilateral. Gonioscopy may reveal blood in the Schlemm canal (see Chapter 4, Fig 4-6). In rare instances, signs of ocular ischemia or venous stasis may be present. Sudden, severe carotid-cavernous fistulas may be accompanied by proptosis and other orbital or neurologic signs. Magnetic resonance imaging or angiography to rule out a vascular malformation may be appropriate for these patients. If these tests fail to show an abnormality and the clinical suspicion is high, traditional angiography with neuroradiologic intervention (eg, coiling of fistula) can be considered when the benefits to the patient outweigh the risks.

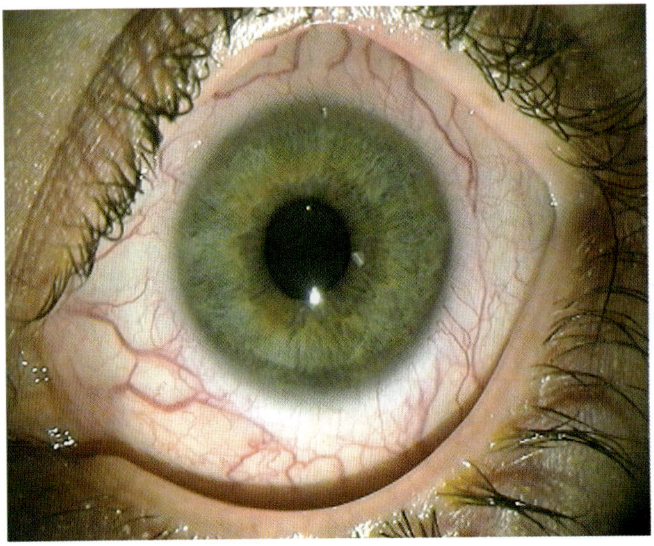

Figure 8-14 Prominent episcleral vessels in a patient with idiopathic elevated episcleral venous pressure. *(Courtesy of Keith Barton, MD.)*

Topical ocular hypotensive medications, particularly those that reduce aqueous production, may be effective in some patients. Because of the etiology of the condition, laser trabeculoplasty is not effective. Glaucoma filtering surgery may be indicated. However, given the risk of a ciliochoroidal effusion or suprachoroidal hemorrhage, prophylactic sclerotomies or scleral windows should be considered.

Trauma and Surgery

Nonpenetrating, or blunt, trauma to the eye may cause a variety of anterior segment conditions that can then lead to secondary glaucoma, including

- inflammation
- hyphema
- angle recession
- lens subluxation (see the discussion of ectopia lentis in Chapter 10)

These findings, particularly when in combination, often lead to elevated IOP initially after trauma. This elevation tends to be brief but may be protracted and result in glaucoma.

Siderosis or *chalcosis* from a retained intraocular metallic foreign body in penetrating or perforating injuries may lead to IOP elevation and glaucoma. Chemical injuries, particularly those involving alkali, may cause acute IOP elevation as a result of inflammation, shrinkage of scleral collagen, release of chemical mediators such as prostaglandins, direct damage to the anterior chamber angle, or compromised anterior uveal circulation. Recurrent inflammation or damage to the trabecular meshwork may progress to glaucoma over months or years after a chemical injury.

Traumatic hyphema

The risk of elevated IOP after a traumatic hyphema is increased with recurrent hemorrhage, or rebleeding. The average reported frequency of rebleeding after an initial hyphema is 5%–10%, but it varies significantly with different study populations. Rebleeding usually occurs within 3–7 days of the initial hyphema and may be related to normal clot retraction and lysis. In general, the larger the hyphema, the higher the incidence of increased IOP, although small hemorrhages may also be associated with marked elevation of IOP, particularly when the angle is already compromised. Increased IOP occurs as a result of obstruction of the trabecular meshwork with red blood cells (RBCs), inflammatory cells, debris, and fibrin, as well as from direct injury to the trabecular meshwork from the blunt trauma. Gentle gonioscopic examination in individuals with blunt trauma may reveal a subtle hyphema. In addition to glaucomatous damage, prolonged IOP elevation in an eye with a hyphema increases the risk of corneal blood staining (Fig 8-15).

Individuals with sickle cell hemoglobinopathies have an increased risk of elevated IOP following hyphema and are more susceptible to the development of optic neuropathy. Normal RBCs pass through the trabecular meshwork without difficulty. However, in the sickle cell hemoglobinopathies (including sickle cell trait), the low pH of the aqueous humor causes the RBCs to sickle and become rigid. These more rigid cells become trapped in the trabecular meshwork, and even low numbers of sickle-shaped RBCs may cause marked elevations in IOP. In addition, the optic nerves of patients with sickle cell disease are much more sensitive

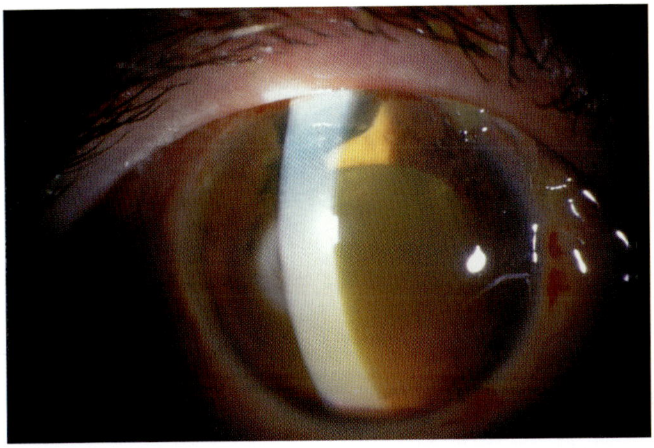

Figure 8-15 Corneal blood staining following trauma. Note the area of layered heme in the inferior angle. *(Courtesy of Wallace L.M. Alward, MD. From the* Iowa Glaucoma Curriculum *[curriculum.iowaglaucoma.org]. © The University of Iowa.)*

to elevated IOP and are prone to development of anterior ischemic optic neuropathy and central retinal artery occlusion, as a result of compromised microvascular perfusion.

In general, conservative management is appropriate for the patient with an uncomplicated hyphema and includes use of an eye shield, limited physical activity, and head elevation. Topical and oral corticosteroids may reduce associated inflammation, although their effect on rebleeding is debatable. If significant ciliary spasm or photophobia occurs, cycloplegic agents may be helpful, but they have no proven benefit for prevention of rebleeding. Oral administration of aminocaproic acid has been shown to reduce rebleeding in some studies. However, this has not been confirmed in all studies, and systemic adverse effects, such as hypotension, syncope, abdominal pain, and nausea, can be significant. Also, discontinuation of aminocaproic acid may be associated with clot lysis and additional IOP elevation.

Treatment of elevated IOP in patients with hyphema includes ocular hypotensive agents, particularly aqueous suppressants, and hyperosmotic agents. It has been suggested that patients with sickle cell hemoglobinopathies avoid carbonic anhydrase inhibitors, because these agents may increase the sickling tendency in the anterior chamber by further lowering the pH; however, this relationship has not been firmly established. The use of systemic carbonic anhydrase inhibitors and hyperosmotic agents may induce a sickle crisis in susceptible individuals who are significantly dehydrated. Adrenergic agonists with significant α_1-agonist effects (apraclonidine, dipivefrin, epinephrine) should also be avoided in patients with sickle cell disease, because of the potential for anterior segment vasoconstriction with their use. Parasympathomimetic agents may not be appropriate in patients with traumatic hyphema as they may increase inflammation and result in more centrally located posterior synechiae.

For patients with sickle cell disease, the threshold for surgical intervention may be lower, given these patients' increased risk of optic neuropathy from elevated IOP. In young children, vision obstruction by the hyphema or corneal blood staining may justify early surgical intervention to reduce the risk of amblyopia. If surgery for elevated IOP becomes necessary, an anterior chamber irrigation is commonly performed first. If a total hyphema is present, pupillary block may occur, and an iridectomy is helpful at the time of the washout. If the IOP remains uncontrolled, filtering surgery may be required. Some surgeons prefer to perform glaucoma filtering surgery with the anterior chamber washout to obtain immediate control of IOP, relieve any pupillary block, and reduce the risk of elevated IOP in the future from damage to the trabecular meshwork.

Campagna JA. Traumatic hyphema: current strategies. *Focal Points: Clinical Modules for Ophthalmologists.* American Academy of Ophthalmology; 2007, module 10.

Gharaibeh A, Savage HI, Scherer RW, Goldberg MF, Lindsley K. Medical interventions for traumatic hyphema. *Cochrane Database Syst Rev.* 2013;12:CD005431. Epub 2013 Dec 3.

Hemolytic and ghost cell glaucoma

Hemolytic glaucoma, ghost cell glaucoma, or both may develop after a vitreous hemorrhage. In *hemolytic glaucoma,* hemoglobin-laden macrophages block the trabecular meshwork. Red-tinged cells can be seen floating in the anterior chamber, and the trabecular meshwork may appear reddish brown. In *ghost cell glaucoma,* degenerated RBCs (ghost cells) obstruct the trabecular meshwork.

Ghost cells are small, khaki-colored RBCs that have lost their intracellular hemoglobin (Fig 8-16). Because they are less pliable than normal RBCs, they obstruct the trabecular meshwork and cause elevated IOP. RBCs degenerate within 1 to 3 months after a vitreous hemorrhage. They gain access to the anterior chamber through a disrupted hyaloid face, which can occur spontaneously or as a result of trauma or previous surgery (eg, pars plana vitrectomy, cataract extraction, capsulotomy).

Patients with ghost cell glaucoma typically present with elevated IOP and a history of or current vitreous hemorrhage from trauma, surgery, or preexisting retinal disease. The IOP may be markedly elevated, with accompanying corneal edema. The anterior chamber may contain degenerated RBCs. The cellular reaction is often out of proportion to the aqueous flare, and the conjunctiva tends not to be inflamed unless the IOP is markedly elevated. On gonioscopy, the angle appears normal except for possible layering of ghost cells in the

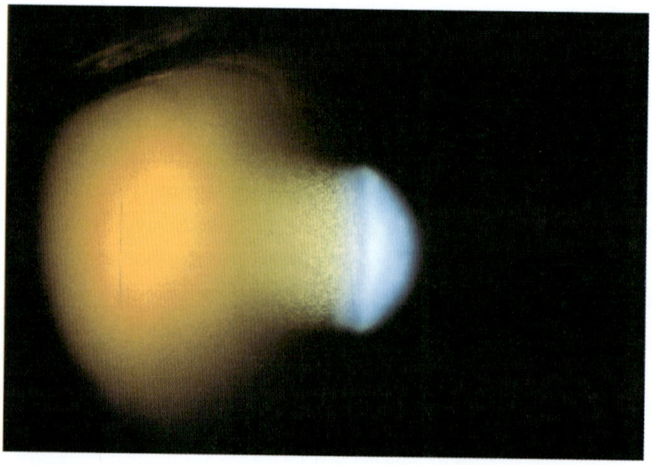

Figure 8-16 Ghost cell glaucoma: the classic appearance of ghost cells in the anterior chamber. These small, khaki-colored cells can become layered, as occurs in a hyphema or hypopyon. *(Courtesy of Ron Gross, MD.)*

inferior angle. A long-standing vitreous hemorrhage may be present, with characteristic khaki coloration and clumps of extracellular pigmentation from degenerated hemoglobin.

In these conditions, IOP typically normalizes once the hemorrhage has cleared. Medical therapy with aqueous suppressants is the preferred initial approach. If medical therapy fails to control the IOP, some patients may require anterior chamber irrigation, pars plana vitrectomy, and/or incisional glaucoma surgery. When a collection of RBCs or ghost cells is present in the vitreous, a pars plana vitrectomy is likely necessary for IOP control.

Traumatic, or angle-recession, glaucoma

Angle recession is a common finding after blunt trauma and involves a tear between the longitudinal and circular muscle fibers of the ciliary body. Although angle recession is not necessarily associated with immediate IOP elevation and glaucoma, it is a sign of probable damage to the trabecular meshwork. Traumatic glaucoma is chronic and usually unilateral and may occur immediately after the ocular trauma or months to years later. It resembles POAG in presentation and clinical course but can be distinguished by its classic gonioscopic findings (Figs 8-17, 8-18):

- widening of the ciliary body band
- absent or torn iris processes

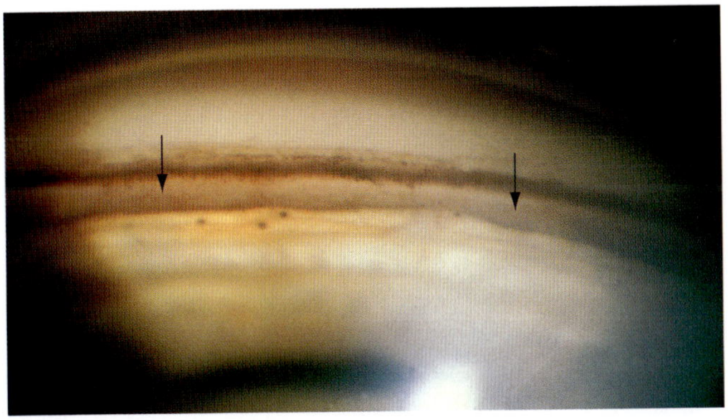

Figure 8-17 Goniophotograph of angle recession. Angle recession occurs when the ciliary body is torn, usually between the longitudinal and circular fibers of the ciliary body, resulting in a deepened angle recess *(arrows)*. The dark circular deposits located on the peripheral iris represent old heme. *(Reproduced from Alward WLM, Longmuir RA.* Color Atlas of Gonioscopy. *2nd ed. American Academy of Ophthalmology; 2008:89. Fig 9-50.)*

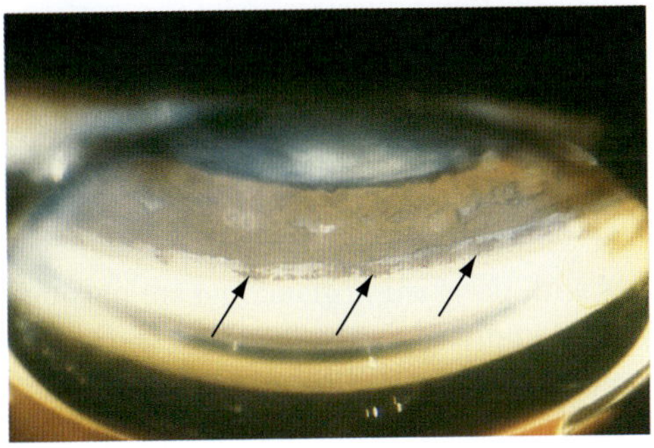

Figure 8-18 Typical gonioscopic appearance of angle recession. Torn iris processes *(arrows)*, a whitened and increasingly visible scleral spur, and a localized depression in the trabecular meshwork are shown. *(Courtesy of Steven T. Simmons, MD.)*

- white, glistening scleral spur
- irregular and dark pigmentation in the angle
- PAS at the border of the recession

Traumatic glaucoma should be considered in a patient with unilateral IOP elevation. The patient's history may reveal the contributing incident, although it may have occurred in the distant past and hence forgotten. Examination may reveal findings consistent with previous trauma, such as corneal scars, iris injury, abnormalities in the angle, focal anterior subcapsular cataracts, and phacodonesis. Comparing gonioscopic findings in the affected eye to those in the fellow eye may help the clinician identify areas of recession.

More extensive angle recession is associated with a greater reduction in outflow facility and an increased risk of glaucoma. However, even with substantial angle recession, this risk is not high. Although the risk of developing glaucoma decreases appreciably after several years, it is still present even 25 years or more after injury. In a significant proportion (up to 50%) of fellow eyes, elevated IOP may occur, suggesting that some eyes with trauma that go on to develop glaucoma may have been predisposed to POAG. Alternatively, it is possible the fellow eyes were more likely to have sustained trauma as well. Because it is not possible to predict which eyes will develop glaucoma, regular monitoring of all eyes with angle recession and their fellow eyes is recommended.

The treatment of traumatic glaucoma is often initiated with aqueous suppressants, prostaglandin analogues, and α_2-adrenergic agonists. Miotics may be useful, but paradoxical responses of increased IOP may occur. Laser trabeculoplasty has reduced efficacy in these patients. Incisional glaucoma surgery may be required to control the IOP in patients not responding to medical therapy.

Surgically induced IOP elevation

Conventional surgical procedures such as cataract extraction are occasionally associated with transient IOP elevation. Similarly, laser surgery—including trabeculoplasty, iridotomy, and posterior capsulotomy—may be complicated by posttreatment IOP elevation. Although the IOP may rise as high as 50 mm Hg or more, these elevations are usually transient, lasting from a few hours to a few days. Other procedures, including vitrectomy and penetrating keratoplasty (PKP), may be followed by a sustained increase in IOP. The exact mechanism of the IOP elevation is not always known. However, the presence of inflammatory cells, RBCs, debris, pigment release, mechanical deformation of the trabecular meshwork, oxidative damage, and angle closure may be involved.

Agents used as adjuncts to intraocular surgery or postoperative treatment (eg, corticosteroids) may also cause secondary IOP elevation. For example, the injection of viscoelastic substances into the anterior chamber may result in a transient and possibly severe postoperative increase in IOP. Cohesive viscoelastic agents, especially in higher-molecular-weight forms, may be more likely to cause an increase in IOP than dispersive viscoelastics.

Postoperative IOP elevation, even over a short period, can cause considerable damage to the optic nerve in susceptible individuals. Eyes with preexisting glaucoma are particularly at risk of further damage; thus, it is extremely important to monitor IOP soon after conventional or laser surgery and to consider treatment with IOP-lowering medications at the time of surgery. If a substantial rise in IOP occurs, IOP-lowering therapy may be required, including the use of topical β-blockers, α_2-adrenergic agonists, or carbonic anhydrase inhibitors. If postoperative inflammation is present, prostaglandin analogues may be deferred until the inflammation has resolved. Paracentesis with release of aqueous fluid (and possibly viscoelastic) can be used to rapidly lower the IOP if it is substantially high. Persistent IOP elevation may require filtering surgery.

The implantation of an intraocular lens (IOL) can lead to a variety of secondary glaucomas, including

- uveitis-glaucoma-hyphema (UGH) syndrome
- secondary pigmentary glaucoma
- pseudophakic pupillary block (see Chapter 10)

UGH syndrome is a secondary inflammatory glaucoma classically caused by chafing of the iris or ciliary body by a malpositioned or rotated anterior chamber IOL. It is characterized by 1 or more of the following:

- chronic inflammation
- elevated IOP
- recurrent hyphemas
- cystoid macular edema
- iris neovascularization

This condition can also occur after implantation of a posterior chamber IOL in the ciliary sulcus or one that is suture-fixated to the iris or sclera. Implantation of single-piece acrylic IOLs in the sulcus is a particular risk factor for this condition and should be avoided. Gonioscopy and ultrasound biomicroscopy may be helpful in revealing the IOL's exact position in relation to the iris and ciliary body. Persistent or recurrent cases often require IOL repositioning or IOL exchange, which can be technically challenging because of possible synechiae and/or an open posterior capsule. This syndrome may be mimicked in patients with neovascularization of the internal lip of a corneoscleral wound, which may result in recurrent spontaneous hyphemas and elevated IOP. Laser ablation of the vessels may successfully resolve these cases.

Secondary glaucoma is a common complication after PKP and occurs with greater frequency in aphakic and pseudophakic patients and after a second graft. Wound-induced distortion of the trabecular meshwork and progressive angle closure are the most common causes of glaucoma after PKP. Attempts to minimize these changes with different-sized donor grafts, peripheral iridectomies, and surgical repair of the iris sphincter have been only partially successful. Alternative procedures, such as lamellar stromal or endothelial grafts, may have a lower risk of elevated IOP. Long-term use of topical corticosteroids after PKP is another potential cause of elevated IOP and secondary glaucoma in these patients. Surgical interventions to treat glaucoma after PKP are associated with an increased risk of graft rejection and failure. See BCSC Section 8, *External Disease and Cornea,* for further discussion of PKP.

Schwartz Syndrome (Schwartz-Matsuo Syndrome)

Individuals with a rhegmatogenous retinal detachment (RRD) typically have lower IOP, presumably because of increased outflow of fluid through the exposed retinal pigment epithelium. Schwartz was the first to describe elevated IOP associated with an RRD. Matsuo later demonstrated the presence of photoreceptor outer segments in the aqueous humor of patients with RRDs. The postulated mechanism of IOP elevation is the liberation of photoreceptor outer segments, which migrate through the vitreous into the anterior chamber and trabecular meshwork, where they impede aqueous outflow. The photoreceptor segments may be mistaken for an anterior chamber inflammatory reaction or pigment. The IOP tends to normalize after successful surgery to reattach the retina.

Drugs and Glaucoma

Corticosteroid-induced glaucoma is an OAG caused by prolonged use of topical, periocular, intravitreous, inhaled, or oral corticosteroids. It mimics POAG in its presentation and clinical course. Approximately one-third of the population without glaucoma demonstrates an IOP elevation between 6 and 15 mm Hg in response to corticosteroids, and only a small percentage (4%–6%) has a significant IOP elevation of more than 15 mm Hg. A high percentage (up to 95%) of patients with POAG experience an ocular hypertensive response to long-term topical corticosteroids. The type and potency of the agent, the means and frequency of its administration, and the susceptibility of the patient all affect the timing and extent of the IOP rise. Risk factors for corticosteroid-induced glaucoma include a history of POAG, a first-degree relative with POAG, very young age (<6 years) or older age, connective tissue disease, type 1 diabetes mellitus, and myopia. The elevated IOP is a result of increased resistance to aqueous outflow in the trabecular meshwork. See also BCSC Section 9, *Uveitis and Ocular Inflammation,* for further discussion of corticosteroids.

Corticosteroid-induced IOP elevation may develop within weeks, months, or years of the drug's use; thus, regular monitoring of IOP is recommended in patients receiving these agents. In general, the risk of IOP elevation is correlated with the glucocorticoid potency of the drug and its ability to penetrate the ocular surface. For example, some corticosteroid preparations, such as fluorometholone, rimexolone, medrysone, or loteprednol, are less likely to raise IOP than are prednisolone, dexamethasone, or difluprednate (see Table 16-15 in BCSC Section 2, *Fundamentals and Principles of Ophthalmology*). However, even weaker corticosteroids or lower concentrations of stronger drugs can raise IOP in susceptible individuals. A corticosteroid-induced rise in IOP may cause glaucomatous optic nerve damage in some patients.

The cause of the elevation in IOP may be related to an underlying ocular disease, such as anterior uveitis, as opposed to corticosteroid use. After the corticosteroid is discontinued, the IOP usually decreases with a time course similar to or slightly longer than that of the onset of elevation. However, elevated IOP may persist in some cases.

IOP may also become elevated in patients who have excessive levels of endogenous corticosteroids (eg, Cushing syndrome). When the corticosteroid-producing tissue is excised, IOP generally returns to normal.

Periocular injection of a corticosteroid, particularly triamcinolone acetonide, may result in elevated IOP. Medical therapy may lower the IOP, but some patients require excision of the corticosteroid depot or glaucoma surgery.

Intravitreous corticosteroid injection may be associated with transient elevations in IOP in more than 50% of patients. Up to 25% of these patients may require topical medications to control IOP, and 1%–2% may require incisional glaucoma surgery. In contrast, intravitreous implants that release corticosteroid are frequently associated with elevated IOP, often requiring patients to undergo incisional glaucoma surgery for IOP control. Surgical treatment has a high success rate in lowering IOP in these patients; laser trabeculoplasty may also be of benefit.

Cycloplegic drugs can increase IOP in individuals with open angles. Routine dilation for ophthalmoscopy may increase IOP; those at greater risk include patients with POAG, pseudoexfoliation syndrome, or pigment dispersion syndrome, as well as those receiving miotic therapy.

Intravitreous injection of anti–vascular endothelial growth factor (anti-VEGF) agents is a common treatment for choroidal neovascularization and macular edema. Intravitreous injection may result in a transient rise in IOP. Over time, repeated injections may result in sustained IOP elevation. The etiology of the elevated IOP is unknown, but theories include increased inflammation and injury to or mechanical blockage of the trabecular meshwork.

Dedania VS, Bakri SJ. Sustained elevation of intraocular pressure after intravitreal anti-VEGF agents: what is the evidence? *Retina.* 2015;35(5):841–858.

CHAPTER 9

Primary Angle Closure

This chapter includes related videos. Go to www.aao.org/bcscvideo_section10 or scan the QR codes in the text to access this content.

Highlights

- Primary angle-closure disease is a common cause of glaucoma, particularly in Asian populations.
- Although pupillary block is the most common mechanism, other causes, including plateau iris and lens-associated factors, often play a role.
- Gonioscopy should be performed in all patients whom the clinician suspects of having glaucoma or narrow angles, including those with hyperopia and older phakic patients.
- Treatment is tailored to the individual patient and can include medical therapy, laser iridotomy, laser iridoplasty, and lensectomy.

Introduction

Angle closure refers to an anatomic configuration in which there is mechanical blockage of the trabecular meshwork by the peripheral iris. Anatomic alterations in anterior segment structures result in obstruction of the iridocorneal drainage angle through apposition *(iridotrabecular contact)* or consequent to the formation of peripheral anterior synechiae (PAS; adhesions of the peripheral iris to the trabecular meshwork). The term *angle-closure disease* refers to the presence of PAS, ocular hypertension associated with angle closure, acute primary angle closure, or glaucomatous optic neuropathy attributable to primary angle closure.

Angle closure is divided into 2 main categories—(1) primary angle closure and (2) secondary angle closure—according to the etiology of the disease. In *primary angle closure,* no secondary pathologic condition can be identified; there is only an anatomic predisposition. In *secondary angle closure,* an identifiable pathologic cause—such as an intumescent lens, iris neovascularization, chronic inflammation, corneal endothelial migration into the angle, or epithelial ingrowth—initiates the angle closure. See Chapter 10 in this volume for discussion of secondary angle closure.

Table 9-1 European Glaucoma Society Classification of Angle Closure

Stage	Definition
Primary angle-closure suspect (PACS)	Iridotrabecular contact ≥180° but no evidence of trabecular meshwork or optic nerve damage
Primary angle closure (PAC)	Iridotrabecular contact ≥180° with elevated IOP or PAS but no optic nerve damage
Primary angle-closure glaucoma (PACG)	PAC with glaucomatous optic neuropathy

IOP = intraocular pressure; PAS = peripheral anterior synechiae.

Current nomenclature further classifies eyes on the primary angle-closure spectrum into 3 categories based on the severity of the condition:

- *primary angle-closure suspect (PACS),* in which the eye has an anatomic configuration that increases the risk of developing angle-closure disease
- *primary angle closure (PAC),* in which trabecular meshwork damage or dysfunction is already present, characterized by PAS or elevated intraocular pressure (IOP)
- *primary angle-closure glaucoma (PACG),* which is characterized by PAS or elevated IOP and glaucomatous optic neuropathy (Table 9-1)

Worldwide prevalence of angle-closure glaucoma (ACG) is estimated to reach over 23 million in 2020 and over 32 million in 2040. ACG is more common in females and in certain ethnic groups, such as particular Asian populations and the Inuit. Prevalence rates in European and African populations are generally lower, but genetic heterogeneity can result in widely varying prevalence within populations of the same continent. ACG has been estimated to account for over 90% of blindness due to glaucoma in the Chinese population.

The angle-closure–related disorders are a diverse group of diseases. Although the various forms of angle closure are united by the presence of PAS and/or iridotrabecular apposition, different mechanisms are responsible for these features. Moreover, the clinical presentation of angle closure varies from the abrupt and dramatic onset of acute angle closure to the insidious and asymptomatic presentation of chronic disease.

To initiate the appropriate therapy, the physician must identify the anatomic changes in the angle and the underlying pathophysiology that has precipitated the disease. Early diagnosis and treatment of most forms of angle closure or narrowing can be invaluable and sometimes curative. Screening patients at greatest risk for angle closure can be beneficial in reducing both the number of patients who develop these diseases and the risk of blindness.

American Academy of Ophthalmology Glaucoma Panel. Preferred Practice Pattern® Guidelines. *Primary Angle Closure.* American Academy of Ophthalmology; 2016. www.aao.org/ppp

Chan EW, Li X, Tham YC, et al. Glaucoma in Asia: regional prevalence variations and future projections. *Br J Ophthalmol.* 2016;100(1):78–85.

Tham YC, Li X, Wong TY, Quigley HA, Aung T, Cheng CY. Global prevalence of glaucoma and projections of glaucoma burden through 2040: a systematic review and meta-analysis. *Ophthalmology.* 2014;121(11):2081–2090.

Yip JL, Foster PJ. Ethnic differences in primary angle-closure glaucoma. *Curr Opin Ophthalmol.* 2006;17(2):175–180.

Pathogenesis and Pathophysiology

The hallmark of angle closure is the apposition or adhesion of the peripheral iris to the trabecular meshwork. The portion of the anterior chamber angle affected by such apposition is described as "closed," and drainage of aqueous humor through the angle is reduced as a result. Such closure may be transient and intermittent *(appositional)* or permanent *(synechial)*. These 2 forms of angle closure can be distinguished by means of indentation gonioscopy. The IOP becomes elevated as a result of reduced aqueous humor outflow through the trabecular meshwork.

In addition to these traditional mechanisms of angle closure, more recent work suggests that the dynamic changes in iris volume and water content normally occurring in the human eye are dysfunctional in patients with angle-closure disease and may play an important role in its pathogenesis. In unaffected eyes, iris volume is reduced with pupillary dilation, much like a sponge being squeezed; however, eyes with angle closure demonstrate paradoxical expansion of volume, likely contributing to the crowding and closure of the angle. A variety of factors that cause pupillary dilation—certain drugs, pain, emotional upset, and fright, among others—may precipitate acute angle closure.

In the primary angle-closure spectrum, the major mechanism is pupillary block. In up to one-third of eyes with angle closure, plateau iris is at least a contributing factor to the anatomic abnormality.

Aptel F, Denis P. Optical coherence tomography quantitative analysis of iris volume changes after pharmacologic mydriasis. *Ophthalmology.* 2010;117(1):3–10.

Quigley HA. The iris is a sponge: a cause of angle closure. *Ophthalmology.* 2010;117(1):1–2.

Pupillary Block

Pupillary block is the most frequent cause of angle closure. Although the pathophysiology of the PAC spectrum is complex and not completely understood, pupillary block is the main or a contributing cause in most cases. The flow of aqueous humor from the posterior chamber through the pupil is impeded at the level of the lens–iris interface, and this obstruction creates a pressure gradient between the posterior and anterior chambers, causing the peripheral iris to bow forward against the trabecular meshwork (Fig 9-1). Pupillary block is maximal when the pupil is in the mid-dilated position. In most cases of angle closure, pupillary block results from anatomic factors at the lens–iris interface. Pupillary block may be broken by an unobstructed peripheral iridectomy or iridotomy.

In phakic eyes, the lens (and its alteration with age) plays a critical role in pupillary block. Recent studies have found that a high lens vault (defined as how far the lens protrudes anterior to the plane of the scleral spur) is a major risk factor for angle-closure disease. Iris thickness, area, and volume have also been strongly correlated with narrower angle and risk for angle closure. Smaller anterior chamber dimensions, including anterior chamber depth (ACD), width (ACW), area (ACA), and volume (ACV), are also risk factors.

Plateau Iris and Iris-Induced Angle Closure

In plateau iris and iris-induced angle closure, the peripheral iris is the cause of the iridotrabecular apposition. Iris-induced angle closure can be the direct result of developmental

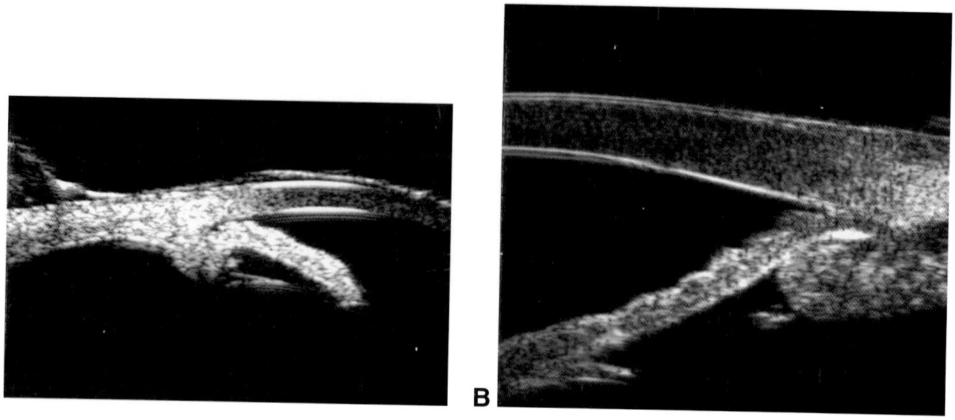

A B

Figure 9-1 Ultrasound biomicroscopy imaging. **A,** Eye with pupillary block showing anterior bowing of the iris. **B,** Eye with plateau iris anatomy showing a large, anteriorly rotated ciliary process causing appositional angle closure. *(Part A courtesy of Shan Lin, MD; part B courtesy of Sunita Radhakrishnan, MD, from the Glaucoma Center of San Francisco archives.)*

anomalies such as anterior cleavage abnormalities, in which the iris insertion into the scleral spur or meshwork is more anterior; a thick peripheral iris, which on dilation "rolls" into the trabecular meshwork; and/or anteriorly displaced ciliary processes (see Fig 9-1), which may secondarily rotate the peripheral iris forward *(plateau iris)* into the trabecular meshwork (see the section Plateau Iris later in this chapter). Though it was thought that iris-induced angle closure occurs in aniridia due to rotation of the rudimentary iris leaflets into the angle, new evidence suggests that this phenomenon occurs as a result of intraocular surgery rather than spontaneously.

Role of Medications in Angle Closure

In predisposed eyes with shallow anterior chambers, either mydriatic or miotic agents can precipitate acute angle closure. Mydriatic agents include not only dilating drops but also systemic medications with sympathomimetic or anticholinergic activity that may cause mild pupillary dilation. The effect of miotics is to pull the peripheral iris away from the anterior chamber angle. However, strong miotics may also cause the zonular fibers of the lens to relax, allowing the lens–iris interface to move forward. Furthermore, their use results in greater iris–lens contact, thus potentially increasing pupillary block. For these reasons, miotics, especially the cholinesterase inhibitors, may induce or worsen angle closure. Gonioscopy should be repeated soon after miotic drugs are administered to patients with narrow angles.

Systemic drugs with adrenergic (sympathomimetic) or anticholinergic (parasympatholytic) activity have the potential to cause angle closure. They include

- allergy and cold medications
  - adrenergic agents, including ephedrine
  - antihistamines such as diphenhydramine

- bronchodilator medications (for asthma and chronic obstructive pulmonary disease) such as ipratropium bromide and tiotropium bromide
- antidepressants, anxiolytics, and antipsychotics
  - selective serotonin reuptake inhibitors (SSRIs) such as fluoxetine and paroxetine
  - tricyclic antidepressants such as amitriptyline and imipramine
  - antihistamine-anxiolytics such as hydroxyzine
  - phenothiazines such as chlorpromazine
- antispasmodics used in urology such as tolterodine and oxybutynin
- gastrointestinal drugs
  - antihistamines, including cimetidine and ranitidine
- muscle relaxants such as orphenadrine and trihexyphenidyl
- antinausea mediations, including promethazine

Although systemic administration generally does not raise intraocular drug levels as much as topical administration, even slight mydriasis in a patient with a critically narrow angle can induce angle closure. When such drugs are administered to patients with potentially occludable angles, it is important to inform the patient of the risk and consider iridotomy.

Risk Factors

Race and Ethnicity

The prevalence of PACG in patients older than 40 years varies greatly, depending on race and ethnicity; for example, it is 0.1%–0.6% in people of African ancestry, 0.1%–0.4% in European-derived populations, 0.3%–2.2% in Japanese individuals, 0.4%–1.7% in Chinese individuals, and 2.1%–4.8% in Inuit persons. Some of this variation in prevalence—for example, between White individuals and Inuit individuals—can be explained by differences in the biometric parameters (anterior chamber depth, axial length) of these groups; however, the increased prevalence of PACG in Chinese and in other East Asian populations cannot be explained by major biometric parameters alone. Recent anterior segment anatomic studies suggest that differences in other parameters such as iris thickness and area; dynamic changes in the iris; lens vault; and anterior chamber width can be significant contributing factors. It has become increasingly clear that the burden of PACG is greater in Asian countries. However, recent increases in the prevalence of myopia (with associated axial elongation) in Asian countries—particularly urban areas—may counterbalance these trends in PACG.

Day AC, Baio G, Gazzard G, et al. The prevalence of primary angle closure glaucoma in European derived populations: a systematic review. *Br J Ophthalmol.* 2012;96(9):1162–1167.

Quigley HA. Angle-closure glaucoma—simpler answers to complex mechanisms: LXVI Edward Jackson Memorial Lecture. *Am J Ophthalmol.* 2009;148(5):657–669.

Tham YC, Li X, Wong TY, Quigley HA, Aung T, Cheng CY. Global prevalence of glaucoma and projections of glaucoma burden through 2040: a systemic review and meta-analysis. *Ophthalmology.* 2014;121(11):2081–2090.

Ocular Biometrics

Eyes on the primary angle-closure spectrum tend to have a small, "crowded" anterior segment and short axial length (AL). The most important factors predisposing an eye to angle closure are a shallow anterior chamber, a thick lens, increased anterior curvature of the lens, a short AL, and a small corneal diameter and radius of curvature. Studies using anterior segment imaging have contributed additional parameters that are risk factors for angle closure, including increased iris thickness and area and greater lens vault (see the discussion in Chapter 4 on anterior segment imaging). An ACD of <2.5 mm predisposes patients to PAC; in most patients with PAC, the ACD is <2.1 mm. Improvements in ocular biometry techniques have allowed researchers to demonstrate a clear association between ACD and development of PAS. While primary PAS seem to be uncommon in eyes with ACD >2.4 mm, there is a strong correlation between increasing PAS formation and an ACD of <2.4 mm. However, in some cases, angle closure can occur in eyes with deep anterior chambers, with plateau iris as a common cause.

Age

The prevalence of angle closure increases with each decade after 40 years of age. This has been explained by the increasing thickness and forward movement of the lens with age and the resultant increase in iridolenticular contact. Angle-closure disease is rare in persons younger than 40 years, and the etiology of angle closure in young individuals is most often related to structural or developmental anomalies such as plateau iris and retinopathy of prematurity rather than pupillary block.

Ritch R, Chang BM, Liebmann JM. Angle closure in younger patients. *Ophthalmology.* 2003;110(10):1880–1889.

Sex

Primary angle closure is 2–4 times more common in women than in men, irrespective of race. Studies assessing ocular biometry data have found that women tend to have smaller anterior segments and shorter ALs than men. These differences, however, do not appear to be large enough to completely explain the sex predilection.

Family History and Genetics

The incidence of PAC is increased in first-degree relatives of affected individuals. In White individuals, the prevalence of PAC in first-degree relatives has been reported to be between 1% and 12%, whereas results from a survey in a Chinese population showed that the risk was 6 times higher in patients with any family history. Among the Inuit, the relative risk in persons with a family history is increased 3.5 times compared with the general Inuit population. These familial associations support a genetic influence in PAC. Recent genome-wide association studies have shown a complex genetic inheritance pattern with variable penetrance of genetic loci.

Rong SS, Tang FY, Chu WK, et al. Genetic associations of primary angle-closure disease: a systematic review and meta-analysis. *Ophthalmology.* 2016;123(6):1211–1221.

Refractive Error

The primary angle-closure spectrum occurs most commonly, but not exclusively, in patients with hyperopia, regardless of race. Nonetheless, angle closure does occur in patients with significant myopia, underscoring the importance of gonioscopy in all patients. Angle closure in a patient with high myopia is a prompt for the clinician to search for secondary mechanisms such as microspherophakia, plateau iris, or phacomorphic angle closure related to nuclear sclerotic cataract. However, the primary angle-closure spectrum may occur in individuals even with simple myopia, particularly those of Asian descent. Axial myopia is primarily the result of elongation of the posterior segment of the eye, while the anterior segment sometimes retains properties that predispose to angle closure. Thus, even though myopia and axial elongation are associated with lower risk for angle closure, there may be some risk in myopic eyes.

Yong KL, Gong T, Nongpiur ME, et al. Myopia in Asian subjects with primary angle closure: implications for glaucoma trends in East Asia. *Ophthalmology.* 2014;121(8):1566–1571.

The Primary Angle-Closure Spectrum

Primary Angle-Closure Suspect

The term *primary angle-closure suspect (PACS)* is defined by the presence of a narrow angle with ≥180° of appositional iridotrabecular contact, without overt signs of PAC (IOP elevation or PAS) or glaucomatous optic nerve damage. PACS eyes are at risk for developing angle-closure disease (acute angle-closure crisis, PAC, or PACG).

Only a small percentage of PACS eyes develop angle-closure disease, and the predictive value of gonioscopy is relatively poor even when performed by experienced clinicians. When performing gonioscopy, the clinician should observe the effect that the examination light has on the angle recess. For example, pupillary constriction stimulated by the slit-lamp beam itself may open the angle, and the narrow recess may go unrecognized (Video 9-1; Fig 9-2).

VIDEO 9-1 Angle apposition when going from light to dark conditions.
Courtesy of Shan Lin, MD.
Scan the QR code or access the video at www.aao.org/bcscvideo_section10.

Provocative tests such as pharmacologic pupillary dilation and the dark-room prone-position test can precipitate a limited form of angle closure and thus have been used in an attempt to predict which patients might develop angle closure and benefit from an iridotomy. However, the recent Zhongshan Angle-Closure Prevention (ZAP) study showed that provocative testing (15-minute dark-room prone position) is not predictive of an angle-closure attack or development of glaucoma (although eyes were excluded from the study if there was a 15 mm Hg elevation in IOP on either mydriatic dilation or dark-room, prone provocative testing). Anterior segment imaging is under investigation in hopes it may be a better predictor of angle-closure disease (see the section Anterior Segment Imaging in Chapter 4).

He M, Jiang Y, Huang S, et al. Laser peripheral iridotomy for the prevention of angle closure: a single-centre, randomized controlled trial. *Lancet.* 2019;393(10181):1609–1618.

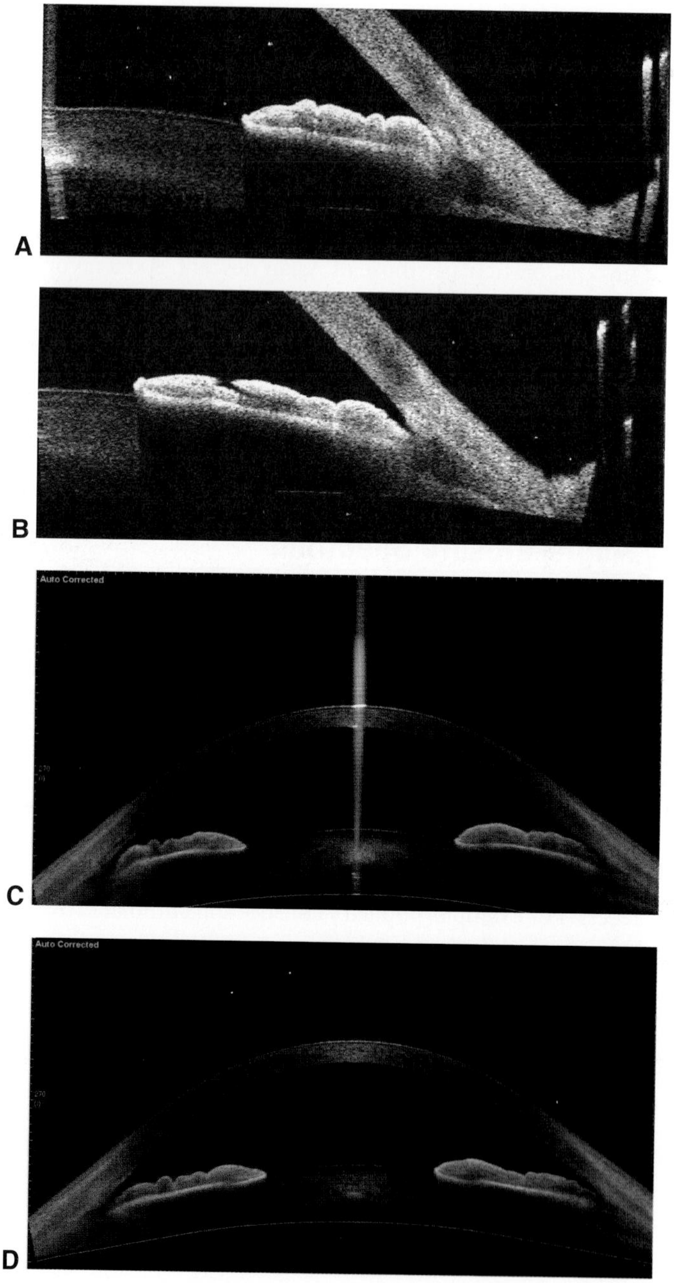

Figure 9-2 Anterior segment optical coherence tomography of a narrow angle. **A,** Angle closure is evident when the angle is imaged with lights off. **B,** The same angle is much more open when it is imaged with lights on. **C,** Narrow angles due to plateau iris (before laser iridotomy). **D,** Same meridian with persistent narrow angles after laser iridotomy. *(Parts A and B courtesy of Yaniv Barkana, MD; parts C and D courtesy of David A. Lee, MD.)*

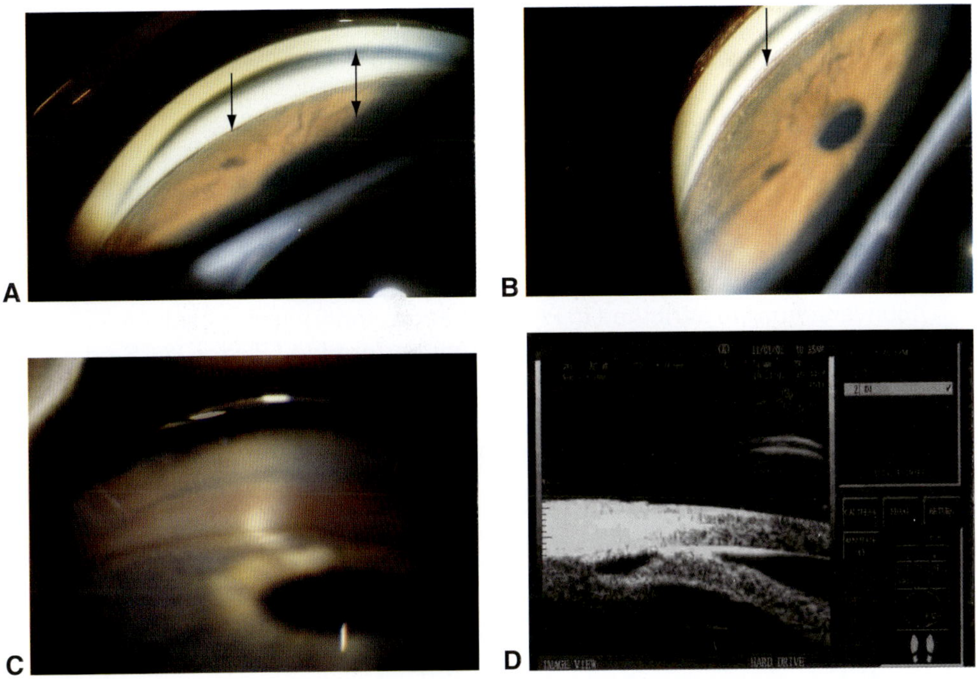

Figure 9-3 Plateau iris syndrome. **A,** Eye with plateau iris has a flat iris plane but shallow angle recess *(arrow).* Note that the midperipheral angle appears deeper *(double arrow)* than the narrow angles associated with pupillary block. **B,** Plateau iris syndrome after laser peripheral iridoplasty, with a much deeper angle recess *(arrow).* **C,** Image shows the classic "double-hump" sign. **D,** Ultrasound biomicroscopy shows peripheral iris contact with Schwalbe line, anterior to the angle recess, in a case of plateau iris configuration *(Parts A and B courtesy of M. Roy Wilson, MD; part C courtesy of Wallace L.M. Alward, MD; part D courtesy of Robert Ritch, MD.)*

Management

It is considered reasonable to perform a laser peripheral iridotomy (LPI; Fig 9-3) in an eye that meets the criteria for PACS (Videos 9-2, 9-3). However, iridotomy is not necessary for all PACS patients, and the decision of whether to treat an asymptomatic individual with narrow angles is based on an accurate assessment of the anterior chamber angle, the clinical judgment of the ophthalmologist, and the patient's preference. (See the sidebar Treatment Controversies for further discussion.) Any patient with narrow angles should be advised of the symptoms of acute angle closure, the need for immediate ophthalmologic attention if symptoms occur, and the value of long-term periodic follow-up.

VIDEO 9-2 Angle apposition before LPI.
Courtesy of Shan Lin, MD.

VIDEO 9-3 Angle apposition after LPI, with angle opening.
Courtesy of Shan Lin, MD.

TREATMENT CONTROVERSIES

Laser Peripheral Iridotomy

Whether to perform an LPI in patients who meet the criteria for PACS remains controversial. The Zhongshan Angle-Closure Prevention (ZAP) trial randomized 1 eye of subjects with PACS to LPI, with the contralateral eye serving as a control. The study showed that very few cases in either group progressed to PACG or an acute attack. There was a significantly lower risk of conversion to PAC with treatment; however, most cases of conversion were attributed to PAS formation alone, without ocular hypertension. Overall, the results suggest that performing LPIs for PACS on a population basis is not recommended. However, on an individual basis, the clinician needs to consider whether an LPI is appropriate based on narrowness of the angle, the presence of symptoms such as eye discomfort in the evening, and other factors relevant to the particular patient, including his or her personal preference given the available evidence.

An LPI should be considered for patients who have a narrow angle with PAS, increased segmental trabecular meshwork pigmentation, a history of previous acute angle closure, or other risk factors for angle closure (ACD <2.0 mm, strong family history). The status of the lens and the potential benefit of cataract surgery should also be taken into consideration.

Furthermore, there is controversy as to whether an LPI should be performed in eyes in which most or all of the angle is closed with PAS. Such eyes have limited outflow facility and may have marked IOP increase as a result of the dispersed pigment and debris. In some cases, the IOP elevation is refractory to medications and requires filtering surgery. Thus, caution should be exercised in such cases, and avoidance of the LPI may be the better course of action.

Iridoplasty

Another controversial area is whether to perform iridoplasty in angle closure. There is evidence that iridoplasty is effective in further widening a narrow angle after iridotomy (Video 9-4). However, there is no strong evidence that iridoplasty is beneficial in preventing development of future glaucoma or progression of existing glaucoma.

VIDEO 9-4 Iridoplasty in the peripheral iris.
Courtesy of Robert Ritch, MD.

Lensectomy

Clear lens extraction (LE) may be beneficial to certain patients with angle closure. The EAGLE study was a prospective randomized trial that evaluated the safety and efficacy of LE in subjects with no or non–visually significant cataracts, compared with standard treatment with LPI and medications. Subjects enrolled were ≥50 years, without visually significant cataracts, and with newly diagnosed PAC with IOP ≥30 mm Hg or PACG. The study found that LE resulted in lower IOP, less medication usage, better quality of life, and similar visual field progression as the control group.

Azuara-Blanco A, Burr J, Ramsay C, et al; EAGLE study group. Effectiveness of early lens extraction for the treatment of primary angle-closure glaucoma (EAGLE): a randomised controlled trial. *Lancet.* 2016;388(10052):1389–1397.

He M, Jiang Y, Huang S, et al. Laser peripheral iridotomy for the prevention of angle closure: a single-centre, randomised controlled trial. *Lancet.* 2019;393(10181):1609–1618.

Lim DK, Chan HW, Zheng C, et al. Quantitative assessment of changes in anterior segment morphology after argon laser peripheral iridoplasty: findings from the EARL study group. *Clin Exp Ophthalmol.* 2019;47(1):33–40.

Ng WS, Ang GS, Azuara-Blanco A. Laser peripheral iridoplasty for angle-closure. *Cochrane Database Syst Rev.* 2012;(2):CD006746.

Primary Angle Closure

Primary angle closure is defined by the presence of a narrow angle, as in PACS, along with PAS and/or elevated IOP (>21 mm Hg). The angle can close gradually, with a slow increase in IOP as angle function progressively becomes compromised. Even in the absence of synechial angle closure, there can be damage to the trabecular meshwork from appositional iridotrabecular contact, leading to increased IOP. The chronic form of PAC, in which there is gradual, asymptomatic synechial angle closure, is the most common presentation of angle-closure disease.

Management

An LPI is usually necessary to relieve the pupillary block component and reduce the potential for further synechial angle closure. However, there is some debate about performing LPI in an eye with extensive synechiae, as IOP elevation may occur (see Treatment Controversies). Without an iridotomy, closure of the angle usually progresses, making the IOP more difficult to control. Even with a patent peripheral iridotomy, progressive angle closure can occur, and repeated periodic gonioscopy is imperative. An iridotomy with or without long-term use of ocular hypotensive medications controls the disease in most patients with PAC. However, the EAGLE study suggests that in PAC cases with IOP of ≥30 mm Hg, lensectomy may be the preferred treatment (see Treatment Controversies).

Azuara-Blanco A, Burr J, Ramsay C, et al; EAGLE study group. Effectiveness of early lens extraction for the treatment of primary angle-closure glaucoma (EAGLE): a randomised controlled trial. *Lancet.* 2016;388(10052):1389–1397.

Primary Angle-Closure Glaucoma

Primary angle-closure glaucoma (PACG) is a form of angle-closure disease in which the conditions of PAC are met, and there is also optic nerve damage and/or visual field loss consistent with glaucomatous optic neuropathy. Because of the insidious nature of this condition, vision loss may be the presenting symptom. Accordingly, this disease tends to be diagnosed in its later stages and is a major cause of blindness in Asia. The clinical course of PACG usually resembles that of open-angle glaucoma in its lack of initial symptoms, modest elevation of IOP, progressive glaucomatous optic nerve damage, and characteristic patterns of visual field loss. Over time, however, IOP can rise precipitously and become more difficult to control. The diagnosis of PACG is frequently overlooked, and this condition is commonly confused with POAG. As previously noted, gonioscopic examination of all glaucoma patients is important to establish an accurate diagnosis.

Management

As with PAC, LPI is considered the standard of care. It has similar precautions related to eyes with extensive PAS in which a paradoxical rise in IOP can occur (see Treatment Controversies).

Medical treatment for PACG can include both aqueous suppressants and outflow drugs. Prostaglandin analogues are very effective for lowering IOP in angle-closure glaucoma, with efficacy similar to or exceeding that of β-blockers. The degree of IOP reduction does not seem to correlate with the amount of permanent angle closure. The efficacy of other outflow drugs, such as Rho kinase inhibitors, has yet to be established.

Cataract surgery alone is beneficial in reducing IOP and use of medications, and it compares favorably to cataract extraction combined with trabeculectomy. The recent EAGLE study showed that lens extraction can be an effective option in treating PACG. (See also Treatment Controversies.)

Chen R, Yang K, Zheng Z, Ong ML, Wang NL, Zhan SY. Meta-analysis of the efficacy and safety of latanoprost monotherapy in patients with angle-closure glaucoma. *J Glaucoma.* 2016;25(3):e134–144.

Tham CC, Kwong YY, Leung DY, et al. Phacoemulsification versus combined phacotrabeculectomy in medically controlled chronic angle closure glaucoma with cataract. *Ophthalmology.* 2008;115(12):2167–2173.e2.

Tham CC, Kwong YY, Leung DY, et al. Phacoemulsification versus combined phacotrabeculectomy in medically uncontrolled chronic angle closure glaucoma with cataracts. *Ophthalmology.* 2009;116(4):725–731, 731.e1–3.

Symptomatic Primary Angle Closure

IOP elevation with acute or subacute blockage of most of the angle can cause symptomatic angle closure.

Subacute primary angle closure

Subacute, or *intermittent, angle closure* is a condition characterized by episodes of blurred vision, halos, and mild pain caused by elevated IOP. Vague symptoms of pain or headache not associated with visual symptoms have a low specificity for angle closure. The visual symptoms resolve spontaneously, especially during sleep-induced miosis, and the IOP is usually normal between episodes, which occur periodically over days, months, or years. These episodes are often confused with headaches or migraines, so obtaining a careful history is required. The correct diagnosis can be made only with a high index of suspicion and gonioscopy. The typical history and the gonioscopic appearance of a narrow angle with or without PAS help establish the diagnosis. The management of subacute primary angle closure is similar to that of PAC.

Acute primary angle closure

In *acute primary angle closure (APAC),* IOP rises rapidly as a result of relatively sudden blockage of the trabecular meshwork by the iris. APAC, which is sometimes called *acute angle-closure crisis,* is typically manifested by ocular pain, headache, blurred vision, and rainbow-colored halos around lights. Acute systemic distress may result in nausea and vomiting. The rise in IOP to relatively high levels causes corneal epithelial edema, which is responsible for the visual symptoms. Signs of acute angle closure include

- high IOP
- mid-dilated, sluggish, and irregularly shaped pupil
- corneal epithelial edema
- congested episcleral and conjunctival blood vessels
- shallow peripheral anterior chamber
- mild amount of aqueous flare and cells

Diagnosis Definitive diagnosis depends on gonioscopic verification of angle closure. Gonioscopy should be possible in almost all cases of APAC, although clearing of corneal edema with topical IOP-lowering therapy, topical glycerin, or paracentesis may be necessary to allow visualization of the angle. Dynamic gonioscopy, with indentation of the central cornea, may help the clinician determine whether the iris–trabecular meshwork blockage is reversible *(appositional closure)* or irreversible *(synechial closure),* and it may also be therapeutic in breaking the attack of acute angle closure. Gonioscopy of the fellow eye in a patient with APAC usually reveals a narrow, occludable angle. The presence of a deep angle in the fellow eye should prompt the clinician to search for secondary causes of elevated IOP, such as a posterior segment mass, zonular insufficiency, anterior segment neovascularization, or the iridocorneal endothelial syndrome, among others. When performing gonioscopy, the clinician should note the effect of the examination light on the angle recess; the slit-lamp beam can cause pupillary constriction, thus artificially opening the inherently narrow angle recess (see Fig 9-2).

During an acute attack, the IOP may be high enough to cause glaucomatous optic nerve damage, ischemic optic neuropathy, and/or retinal vascular occlusion. PAS can form rapidly, and IOP-induced ischemia may produce sector atrophy of the iris, releasing pigment. This causes pigmentary dusting of the iris surface and corneal endothelium. Iris ischemia, specifically of the iris sphincter muscle, may cause the pupil to become permanently fixed and dilated. *Glaukomflecken,* characteristic small anterior subcapsular lens opacities, may also develop as a result of necrosis. These findings are helpful in the detection of previous episodes of APAC.

Management The definitive treatment for APAC associated with pupillary block is usually LPI (discussed in Chapter 13). Once an iridotomy has been performed, the pupillary block is relieved and the pressure gradient between the posterior and anterior chambers is normalized, which in most cases allows the iris to fall away from the trabecular meshwork. As a result, the anterior chamber deepens, and the angle opens. However, corneal edema at presentation may interfere with the creation of a patent LPI, and medications or procedures may be needed to break the attack and clear the cornea until iridotomy can be performed.

If the APAC is mild, it may be broken by cholinergic agents (pilocarpine 1%–2%), which induce miosis that pulls the peripheral iris away from the trabecular meshwork. However, these agents may worsen some types of angle closure without pupillary block and exacerbate pupillary block in some eyes. Stronger miotics are ideally avoided, as they may increase the vascular congestion of the iris or rotate the lens–iris interface more anteriorly, increasing the pupillary block. Moreover, when the IOP is markedly elevated (eg, >40–50 mm Hg), the pupillary sphincter may be ischemic and unresponsive to miotic agents alone. Consequently, in most cases, the patient is treated with other topical agents, including β-adrenergic antagonists, α_2-adrenergic agonists, and/or prostaglandin analogues; and with topical, oral, or intravenous carbonic anhydrase inhibitors. If needed, hyperosmotic agents may be administered orally or intravenously. Nonselective adrenergic agonists or medications with significant α_1-adrenergic activity (apraclonidine) would ideally be avoided to prevent further pupillary dilation and iris ischemia.

Globe compression over the central cornea, dynamic gonioscopy, and careful paracentesis with a 30-gauge needle or sharp blade are all techniques to acutely lower the IOP in order to clear the corneal edema. Care must be taken with these maneuvers, as they can easily injure the lens or iris. A peripheral iridotomy or, in certain circumstances, lens extraction should be performed once the attack is broken and the cornea is of adequate clarity. Following resolution of the acute attack, it is important to reevaluate the angle by gonioscopy to assess the degree of residual synechial angle closure and to confirm the reopening of at least part of the angle. Laser peripheral iridoplasty may also help relieve acute attacks. In rare cases, a surgical iridectomy is required; these procedures are discussed in Chapter 13. Lensectomy is also a viable treatment option, although LPI may be more easily accomplished in the acute setting, especially if the eye is inflamed.

Improved IOP does not necessarily mean that the angle has opened. Because of ciliary body ischemia and reduced aqueous production, the IOP may remain low for weeks following acute angle closure. Thus, IOP may be a poor indicator of angle function or anatomy. A second gonioscopy or serial gonioscopy is therefore essential for follow-up of the patient to be certain that the angle has adequately opened.

In most cases of APAC, the fellow eye shares the anatomic predisposition for increased pupillary block and is at high risk of developing the same condition, especially if the inciting mechanism included a systemic sympathomimetic agent such as a nasal decongestant or an anticholinergic agent. In addition, the pain and emotional upset resulting from the involvement of the first eye may increase sympathetic flow to the fellow eye, resulting in pupillary dilation. It is recommended that a peripheral iridotomy be performed in the fellow eye if a similar angle configuration is present.

Lam DS, Leung DY, Tham CC, et al. Randomized trial of early phacoemulsification versus peripheral iridotomy to prevent intraocular pressure rise after acute primary angle closure. *Ophthalmology.* 2008;115(7):1134–1140.

Plateau Iris

Plateau iris refers to an atypical configuration of the anterior chamber angle that may result in angle-closure disease. It is a common finding in younger subjects with angle closure. Evidence suggests that plateau iris configuration may result from more anteriorly positioned ciliary processes, which can be seen as an absence of the ciliary sulcus on ultrasound biomicroscopy (UBM) imaging. Angle closure in plateau iris is most often caused by these anteriorly positioned ciliary processes severely narrowing the anterior chamber recess by pushing the peripheral iris forward. A component of pupillary block is often present. The angle may be further compromised following dilation of the pupil, as the peripheral iris crowds and obstructs the trabecular meshwork.

Plateau iris may be suspected if the central anterior chamber appears to be of normal depth, and the iris plane appears flat for an eye with angle closure. This suspicion can be confirmed by the presence of the *"double-hump" sign* on gonioscopy (the iris is indented by the anteriorly situated ciliary processes, creating the appearance of a hump in the iris contour during indentation gonioscopy) or by ultrasound biomicroscopy (see Fig 9-3). The condition will be missed if the examiner relies solely on slit-lamp examination or the Van Herick method of angle examination.

Plateau iris configuration is the term used to describe an eye with gonioscopic and/or imaging evidence of plateau iris in which a mydriatic provocative test does not induce IOP elevation. Conversely, in plateau iris syndrome, pharmacologic mydriasis induces IOP elevation of 6 mm Hg or more. In plateau iris syndrome, PAS formation has been reported to begin at the Schwalbe line (see Fig 9-3) and then to extend in a posterior direction over the trabecular meshwork, scleral spur, and angle recess. The reverse is seen in pupillary block–induced angle closure, in which synechiae form in the posterior-to-anterior direction.

Management

The initial management of plateau iris includes either laser iridotomy to remove any component of pupillary block or lensectomy if cataract is present. Eyes with plateau iris configuration may be monitored without further intervention. Eyes with plateau iris syndrome remain predisposed to angle closure—and possible acute attack—despite a patent iridotomy because of the peripheral iris anatomy. Plateau iris syndrome is the most common reason for a persistently narrow or occludable angle after LPI or cataract surgery. Thus, careful assessment of the angle following iridotomy or lensectomy is necessary to determine whether additional treatment is required to further deepen the angle. Combined lensectomy and endoscopic cyclophotocoagulation (ECP) can also be utilized to deepen the angle in plateau iris, as ECP causes the collagen fibers to contract and shrinks the ciliary processes, and may also rotate the ciliary processes posteriorly away from the peripheral iris.

Patients with plateau iris syndrome may be treated with long-term miotic therapy. However, laser peripheral iridoplasty may be more useful in individuals with this condition to flatten and thin the peripheral iris (see Fig 9-3 and Chapter 13). Repeated gonioscopy at regular intervals is necessary because the risk of chronic angle closure remains despite measures to deepen the angle recess. The management of plateau iris syndrome is evolving, and further research is needed to determine the optimal management of this condition.

Li Y, Wang YE, Huang G, et al. Prevalence and characteristics of plateau iris configuration among American Caucasian, American Chinese and mainland Chinese subjects. *Br J Ophthalmol.* 2014;98(4):474–478.

Kumar RS, Tantisevi V, Wong MH, et al. Plateau iris in Asian subjects with primary angle closure glaucoma. *Arch Ophthalmol.* 2009;127(10):1269–1272.

Pavlin CJ, Foster FS. Plateau iris syndrome: changes in angle opening associated with dark, light, and pilocarpine administration. *Am J Ophthalmol.* 1999;128(3):288–291.

Ritch R, Chang BM, Liebmann JM. Angle closure in younger patients. *Ophthalmology.* 2003;110(10):1880–1889.

CHAPTER 10

Secondary Angle Closure

Highlights

- Secondary angle closure can occur in a variety of settings, including anterior segment neovascularization and inflammation and after surgery.
- Secondary angle closure can be divided into types with pupillary block or without pupillary block.
- Detection of iris and angle neovascularization requires careful observation with the slit lamp and gonioscopy.
- Control of neovascular glaucoma has dramatically improved with the use of anti–vascular endothelial growth factor (anti-VEGF) therapy and, when combined with panretinal photocoagulation, can often obviate the need for surgical intervention.
- It is important to ask patients presenting with acute bilateral angle closure about the use of drugs, including topiramate, that can induce secondary angle closure.

Introduction

Secondary angle closure can be divided mechanistically into types with pupillary block and those without pupillary block. Non–pupillary block secondary angle closure can be further categorized as being caused by either "pushing" or "pulling" mechanisms (or possibly both), that is, those that push the iris forward from behind or those that pull the iris forward into contact with the trabecular meshwork. Table 10-1 shows the classification of secondary non–pupillary block angle closure according to pushing or pulling mechanisms.

Secondary Angle Closure With Pupillary Block

Lens-Induced Angle Closure

Phacomorphic glaucoma

The mechanism of phacomorphic glaucoma is typically multifactorial. However, by definition, a significant component of the pathologic angle narrowing is related to the acquired mass effect of the cataractous lens itself. As seen in the primary angle-closure (PAC) spectrum, pupillary block often plays an important role in this condition. Phacomorphic narrowing of the angle generally occurs slowly with formation of the cataract. However, in some cases, the onset may be acute and rapid, precipitated by marked lens

Table 10-1 Underlying Mechanisms of Non–Pupillary Block Angle Closure

Anterior pulling mechanisms	
	Contraction of inflammatory membrane or fibrovascular tissue
	Migration of corneal endothelium (iridocorneal endothelial syndrome)
	Fibrous ingrowth
	Epithelial ingrowth
	Iris incarceration in traumatic wound or surgical incision
Posterior pushing mechanisms	
	Malignant glaucoma (also referred to as aqueous misdirection)
	Ciliary body swelling, inflammation, or cysts
	Anteriorly located ciliary processes (plateau iris configuration/syndrome)
	Choroidal swelling, serous or hemorrhagic choroidal detachments, or effusions
	Posterior segment tumors or space-occupying lesions (silicone oil, gas bubble)
	Contraction of retrolental tissue (persistent fetal vasculature, retinopathy of prematurity)
	Anteriorly displaced lens
	Encircling retinal bands or scleral buckles

swelling *(intumescence)* as a result of cataract formation and the development of pupillary block in an eye that is not otherwise anatomically predisposed to closure (Figs 10-1, 10-2).

Distinguishing between the PAC spectrum and phacomorphic angle closure is not always straightforward, but making the distinction may not be necessary, as the treatment of both conditions is similar. However, the anterior chamber depth (ACD), gonioscopic appearance, and degree of cataract differ between eyes on the PAC spectrum and those with phacomorphic angle closure, and these differences can help the clinician determine the etiology (see also BCSC Section 11, *Lens and Cataract*). Several methods of anterior segment imaging (anterior segment optical coherence tomography [AS-OCT], ultrasound

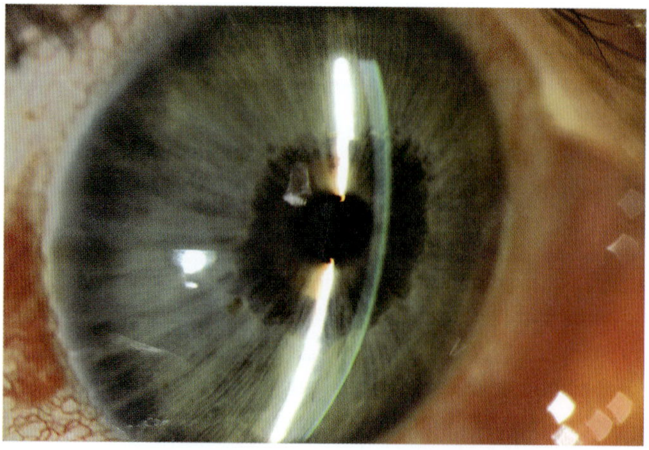

Figure 10-1 Phacomorphic glaucoma. Lens intumescence precipitates pupillary block and secondary angle closure in an eye not anatomically predisposed to angle closure. *(Courtesy of Wallace L.M. Alward, MD. From the* Iowa Glaucoma Curriculum *[curriculum.iowaglaucoma.org]. © The University of Iowa.)*

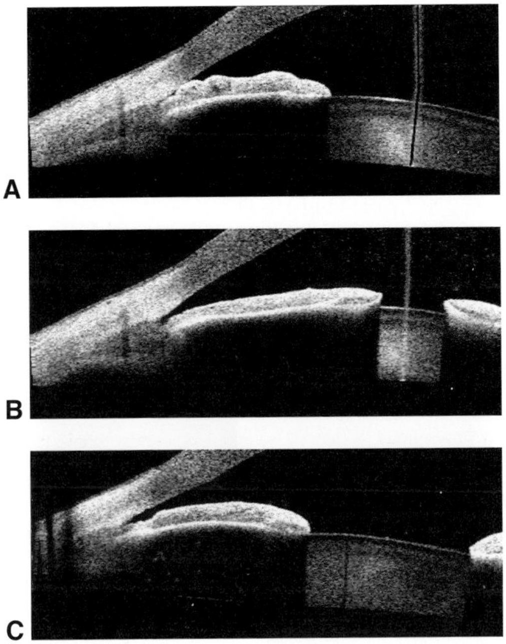

Figure 10-2 Phacomorphic glaucoma. **A,** In this example, the angle remains narrow despite a patent iridotomy. **B,** In bright light, the angle is transiently made deeper by pupil constriction. **C,** In this case, a longer-term solution is provided by thinning the peripheral iris with laser iridoplasty. Lensectomy is also an effective treatment strategy. *(Courtesy of Yaniv Barkana, MD.)*

biomicroscopy [UBM], and Scheimpflug) provide parameters that can assist in the diagnosis. For example, AS-OCT in patients with phacomorphic angle closure showed that the ACD was about half that of control eyes (1.4 mm vs 2.8 mm) and that the lens vault was triple the value of controls (1.4 mm vs 0.4 mm).

Laser peripheral iridotomy (LPI) followed by cataract extraction in a quiet eye is the traditional treatment. However, in many cases, the iridotomy is unnecessary, because cataract surgery is the definitive treatment in eyes that have the potential for improved vision. Cholinergic agents have no role in the treatment of this condition because they may further narrow the angle (by increasing the pupillary block and causing forward movement of the lens–iris interface due to zonular laxity) and worsen vision in the presence of cataract. In addition, the miotic pupil makes subsequent cataract surgery more challenging.

Ectopia lentis

Ectopia lentis is defined as displacement of the crystalline lens from its normal anatomic position (Fig 10-3). With forward displacement, pupillary block may occur, resulting in iris bombé, shallowing of the anterior chamber angle, and secondary angle closure. Common causes of lens subluxation include

- pseudoexfoliation syndrome
- trauma
- Marfan syndrome
- homocystinuria

- microspherophakia
- Weill-Marchesani syndrome
- Ehlers-Danlos syndrome
- sulfite oxidase deficiency

The most common cause of acquired zonular insufficiency and crystalline lens subluxation is *pseudoexfoliation syndrome* (Fig 10-4).

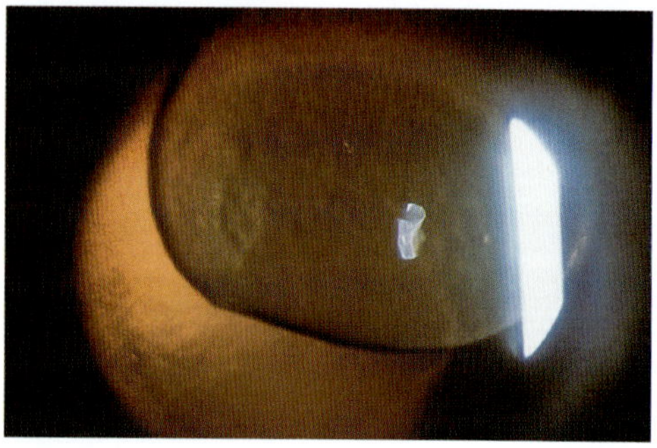

Figure 10-3 Ectopia lentis: dislocation of the lens into the anterior chamber through a dilated pupil. *(Courtesy of Ron Gross, MD.)*

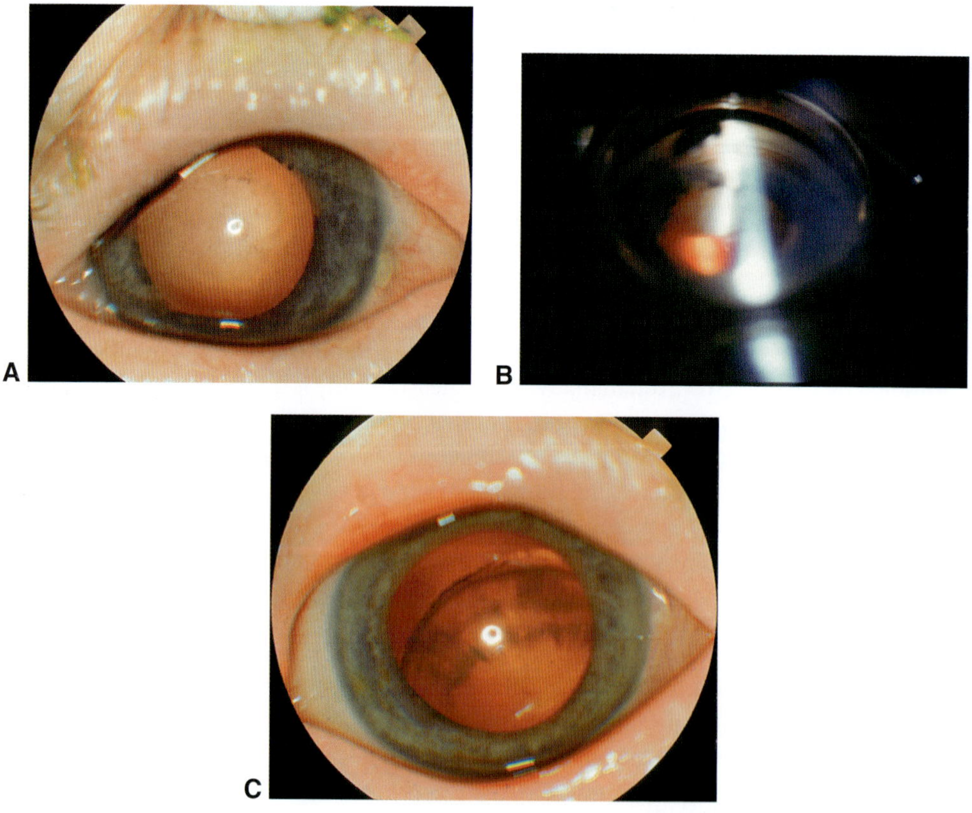

Figure 10-4 Pseudoexfoliation syndrome is a common cause of subluxation of the crystalline lens. **A,** Right eye of a patient with complete dislocation of the lens. **B,** Gonioscopic view of the same eye reveals that the dislocated lens is in the inferior vitreous cavity. **C,** Left eye (same patient) showing subluxation of the lens. *(Courtesy of Thomas W. Samuelson, MD.)*

The treatment of choice is the creation of 2 laser iridotomies 180° apart so that both will not be occluded simultaneously by the lens. This relieves the pupillary block and is a temporizing measure until more definitive lensectomy, if indicated to improve visual function, can be performed. Lens extraction is usually indicated to restore vision and to reduce the risk of recurrent pupillary block and peripheral anterior synechiae (PAS) formation.

Microspherophakia

Microspherophakia, a congenital disorder in which the lens has a spherical or globular shape, may cause ectopia lentis and subsequent pupillary block with resultant angle closure (Fig 10-5). Treatment with cycloplegia may tighten the zonules, flatten the lens, and pull it posteriorly, breaking the pupillary block. Miotics may make the condition worse by increasing the pupillary block and by rotating the ciliary body forward, loosening the zonules and allowing the lens to become more globular. Microspherophakia is often familial and may occur as an isolated condition or as part of Weill-Marchesani or Marfan syndrome.

Aphakic or pseudophakic angle closure

Pupillary block may occur in aphakic and pseudophakic eyes. Vitreous can block the pupil and/or an iridotomy site in aphakic or pseudophakic eyes or in a phakic eye with a dislocated lens. Generally, the anterior chamber shallows, and the iris assumes a bombé configuration. Treatment with mydriatic and cycloplegic agents may restore aqueous flow through the pupil but may also make performing a laser iridotomy difficult initially. Topical β-adrenergic antagonists, α_2-adrenergic agonists, carbonic anhydrase inhibitors, and hyperosmotic agents can be effective in reducing intraocular pressure (IOP) prior to performing an iridotomy. One or more laser iridotomies may be required.

Pupillary block may also occur with anterior chamber intraocular lenses (ACIOLs). An iridectomy or early postoperative iridotomy should be performed when an ACIOL is implanted. This is to prevent pupillary block from developing as a result of apposition of the iris to the ACIOL optic or apposition of the vitreous face to the pupil–optic complex. If pupillary block occurs, the peripheral iris bows forward around the ACIOL and occludes the angle. In this instance, the central chamber remains deep relative to the peripheral chamber because the ACIOL itself prevents the central portions of the iris and vitreous face from moving forward. Laser iridotomies, often multiple, are required to relieve the

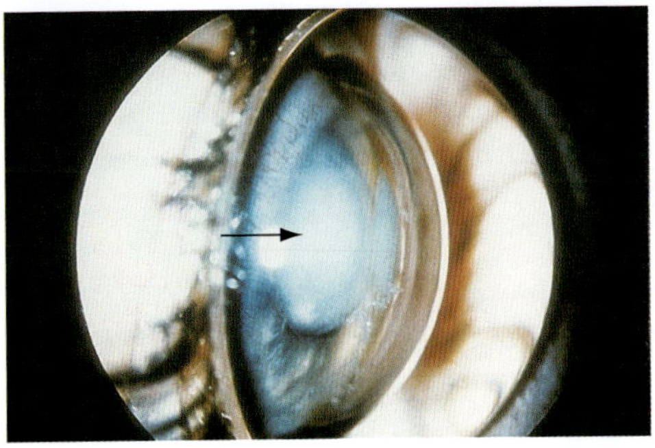

Figure 10-5 Ectopia lentis due to microspherophakia. The lens *(arrow)* is trapped anteriorly by the pupil, resulting in iris bombé and a dramatic shallowing of the anterior chamber. *(Courtesy of G.L. Spaeth, MD.)*

pupillary block. In rare cases, pupillary block can occur in the presence of an iridectomy if the lens haptic or vitreous obstructs the iridectomy site or the pupil.

In addition, pupillary block can occur following posterior capsulotomy when vitreous obstructs the pupil. A condition referred to as *capsular block* may also be seen, wherein retained viscoelastic or fluid in the capsular bag pushes a posterior chamber intraocular lens (IOL) anteriorly, which may narrow the angle.

Secondary Angle Closure Without Pupillary Block

A number of disorders can lead to secondary angle closure without pupillary block. This form of secondary angle closure may occur through 1 of 2 mechanisms (see Table 10-1):

- *a pulling mechanism,* caused by contraction of an inflammatory, hemorrhagic, cellular, or vascular membrane, band, or exudate in the angle, leading to PAS formation
- a *pushing mechanism,* caused by forward displacement of the lens–iris interface, often accompanied by swelling and anterior rotation of the ciliary body

Conditions Associated With a Pulling Mechanism

Neovascular glaucoma

This common, severe type of secondary angle closure is characterized by anterior segment neovascularization along with a fibrovascular membrane on the surface of the iris, pupillary margin, and trabecular meshwork. It is caused by a variety of disorders that involve retinal or ocular ischemia or ocular inflammation (Table 10-2), most commonly diabetic retinopathy, central retinal vein occlusion (CRVO), branch retinal vein occlusion (BRVO), and ocular

Table 10-2 Disorders Predisposing to Neovascularization of the Iris and Angle

Systemic vascular diseases	**Other ocular diseases**
Carotid occlusive disease[a]	Chronic uveitis
Carotid artery ligation	Chronic retinal detachment
Carotid-cavernous fistula	Endophthalmitis
Giant cell arteritis	Stickler syndrome
Takayasu (pulseless) disease	Retinoschisis
	Pseudoexfoliation syndrome
Ocular vascular diseases	**Intraocular tumors**
Diabetic retinopathy[a]	Uveal melanoma
Central retinal vein occlusion[a]	Metastatic carcinoma
Central retinal artery occlusion	Retinoblastoma
Branch retinal vein occlusion	Lymphoma
Sickle cell retinopathy	Reticulum cell sarcoma
Coats disease	**Ocular therapy**
Eales disease	Radiation therapy
Retinopathy of prematurity	**Trauma**
Persistent fetal vasculature	
Syphilitic vasculitis	
Anterior segment ischemia	

[a]Most common causes.

ischemic syndrome. Anterior segment neovascularization can also occur with metastatic or other tumors of the eye, such as retinoblastomas, medulloepitheliomas, and choroidal melanomas, as well as following radiation treatment, resulting in neovascular glaucoma.

The pathophysiology of neovascular glaucoma most often involves secretion of angiogenic factors, especially vascular endothelial growth factor (VEGF), from ischemic retinal tissue. These angiogenic factors can diffuse into the anterior chamber and cause iris and angle neovascularization. In rare instances, anterior segment neovascularization may occur without demonstrable retinal ischemia, as in Fuchs uveitis syndrome and other types of uveitis, pseudoexfoliation syndrome, or isolated iris melanomas. When an ocular cause cannot be found, carotid artery occlusive disease should be considered.

Clinically, patients often present with acute IOP elevation together with reduced vision, ocular pain, conjunctival hyperemia, and microcystic corneal edema. In establishing a diagnosis, the clinician should distinguish dilated iris vessels associated with inflammation from neovascularization. Neovascularization of the anterior segment usually develops in a classic pattern, beginning with fine vascular tufts at the pupillary margin. As these vessels grow, they extend radially over the iris (Fig 10-6). Unlike dilated stromal vessels, these vessels are delicate and lacy and do not adhere to the normal anterior segment vasculature. Further, when they involve the angle, they cross the ciliary body face and scleral spur as fine single vessels that branch as they reach the trabecular meshwork (Fig 10-7). Often, the trabecular meshwork takes on a reddish coloration. With contraction of the fibrovascular membrane, PAS develop and coalesce, gradually closing the angle. Although the fibrovascular membrane can cause ectropion uveae, it typically does not grow over healthy corneal endothelium (Figs 10-8, 10-9). Thus, the PAS end at the Schwalbe line, distinguishing this condition from iridocorneal endothelial syndrome, which also features ectropion uveae. When performing gonioscopy in patients with possible neovascularization, the clinician may find it helpful to use a bright slit-lamp beam and high magnification to better visualize the fine vessels.

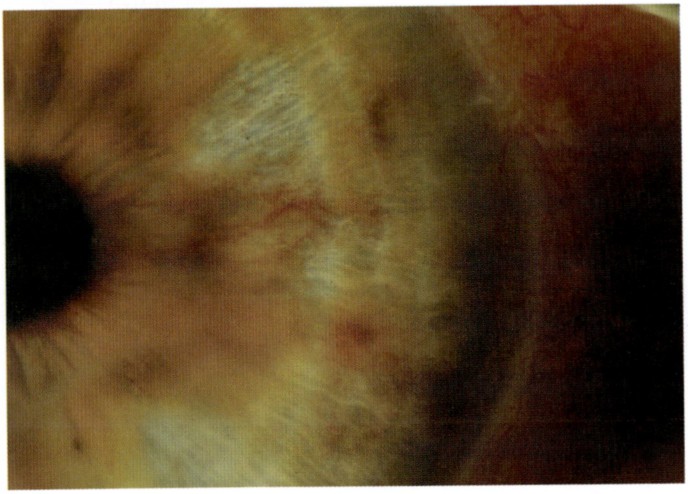

Figure 10-6 Iris neovascularization usually begins at the pupillary margin. Here there is more extensive iris neovascularization with radial extension along the iris surface. *(Courtesy of Angelo P. Tanna, MD.)*

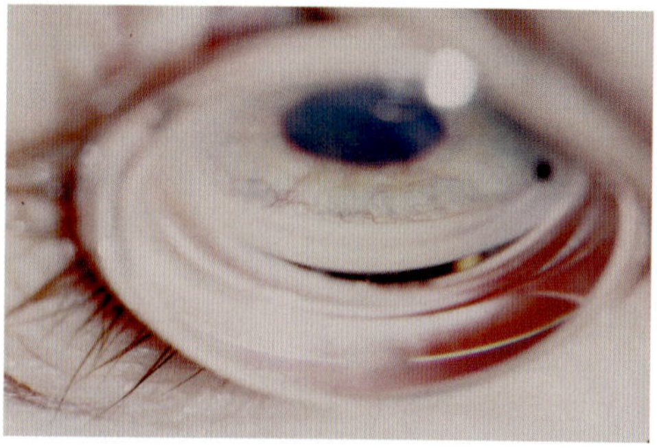

Figure 10-7 Iris neovascularization. With progressive angle involvement, peripheral anterior synechiae (PAS) develop with contraction of the fibrovascular membrane, resulting in secondary neovascular glaucoma. *(Courtesy of H. Dunbar Hoskins, MD. From the Glaucoma Center of San Francisco archives.)*

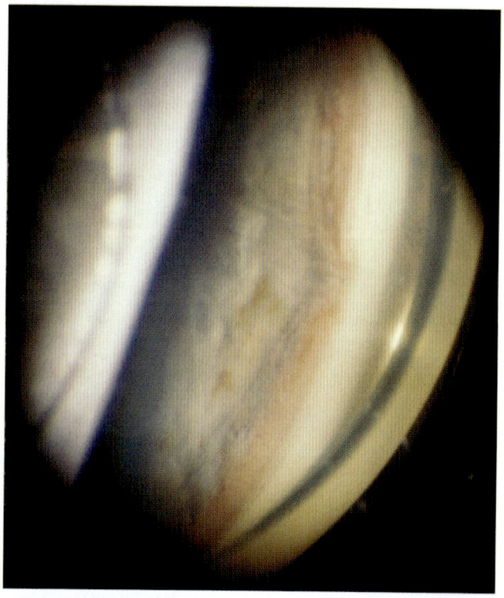

Figure 10-8 With end-stage neovascular glaucoma, total angle closure occurs, obscuring the iris neovascularization. The PAS end at the Schwalbe line because the fibrovascular membrane does not grow over healthy corneal endothelium. *(Courtesy of Wallace L.M. Alward, MD. From the* Iowa Glaucoma Curriculum *[curriculum.iowaglaucoma.org]. © The University of Iowa.)*

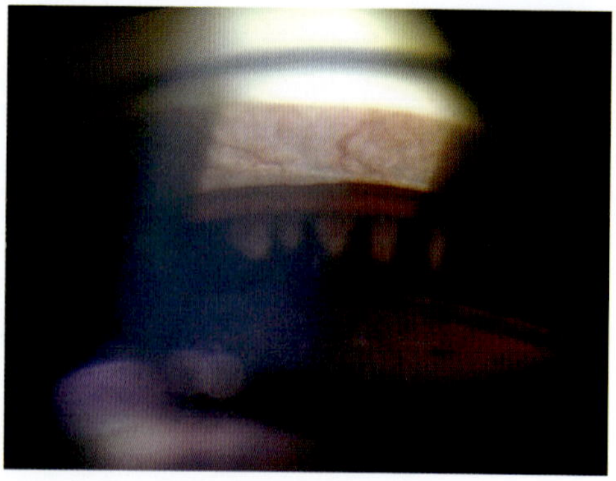

Figure 10-9 With vessel growth, iris neovascularization extends from the pupillary margin radially toward the anterior chamber angle. *(Courtesy of Wallace L.M. Alward, MD. From the* Iowa Glaucoma Curriculum *[curriculum.iowaglaucoma.org]. © The University of Iowa.)*

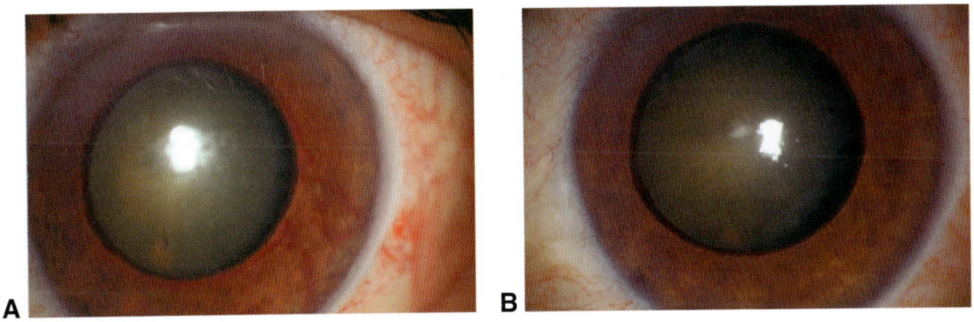

Figure 10-10 Effect of bevacizumab on iris neovascularization. **A,** Slit-lamp photograph of florid iris neovascularization taken prior to injection of bevacizumab. **B,** Regression of iris neovascularization 4 days after treatment with bevacizumab. *(Courtesy of Nicholas P. Bell, MD.)*

Because the prognosis for neovascular glaucoma is typically poor, prevention and early diagnosis are essential. In CRVO, angle neovascularization develops without iris neovascularization in approximately 4% of patients. Thus, gonioscopy is important for early diagnosis. Since the most common cause of iris neovascularization is ischemic retinopathy, the definitive treatment when the ocular media are clear is panretinal photocoagulation (PRP). However, intravitreal anti-VEGF therapy can be used to acutely reduce the neovascular stimulus. The regression of neovascularization after PRP, anti-VEGF therapy, or both may reduce or normalize IOP, depending on the extent of PAS. Even in the presence of total synechial angle closure, PRP may improve the success rate of subsequent glaucoma surgery by eliminating the angiogenic stimulus and may decrease the risk of hemorrhage at the time of surgery. More recently, anti-VEGF agents have been successfully employed to promote regression of the neovascular tissue prior to filtering surgery (Fig 10-10) and to improve outcomes. Although anti-VEGF treatment can substantially delay surgery, studies have shown that PRP is the most important factor in obviating the need for IOP-lowering surgery for neovascular glaucoma.

Medical management of neovascular glaucoma yields variable success and is sometimes only a temporizing measure until more definitive incisional or laser surgery is undertaken. Topical β-adrenergic antagonists, α_2-adrenergic agonists, carbonic anhydrase inhibitors, cycloplegics, and corticosteroids may be useful in reducing IOP and decreasing inflammation, either as a long-term therapy or prior to filtering surgery. Incisional glaucoma surgery is more likely to be successful if performed after the neovascularization has regressed following PRP or anti-VEGF therapy. In many cases, tube shunt surgery, usually with a valved device, is the surgical procedure of choice. If these therapies fail or if the eye has poor visual potential, either endoscopic or transscleral cyclophotocoagulation can be considered as an alternative. See Chapter 13 for discussion of these procedures.

Havens SJ, Gulati V. Neovascular glaucoma. *Dev Ophthalmol.* 2016;55:196–204.

Iridocorneal endothelial syndrome

Iridocorneal endothelial (ICE) syndrome is a group of disorders characterized by abnormal corneal endothelial cells that behave like epithelial cells in that they proliferate, migrate, and fail to exhibit contact inhibition. These abnormal endothelial cells cause variable degrees of iris atrophy, secondary angle closure, and corneal edema. (See also BCSC Section 8, *External Disease and Cornea.*) Three clinical variants have been described:

- Chandler syndrome
- essential (progressive) iris atrophy
- Cogan-Reese syndrome (sometimes called *iris nevus syndrome*)

Chandler syndrome is the most common type, accounting for approximately 50% of the cases of ICE syndrome.

ICE syndrome is clinically unilateral, occurs more often in women, and most commonly presents between 20 and 50 years of age. No consistent association has been found with other ocular or systemic diseases, and familial cases are very rare. A viral etiology has been postulated for ICE syndrome after lymphocytes were observed on the corneal endothelium of affected individuals. Patients typically present with elevated IOP, decreased vision due to corneal edema, secondary chronic angle-closure glaucoma, or an abnormal iris appearance. In each of the 3 clinical variants, the abnormal corneal endothelium takes on a "beaten bronze" appearance similar to cornea guttata, as seen in Fuchs corneal endothelial dystrophy. Microcystic corneal edema may be present without elevated IOP, especially in Chandler syndrome. The unaffected eye may have subclinical irregularities of the corneal endothelium detectable with confocal or specular microscopy without other manifestations of the disease.

High PAS are characteristic of ICE syndrome (Fig 10-11), and they often extend anterior to the Schwalbe line. The extent of angle closure does not always correlate with the IOP because some angles may be functionally closed by the endothelial membrane without overt PAS formation.

Various degrees of iris atrophy and corneal changes distinguish the specific clinical entities. The *essential iris atrophy variant* of ICE syndrome is characterized by severe progressive iris atrophy resulting in heterochromia, corectopia, ectropion uveae, iris stromal and pigment epithelial atrophy, and hole formation (Fig 10-12). In *Chandler syndrome,* minimal iris atrophy and corectopia occur, and the corneal and angle findings predominate (Fig 10-13). Iris atrophy also tends to be less severe in *Cogan-Reese syndrome,* a condition distinguished by tan pedunculated nodules or diffuse pigmented lesions on the anterior iris surface.

Glaucoma develops in approximately 50% of patients with ICE syndrome and may be more severe in those with essential iris atrophy or Cogan-Reese syndrome. In ICE, the

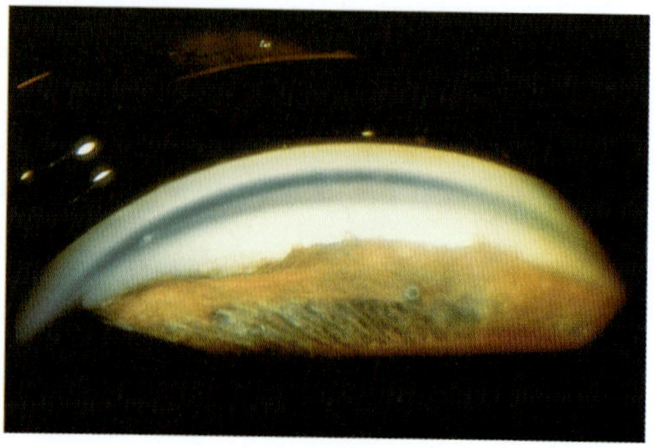

Figure 10-11 The classic high PAS of iridocorneal endothelial syndrome. These PAS extend anterior to the Schwalbe line in this patient with essential iris atrophy. *(Courtesy of Steven T. Simmons, MD.)*

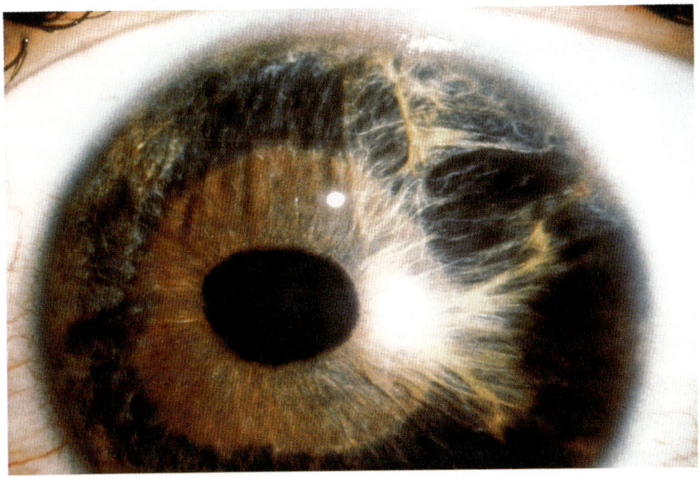

Figure 10-12 Clinical photograph showing corectopia and hole formation, typical findings in essential iris atrophy. *(Courtesy of Steven T. Simmons, MD.)*

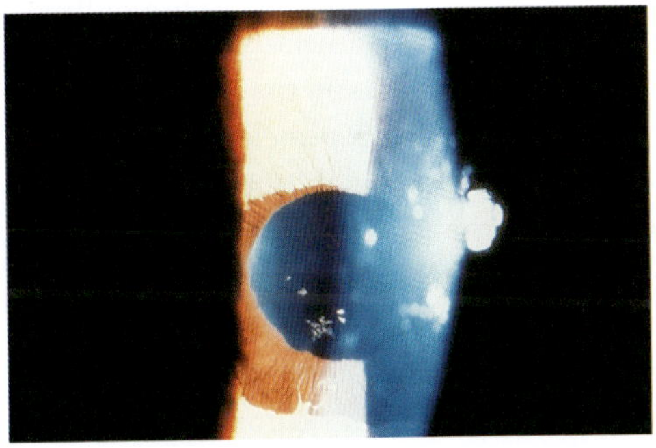

Figure 10-13 Clinical photograph showing ectropion uveae in a patient with Chandler syndrome. *(Courtesy of Steven T. Simmons, MD.)*

corneal endothelium migrates posterior to the Schwalbe line, onto the trabecular meshwork and iris. Electron microscopy has shown the endothelium to vary in thickness, with areas of single and multiple endothelial cell layers and surrounding collagenous and fibrillar tissue. Unlike normal corneal endothelium, filopodial processes and cytoplasmic actin filaments are present, allowing cellular motility. PAS are formed when this migratory endothelium and its surrounding collagenous fibrillar tissue contract.

The diagnosis of ICE syndrome must always be considered in young to middle-aged patients who present with unilateral secondary angle closure. It is particularly important to maintain a high index of suspicion for this condition because it can mimic primary open-angle glaucoma when the iris and corneal features are subtle. Specular microscopy can confirm the diagnosis by demonstrating an asymmetric loss of endothelial cells and atypical endothelial cell morphology in the involved eye.

Therapy is directed toward the corneal edema and IOP reduction. Hypertonic saline solution and medications to reduce the IOP, when elevated, can be effective in controlling the corneal edema. IOP can be lowered with aqueous suppressants and prostaglandin analogues. Miotics are often ineffective. When medical therapy fails, trabeculectomy or tube shunt surgery can be effective. Late failures have been reported with trabeculectomy secondary to endothelialization of the fistula. The fistula can be reopened with the Nd:YAG laser in some cases. Laser trabeculoplasty has no therapeutic role in ICE syndrome.

Epithelial and fibrous ingrowth

Epithelial and fibrous proliferations are rare surgical complications that can cause severe secondary glaucoma. Epithelial and fibrous ingrowth occurs when epithelium, fibroblasts, or both invade the anterior chamber through a defect in a wound site. Fortunately, improved surgical and wound closure techniques have greatly reduced the incidence of these entities. Although both types are potential causes of corneal graft failure, fibrous ingrowth is more common than epithelial ingrowth. Risk factors for developing ingrowth include prolonged inflammation, wound dehiscence, delayed wound closure, and a Descemet membrane tear. Epithelial ingrowth has also been reported following Descemet-stripping automated endothelial keratoplasty.

Epithelial ingrowth presents as a grayish, sheetlike membrane on the trabecular meshwork, iris, ciliary body, and posterior surface of the cornea. It is often associated with vitreous incarceration, wound gape, ocular inflammation, hypotony secondary to choroidal effusions, and corneal edema (Figs 10-14, 10-15). The ingrowth consists of nonkeratinized stratified squamous epithelium with an avascular subepithelial connective tissue layer.

Application of green laser produces characteristic white burns on the epithelial membrane on the iris surface and can help to confirm the diagnosis of epithelial ingrowth and to determine the extent of involvement. If the diagnosis remains in question, cytologic examination of an aqueous humor aspirate can be performed. Cryotherapy is an option for the treatment of epithelial ingrowth. Radical surgery is sometimes necessary to remove the intraocular epithelial membrane and affected tissues and to repair the fistula, but the prognosis remains poor. Thus, the decision to intervene is based on the extent of disease, the visual potential, the status of the fellow eye, and sociomedical circumstances relevant to the affected individual.

Fibrovascular tissue may also proliferate into an eye from a penetrating wound. Unlike epithelial proliferation, *fibrous ingrowth* progresses slowly and is often self-limited. Fibrous ingrowth appears as a thick, gray-white, vascular retrocorneal membrane with an irregular border. The ingrowth often involves the angle, resulting in PAS formation with destruction of the trabecular meshwork (Fig 10-16) and ectropion uveae.

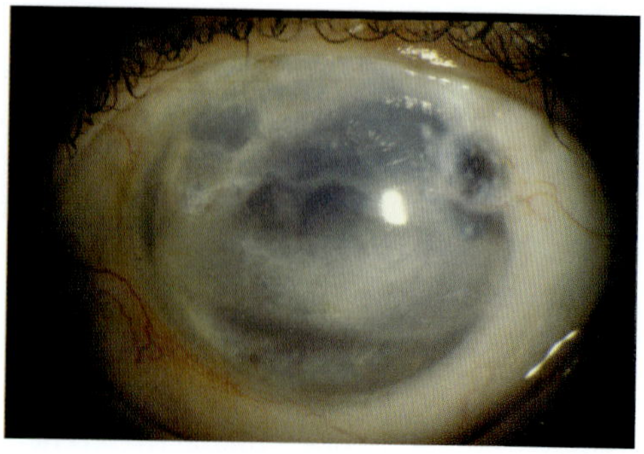

Figure 10-14 Epithelial ingrowth appears as a grayish, sheetlike growth on the endothelial surface of the cornea, usually originating from a surgical incision or traumatic wound. The epithelial ingrowth shown here originated from a glaucoma surgery incision, causing peripheral anterior synechiae. *(Courtesy of Robert Ritch, MD.)*

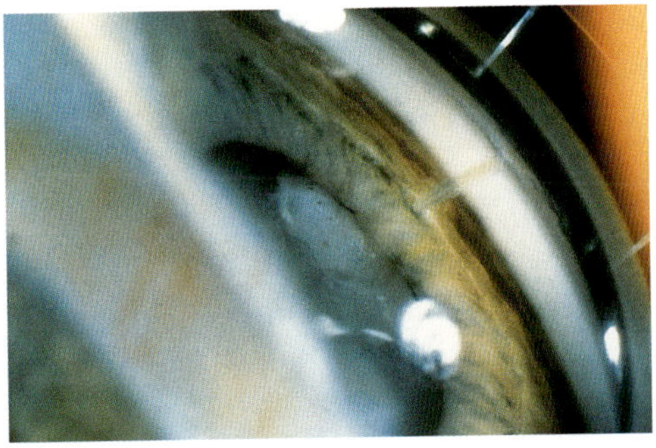

Figure 10-15 Epithelial ingrowth. The precipitating causes of epithelial ingrowth include vitreous incarceration in corneal and scleral wounds, as seen in this photograph, as well as wound gape, ocular inflammation, and hypotony secondary to choroidal effusions. *(Courtesy of Steven T. Simmons, MD.)*

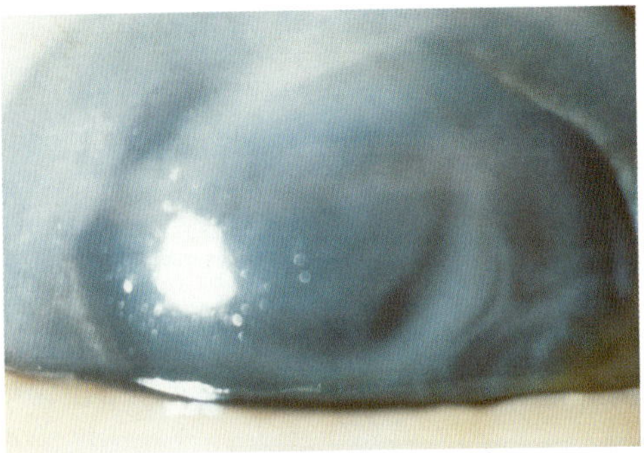

Figure 10-16 Fibrous ingrowth appears as a thick, grayish, retrocorneal membrane that results in high PAS and obstruction of the trabecular meshwork. *(Courtesy of Steven T. Simmons, MD.)*

Trauma

Angle closure without pupillary block may develop after trauma, as a result of PAS formation associated with angle recession or from contusion, hyphema, and inflammation. See Chapter 8 for discussion of trauma.

Conditions Associated With a Pushing Mechanism

Tumors

Tumors in the posterior segment of the eye or anterior uveal cysts may cause unilateral secondary angle closure. Primary choroidal melanomas, ocular metastases, and retinoblastoma are the tumors most commonly responsible. The mechanism of the angle closure is determined by the size, location, and pathology of the tumor. For example, choroidal and retinal tumors tend to shift the lens–iris interface forward as the tumors enlarge, whereas breakdown of the blood–aqueous barrier and inflammation from tissue necrosis can result in posterior synechiae and PAS formation, further exacerbating other underlying mechanisms of angle closure.

Ocular tumors can also cause anterior segment neovascularization leading to angle closure (see the section "Neovascular glaucoma").

Malignant glaucoma

Malignant glaucoma (also called *aqueous misdirection* or *ciliary block glaucoma*) is a rare but potentially devastating form of glaucoma that usually presents following ocular surgery in patients with a history of angle closure. In rare instances, it can occur spontaneously in eyes with an open angle or following cataract surgery or various laser procedures. The disease presents with uniform flattening of both the central and peripheral anterior chamber (Fig 10-17). This is in contrast to acute PAC, which presents with iris bombé and a shallow peripheral anterior chamber (Fig 10-18). In malignant glaucoma, there is typically marked asymmetry between the affected anterior chamber and that of the fellow eye. Classically, the condition has been thought to result from anterior rotation of the ciliary body and posterior misdirection of the aqueous, in association with a relative block to forward aqueous movement at the level of the lens equator, vitreous face, and ciliary processes. However, this historical explanation is a matter of controversy, and some have proposed that it is not physically plausible but, rather, that malignant glaucoma may result from the simultaneous presence of several factors, including a small, anatomically predisposed eye, a propensity for choroidal expansion, and reduced vitreous fluid conductivity.

Clinically, the anterior chamber is shallow or flat, with anterior displacement of the lens, IOL, or vitreous face. Optically clear zones may be seen in the vitreous. Some experts argue this represents aqueous humor trapped in the vitreous cavity; however, this is controversial. In the early postoperative setting, malignant glaucoma is often difficult to distinguish from choroidal effusion, pupillary block, or suprachoroidal hemorrhage. Often, the level of IOP, time frame following surgery, patency of an iridotomy, or presence of a

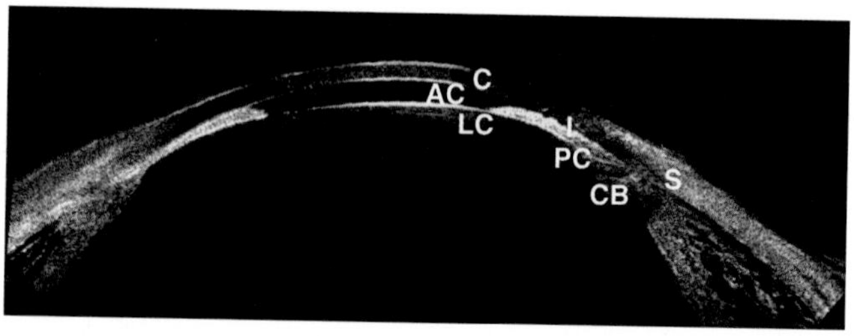

Figure 10-17 Ultrasound biomicroscopy (UBM) of an eye with malignant glaucoma. The lens–iris diaphragm is pushed forward, causing a uniform shallowing of the anterior chamber (AC). The central portion of the anterior lens capsule (LC) is nearly in contact with the cornea (C). Note ciliary body (CB) detachment, which is commonly seen in malignant glaucoma. I=iris; PC=posterior chamber; S=sclera. *(Courtesy of Robert Ritch, MD.)*

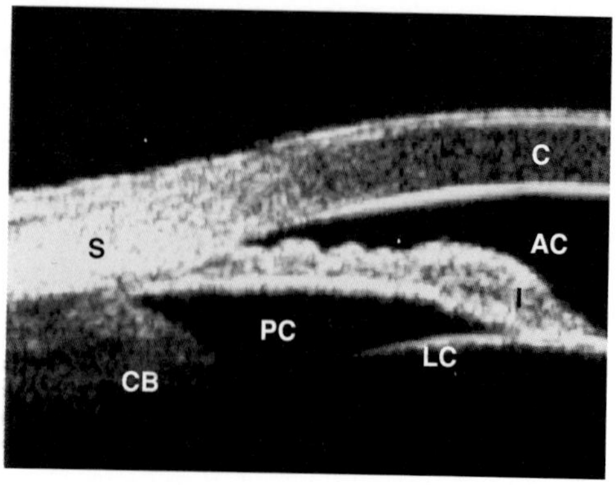

Figure 10-18 UBM of an eye with acute primary angle closure. Pupillary block leads to forward bowing of the peripheral iris. The peripheral chamber is shallow, whereas the central chamber is relatively deep by comparison. AC=anterior chamber; C=cornea; CB=ciliary body; I=iris; LC=lens capsule; PC=posterior chamber; S=sclera. *(From Lundy DC. Ciliary block glaucoma.* Focal Points: Clinical Modules for Ophthalmologists. *American Academy of Ophthalmology; 1999, module 3. Courtesy of Jeffrey M. Liebmann, MD.)*

choroidal effusion or suprachoroidal hemorrhage helps the clinician make the appropriate diagnosis. In some cases, the clinical picture is difficult to interpret, and surgical intervention may be required in order to establish the diagnosis.

Medical management includes the triad of intensive cycloplegic therapy; aggressive aqueous suppression with β-adrenergic antagonists, α_2-adrenergic agonists, and carbonic anhydrase inhibitors; and dehydration of the vitreous with hyperosmotic agents. Miotics can make malignant glaucoma worse and should not be used. In aphakic and pseudophakic eyes, the anterior vitreous can be disrupted with the Nd:YAG laser. Laser photocoagulation of the ciliary processes reportedly has been helpful in treating this condition; this procedure may alter the adjacent vitreous face. In approximately half of patients, malignant glaucoma can be controlled with laser iridotomy and medical management; the other half require surgical intervention alone. The definitive surgical treatment is pars plana vitrectomy with anterior hyaloido-zonulectomy combined with iridectomy and an anterior chamber–deepening procedure. BCSC Section 12, *Retina and Vitreous,* discusses vitrectomy in detail.

Foreman-Larkin J, Netland PA, Salim S. Clinical management of malignant glaucoma [epub ahead of print December 24, 2015]. *J Ophthalmol.* 2015;2015:283707. doi:10.1155/2015/283707

Uveal and ciliary body effusions

Uveal effusion or *uveal hemorrhage* refers to fluid or blood in the potential space between the uvea (choroid and ciliary body) and the sclera. Causes include certain sulfonamide medications (see the section "Drug-induced secondary angle-closure glaucoma"), panretinal photocoagulation, inflammation, infection, penetrating surgery, scleral buckle surgery (see the section "Vitreoretinal surgery"), trauma, retinal vein occlusion, tumor, and uveal effusion syndrome. The suprachoroidal or supraciliary mass effect may result in secondary angle closure related to forward displacement of the lens–iris interface. In addition, exudative retinal detachments can act as space-occupying lesions in the vitreous, which may progressively push the retina forward toward the lens and cause angle closure. Potential causes of exudative retinal detachment include retinoblastoma, Coats disease, metastatic carcinoma, choroidal melanoma, suprachoroidal hemorrhage, choroidal effusion or detachment, infections (eg, HIV), and subretinal neovascularization in age-related macular degeneration with extensive effusion or hemorrhage.

Vitreoretinal surgery

Scleral buckles (especially the encircling bands) used to repair retinal detachments can produce shallowing of the anterior chamber angle and frank angle closure, often accompanied by choroidal effusion and anterior rotation of the ciliary body, causing a flattening of the peripheral iris with a relatively deep central anterior chamber. Vortex vein compression may be responsible for the choroidal effusion. Usually, the anterior chamber deepens with opening of the anterior chamber angle over days to weeks with medical therapy consisting of cycloplegics, anti-inflammatory agents, β-adrenergic antagonists, carbonic anhydrase inhibitors, and hyperosmotic agents. If medical management is unsuccessful, laser iridoplasty, drainage of suprachoroidal fluid, or adjustment of the scleral buckle may be required. The scleral buckle can impede venous drainage by compressing a vortex vein and thus elevating episcleral venous pressure and IOP. Such cases may respond only to moving the scleral buckle or releasing tension on the encircling band. Iridectomy is usually of no benefit in this condition.

Pars plana vitrectomy may lead to angle closure as a result of injection of air, long-acting gases such as sulfur hexafluoride and perfluorocarbon gases (perfluoropropane and perfluoroethane), or silicone oil into the eye. These substances are less dense than water and rise to the top of the eye. An iridotomy may be beneficial and should be located inferiorly to prevent obstruction of the iridotomy site by the gas or oil.

Eyes that have undergone complicated vitreoretinal surgery and have elevated IOP require individualized treatment plans. Therapeutic options include the following: removal of the silicone oil; release of the encircling element; removal of expansile gases; and primary glaucoma surgery, such as trabeculectomy, tube shunt surgery, or a cyclodestructive procedure.

Following *panretinal photocoagulation,* IOP may become elevated by an angle-closure mechanism. The ciliary body is thickened and rotated anteriorly, and, often, an anterior annular choroidal detachment occurs. Generally, this secondary angle closure is self-limited, and therapy consists of temporary medical management with cycloplegic agents, topical corticosteroids, and aqueous suppressants.

Nanophthalmos

A nanophthalmic eye is normal in shape but unusually small, with a shortened axial length (<20 mm), a small corneal diameter, and a relatively large lens for the volume of the eye. Thickened sclera may impede drainage from the vortex veins. These eyes are markedly hyperopic and highly susceptible to angle closure, which occurs at an earlier age than in PAC. Intraocular surgery is frequently complicated by choroidal effusion and nonrhegmatogenous retinal detachment. Choroidal effusion may occur spontaneously and may induce angle closure.

Laser iridotomy, laser peripheral iridoplasty, and medical therapy are the safest ways to manage IOP elevation in these patients. Surgery should be avoided if possible because of the high rate of complications. When intraocular surgery is performed, prophylactic posterior sclerotomies may reduce the severity of intraoperative choroidal effusion. If the angles remain compromised despite a patent iridotomy, lensectomy is an additional treatment option. In such cases, a limited core vitrectomy is sometimes necessary to provide adequate anterior chamber depth for safe lens removal. Many clinicians consider early lens extraction in patients with nanophthalmos to avoid the development of angle closure. In such cases, the surgeon should consider prophylactic measures to reduce the risk for clinically significant choroidal effusion, including sclerotomies, decompression of the eye with a Honan balloon, and systemic hyperosmotic agents such as mannitol.

Persistent fetal vasculature and retinopathy of prematurity

The contraction of retrolental fibrovascular tissue seen in *persistent fetal vasculature* (PFV; formerly known as *persistent hyperplastic primary vitreous*) and in retinopathy of prematurity can cause progressive shallowing of the anterior chamber angle with subsequent angle closure. In PFV, the onset of this complication usually occurs at 3–6 months of age during the cicatricial phase of the disease, although angle closure may occur later in childhood. Cataractous swelling of the lens can also cause angle closure. PFV is usually unilateral and often associated with microphthalmos and elongated ciliary processes. These conditions are discussed in more detail in BCSC Section 6, *Pediatric Ophthalmology and Strabismus,* and Section 12, *Retina and Vitreous.*

In retinopathy of prematurity, angle closure can also be related to a steeper cornea and a higher lens thickness to axial length ratio compared to normal eyes. Neovascularization of the iris is also occasionally associated with retinopathy of prematurity and may contribute to the development of angle closure. LPI can be performed as the first-line treatment of the angle closure. However, lens extraction, trabeculectomy, or tube shunt surgery may be necessary if the IOP cannot be controlled medically.

Drug-induced secondary angle-closure glaucoma

Topiramate, a sulfamate-substituted monosaccharide, is an oral medication prescribed in the treatment of epilepsy, depression, headaches, and idiopathic intracranial hypertension. In some patients, this medication may cause a syndrome characterized by acute myopic shift and acute bilateral angle closure. Patients with this syndrome experience sudden bilateral vision loss with acute myopia, bilateral ocular pain, and headache, usually within 1 month of starting topiramate. In addition to myopia, ocular findings in this syndrome include a uniformly shallow anterior chamber with anterior displacement of the iris and lens, microcystic corneal edema, elevated IOP (40–70 mm Hg), a closed anterior chamber angle, and ciliochoroidal effusion (Fig 10-19). Other medications associated with uveal effusion and secondary angle closure include *acetazolamide, methazolamide, buproprion,* and *trimethoprim-sulfamethoxazole.* Some recreational drugs, including *MDMA ("ecstasy"),* can also cause bilateral secondary angle closure.

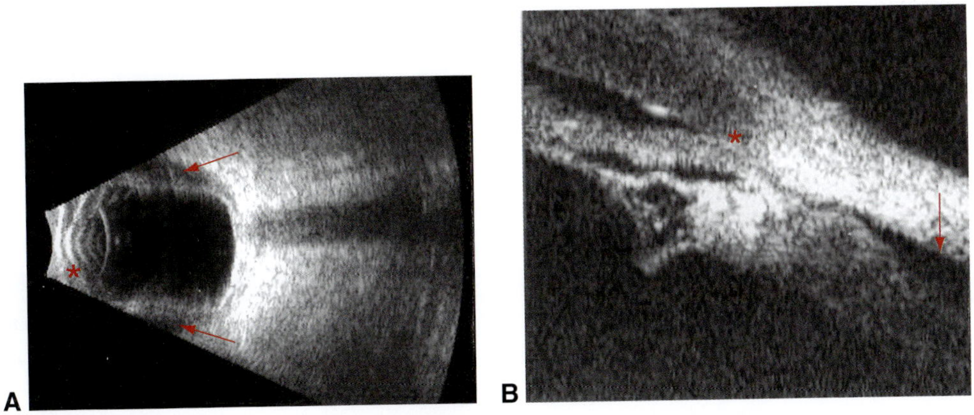

Figure 10-19 Topiramate-induced angle closure. **A,** B-scan ultrasonogram of an eye with a very shallow anterior chamber *(asterisk)* and topiramate-induced angle closure. The choroidal effusion is clearly evident *(arrows).* **B,** Ultrasonographic view of an extremely shallow anterior chamber and closed angle *(asterisk).* The posterior choroidal effusion is clearly visible *(arrow).* *(Courtesy of Jonathan Eisengart, MD.)*

The bilateral presentation of this type of angle closure should alert the clinician to the possibility of an idiosyncratic response to topiramate or other drugs. Treatment of this syndrome involves immediate discontinuation of the inciting medication and initiation of medical therapy, generally in the form of aqueous suppressants, to decrease the IOP. In addition, systemic corticosteroids may hasten recovery. Aggressive cycloplegia may help deepen the anterior chamber and relieve the attack. The secondary angle closure usually resolves within 24–48 hours with medical treatment, and the myopia resolves within 1–2 weeks of discontinuing topiramate. Because pupillary block is not an underlying mechanism of this syndrome, a peripheral iridotomy is not indicated.

Murphy RM, Bakir B, O'Brien C, Wiggs JL, Pasquale LR. Drug-induced bilateral secondary angle-closure glaucoma: a literature synthesis. *J Glaucoma.* 2016;25(2):e99–105.

Conditions Associated With Combined Pushing and Pulling or Other Mechanisms

Ocular inflammation

Secondary angle closure can occur as a result of ocular inflammation. Fibrin and increased aqueous proteins released due to the breakdown of the blood–aqueous barrier may predispose to formation of posterior synechiae (Fig 10-20) and PAS. If left untreated, these posterior synechiae can lead to a secluded pupil, iris bombé, and secondary angle closure (Fig 10-21).

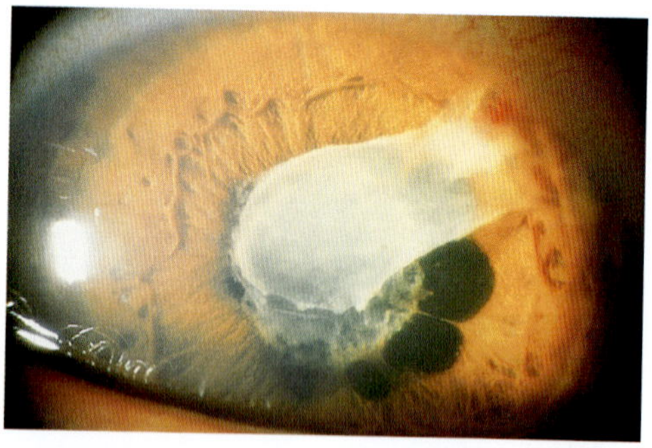

Figure 10-20 Inflammatory glaucoma in a patient with ankylosing spondylitis. A fibrinous anterior chamber reaction and posterior synechiae formation are evident. *(Courtesy of Steven T. Simmons, MD.)*

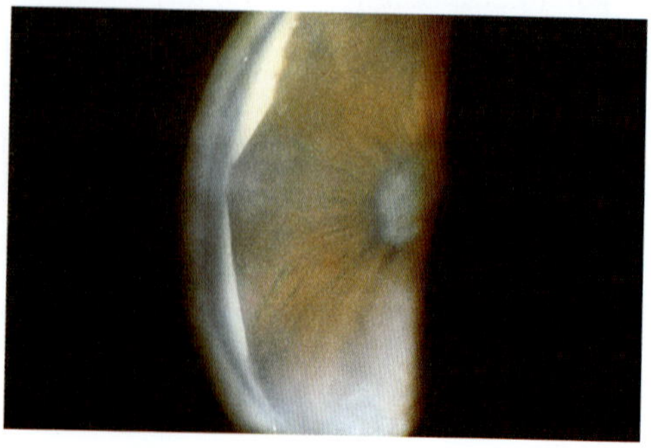

Figure 10-21 Clinical photograph showing inflammatory glaucoma. A secluded pupil is seen in a patient with long-standing uveitis with classic iris bombé and secondary angle closure. *(Courtesy of Steven T. Simmons, MD.)*

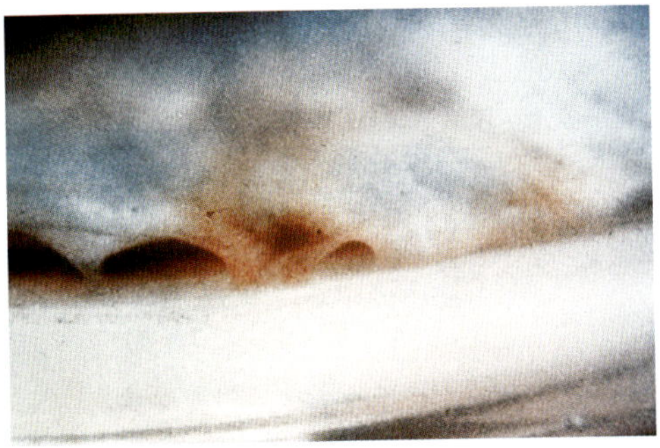

Figure 10-22 Inflammatory glaucoma. PAS in uveitis occur typically in the inferior anterior chamber angle and are nonuniform in height and shape, as shown in this photograph. *(Courtesy of Joseph Krug, MD.)*

Peripheral iris edema, organization of inflammatory debris in the angle, and bridging of the angle by large keratic precipitates (seen in sarcoidosis) can accompany the ocular inflammation and lead to formation of PAS. These PAS most often form in the inferior anterior chamber angle, unlike the PAS in PAC, which typically occur in the superior angle. The PAS are usually not uniform in shape or height, further distinguishing inflammatory disease from PAC (Fig 10-22). In rare instances, ischemia secondary to inflammation may cause rubeosis iridis and neovascular glaucoma.

Ocular inflammation can lead to the shallowing and closure of the anterior chamber angle by other mechanisms as well, such as uveal effusion and subsequent anterior rotation of the ciliary body. Significant posterior uveitis can cause massive exudative retinal detachment or choroidal effusions that push the lens–iris interface forward, resulting in secondary angle closure. Treatment is primarily directed at the underlying cause of the uveitis. Aqueous suppressants and corticosteroids are the primary agents for reducing IOP and preventing synechial angle closure in this situation. Although prostaglandin analogues can cause increased inflammation in some eyes, they may be considered if needed to control IOP.

Interstitial keratitis may be associated with open-angle glaucoma or angle closure. The angle-closure component may be caused by chronic inflammation and PAS formation or by multiple cysts of the iris pigment epithelium.

Sng CC, Barton K. Mechanism and management of angle closure in uveitis. *Curr Opin Ophthalmol.* 2015;26(2):121–127.

Shallow or flat anterior chamber after surgery

A flat anterior chamber from any cause can result in the formation of PAS. Hypotony in an eye with a flat chamber after cataract surgery or filtering surgery indicates the presence of a wound leak unless proven otherwise. A Seidel test should be performed to locate the leak. Simple pressure patching or bandage contact lens application will often seal the leak and allow the chamber to re-form. If the chamber does not re-form, the leak should be repaired surgically to prevent synechial angle closure or other complications of hypotony.

Debate continues concerning how long a postoperative flat chamber should be managed conservatively before surgical intervention is undertaken. Some ophthalmologists repair the wound leak and re-form a flat chamber following cataract surgery within 24 hours. Others prefer observation in conjunction with corticosteroid therapy for several days to prevent formation of synechiae. Although iridocorneal contact is well tolerated, contact between the cornea and the hyaloid face or an IOL requires re-formation of the chamber without delay to minimize corneal endothelial damage. Early intervention should also be considered in the presence of corneal edema, excessive inflammation, or posterior synechiae formation.

CHAPTER 11

Glaucoma in Children and Adolescents

This chapter includes related videos. Go to www.aao.org/bcscvideo_section10 or scan the QR codes in the text to access this content.

Highlights

- Pediatric glaucomas affecting children up to approximately 4 years of age can be associated with significant ocular abnormalities due to the elastic tissue properties in individuals of a young age.
- Examination of a child can be challenging, but good results can be obtained with a systematic and organized approach that includes the use of anesthesia.
- Treatment of pediatric glaucomas more frequently involves surgery than does treatment in adults. The angle is usually the first site of surgical intervention.

Classification

The glaucomas of childhood and adolescence (herein called pediatric glaucomas) are a heterogeneous group of disorders associated with elevated intraocular pressure (IOP). These disorders can cause damage to the optic nerve, visual field, and, up to about age 4, the cornea and other structures. Various presentations and etiologies characterize these rare glaucomas. The Childhood Glaucoma Research Network has defined both glaucoma and glaucoma suspect for pediatric populations (Table 11-1). Although pediatric glaucomas share many characteristics with adult-onset glaucomas, there are numerous management issues that are unique to the pediatric and adolescent populations.

Pediatric glaucoma is typically classified as primary or secondary (Table 11-2). Isolated angle abnormalities are seen in the primary pediatric glaucomas. In *primary congenital glaucoma (PCG),* angle dysgenesis leads to outflow resistance and elevated IOP, which in turn leads to the classic features of PCG: enlarged and/or cloudy corneas, Haab striae, and an enlarged globe (buphthalmos). In *juvenile open-angle glaucoma (JOAG),* another high-pressure primary glaucoma, an isolated angle abnormality may be present; this glaucoma develops later in childhood (generally after age 4) or in early adulthood (Table 11-3).

Secondary pediatric glaucomas are associated with other ocular or systemic conditions. These glaucomas are further classified according to whether the condition is acquired after

Table 11-1 Definitions of Pediatric Glaucoma and Glaucoma Suspect

Finding	Pediatric Glaucoma: IOP-Related Damage to the Eye; at Least 2 of the Following Criteria Required for Diagnosis	Pediatric Glaucoma Suspect: No IOP-Related Damage; at Least 1 of the Following Criteria Required for Diagnosis
IOP	IOP > 21 mm Hg	IOP > 21 mm Hg on 2 separate occasions
Optic disc	Optic disc cupping: progressive increase in cup–disc ratio	Suspicious optic disc appearance for glaucoma, ie, increased cup–disc ratio for size of optic disc
	Cup–disc asymmetry of ≥ 0.2 when the optic discs are a similar size	
	Focal rim thinning	
Cornea	Haab striae	Increased corneal diameter or axial length in eyes with normal IOP
	Diameter ≥ 11 mm in newborns, > 12 mm in children < 1 year, or > 13 mm at any age	
Visual field	Reproducible visual-field defect consistent with glaucomatous optic neuropathy with no other observable reason for defect	Suspicious visual field for glaucoma
Myopia	Progressive myopia, myopic shift, or an increase in ocular dimensions out of keeping with normal growth	–

IOP = intraocular pressure.

Information from Beck AD, Chang TCP, Freedman SF. Definition, classification, differential diagnosis. In: Weinreb RN, Grajewski AL, Papadopoulos M, Grigg J, Freedman S, eds. *Childhood Glaucoma.* Kugler Publications; 2013:3–10. *World Glaucoma Association Consensus Series—9.*

Table 11-2 Classification of Pediatric Glaucoma

Primary pediatric glaucoma

Primary congenital glaucoma

- Neonatal or newborn onset (age 0–1 month)
- Infantile onset (1–24 months)
- Late onset or late recognized (age ≥24 months)

Juvenile open-angle glaucoma (up to 40 years)

Secondary pediatric glaucoma

Glaucoma associated with nonacquired ocular anomalies

Glaucoma associated with nonacquired systemic disease

Glaucoma associated with acquired condition

Glaucoma following cataract surgery

Information from Beck AD, Chang TCP, Freedman SF. Definition, classification, differential diagnosis. In: Weinreb RN, Grajewski AL, Papadopoulos M, Grigg J, Freedman S, eds. *Childhood Glaucoma.* Kugler Publications; 2013:3–10. *World Glaucoma Association Consensus Series—9.*

Table 11-3 Features of Primary Pediatric Glaucomas

Primary congenital glaucoma (PCG)
Isolated angle anomalies, +/– mild congenital iris anomalies
Meets glaucoma definition, usually with ocular enlargement
Spontaneously arrested cases with normal IOP but typical signs of PCG
Juvenile open-angle glaucoma (JOAG)
No ocular enlargement
No congenital ocular anomalies or syndromes
Open angle, normal appearance
Meets glaucoma definition

IOP = intraocular pressure.

Information from Beck AD, Chang TCP, Freedman SF. Definition, classification, differential diagnosis. In: Weinreb RN, Grajewski AL, Papadopoulos M, Grigg J, Freedman S, eds. *Childhood Glaucoma.* Kugler Publications; 2013:3–10. *World Glaucoma Association Consensus Series—9.*

Table 11-4 Features of Secondary Pediatric Glaucomas

Glaucoma Associated With Nonacquired Ocular Anomalies	Glaucoma Associated With Acquired Conditions[a]	Glaucoma Following Cataract Surgery
Includes conditions of predominantly ocular anomalies present at birth that might or might not be associated with systemic signs Meets glaucoma definition	Meets glaucoma definition after acquired condition is recognized	Meets glaucoma definition only after cataract surgery is performed and is subdivided into 3 categories: 1. Congenital idiopathic cataract 2. Congenital cataract associated with ocular anomalies/systemic disease, no previous glaucoma 3. Acquired cataract, no previous glaucoma
	Based on gonioscopy results: Open-angle glaucoma: ≥50% open Angle-closure glaucoma: <50% open or acute angle closure	Based on gonioscopy results: Open-angle glaucoma: ≥50% open Angle-closure glaucoma: <50% open or acute angle closure

[a]An acquired condition is one that is not inherited or present at birth.

Information from Beck A, Chang TCP. Glaucoma: definitions and classification. *Disease Reviews.* Pediatric Ophthalmology Education Center. American Academy of Ophthalmology; 2015. www.aao.org/disease-review/glaucoma-definitions-classification

birth or is present at birth (nonacquired). Nonacquired pediatric glaucoma is categorized according to whether the signs are mainly ocular or systemic (Tables 11-4 through 11-7). Glaucoma following extraction of a congenital cataract comprises its own separate category, outside the nonacquired group. See BCSC Section 6, *Pediatric Ophthalmology and Strabismus,* for additional discussion of many of the topics covered in this chapter.

Table 11-5 Features of Glaucoma Associated With Nonacquired Ocular Anomalies

Conditions with predominantly ocular anomalies present at birth that might or might not be associated with systemic signs
Axenfeld-Rieger anomaly (syndrome if systemic associations)
Peters anomaly (syndrome if systemic associations)
Ectropion uveae
Congenital iris hypoplasia
Aniridia
Persistent fetal vasculature (if glaucoma present before cataract surgery)
Oculodermal melanocytosis (nevus of Ota)
Posterior polymorphous dystrophy
Microphthalmos
Microcornea
Ectopia lentis
Simple ectopia lentis (no systemic associations, possible Type 1 fibrillin *[FBN1]* mutation)
Ectopia lentis et pupillae

Information from Beck AD, Chang TCP, Freedman SF. Definition, classification, differential diagnosis. In: Weinreb RN, Grajewski AL, Papadopoulos M, Grigg J, Freedman S, eds. *Childhood Glaucoma.* Kugler Publications; 2013:3–10. *World Glaucoma Association Consensus Series—9.*

Table 11-6 Features of Glaucoma Associated With Nonacquired Systemic Disease or Syndrome

Conditions with predominantly known syndromes, systemic anomalies, or systemic disease present at birth that might be associated with ocular signs
Chromosomal disorders such as trisomy 21 (Down syndrome)
Connective tissue disorders
Marfan syndrome
Weill-Marchesani syndrome
Stickler syndrome
Metabolic disorders
Homocystinuria
Lowe syndrome
Mucopolysaccharidoses
Phacomatoses
Neurofibromatosis type 1 (NF1)
Sturge-Weber syndrome
Klippel-Trénaunay-Weber syndrome
Rubinstein-Taybi syndrome
Congenital rubella

Information from Beck AD, Chang TCP, Freedman SF. Definition, classification, differential diagnosis. In: Weinreb RN, Grajewski AL, Papadopoulos M, Grigg J, Freedman S, eds. *Childhood Glaucoma.* Kugler Publications; 2013:3–10. *World Glaucoma Association Consensus Series—9.*

Table 11-7 Features of Glaucoma Associated With Acquired Conditions

Uveitis
Trauma (hyphema, angle recession, ectopia lentis)
Steroid induced
Tumors (benign/malignant, ocular/orbital)
Retinopathy of prematurity
Prior ocular surgery other than cataract surgery

Information from Beck AD, Chang TCP, Freedman SF. Definition, classification, differential diagnosis. In: Weinreb RN, Grajewski AL, Papadopoulos M, Grigg J, Freedman S, eds. *Childhood Glaucoma.* Kugler Publications; 2013:3–10. *World Glaucoma Association Consensus Series—9.*

Thau A, Lloyd M, Freedman S, Beck A, Grajewski A, Levin AV. New classification system for pediatric glaucoma: implications for clinical care and research registry. *Curr Opin Ophthalmol.* 2018;29(5):385–394.

Genetics

Some pediatric glaucomas are inherited and have known genetic mutations associated with them. Genetic testing and counseling should be considered for parents of pediatric glaucoma patients and for adults with onset of glaucoma in childhood or early adulthood (see Table 1-2 in Chapter 1 of this volume).

Primary Congenital Glaucoma

Although most cases of PCG occur sporadically, a familial pattern of inheritance is seen in 10%–40% of cases. The inheritance is usually autosomal recessive with incomplete or variable penetrance. Higher rates of familial inheritance are seen in children from the Middle East and central Europe. Patients with a family history consistent with autosomal recessive inheritance should be screened for mutations in *CYP1B1* (cytochrome P450, family 1, subfamily B, polypeptide 1), especially if there is a history of consanguinity in the family. Small families also should be considered for screening; the case may only appear to be "sporadic" because there are too few family members to discern the inheritance pattern. The *CYP1B1* gene encodes an enzyme thought to be important in anterior segment development and regulation of aqueous humor secretion.

Another gene that has been associated with PCG is *LTBP2* (latent transforming growth factor beta-binding protein 2) within the GLC3C locus. Other mutations of this gene are associated with Weill-Marchesani syndrome and microspherophakia. Mutations in *ANGPT1* (angiopoietin-1) or *TEK* (tunica interna endothelial cell kinase, the receptor for *ANGPT1,* also known as *TIE2*) are inherited in an autosomal dominant pattern, result in loss of protein function that affects the development of Schlemm canal, and can lead to PCG.

Pediatric Glaucoma Without Anterior Segment Dysgenesis

Families with autosomal dominant inheritance of early-onset glaucoma without anterior segment dysgenesis (eg, JOAG) can be tested for mutations in *MYOC* (*GLC1A*), the gene coding for myocilin. Aggregation of abnormal myocilin, a protein found in the trabecular meshwork and ciliary body, is thought to cause trabecular meshwork dysfunction. This protein was formerly called TIGR (trabecular meshwork–inducible glucocorticoid response protein). Approximately 20% of these families will have *MYOC* mutations. The confirmed presence of a *MYOC* mutation can prompt earlier screening and monitoring of other family members.

Pediatric Glaucoma With Anterior Segment Dysgenesis

For patients with conditions involving anterior segment dysgenesis (eg, aniridia, Axenfeld-Rieger syndrome, Peters anomaly, nail-patella syndrome), the proband should be tested for mutations in *FOXC1* (forkhead box C1), *PITX2* (paired-like homeodomain transcription factor 2), *PAX6* (paired box 6), and *LMX1B* (LIM homeobox transcription factor 1 beta). These genes are all important in the development of the eye and other structures. The order of the genetic testing is prioritized according to the patient's clinical features. Once a mutation has been identified, the entire family (both affected and unaffected members) can be screened. Unaffected family members may be identified as carriers of the mutation and informed of the potential risk to any future offspring. Together, *PITX2* and *FOXC1* mutations account for 50% of the glaucoma cases associated with anterior segment dysgenesis. The variable interaction between these 2 genes may underlie the diverse phenotypic expression associated with Axenfeld-Rieger syndrome. Over 80% of patients with aniridia have mutations in *PAX6*. Peters anomaly has been linked to mutations in *PITX2, FOXC1, CYP1B1,* and *PAX6.*

Lewis CJ, Hedberg-Buenz A, DeLuca AP, Stone EM, Alward WLM, Fingert JH. Primary congenital and developmental glaucomas. *Hum Mol Genet.* 2017;26(R1):R28–36.

Zhao Y, Sorenson CM, Sheibani N. Cytochrome P450 1B1 and primary congenital glaucoma. *J Ophthalmic Vis Res.* 2015;10(1):60–67.

Primary Congenital Glaucoma

Incidence

Primary congenital glaucoma (PCG) accounts for the majority of primary pediatric glaucomas, and newborn PCG accounts for approximately 25% of PCG cases. Most cases are bilateral (70%) and are diagnosed within the first year of life (>75%). PCG occurs more frequently in males (65%) than females. The incidence varies with ethnicity, and consanguinity greatly increases the risk. Without a family history of PCG, an affected patient has a 2% chance of having a child with PCG.

Pathophysiology

The pathogenesis of PCG is uncertain. Clinically, the angle appears immature, which is thought to result from arrested maturation of tissues from neural crest–derived cells. This in turn is thought to cause increased resistance to aqueous outflow through the trabecular meshwork. Ophthalmologist Otto Barkan hypothesized that this resistance was caused by a membrane covering the anterior chamber angle. Although this membrane has never been identified, individuals with PCG have a developmental anomaly of the anterior chamber angle, with dysgenesis and compression of the trabecular meshwork and an anterior insertion of the iris root (Fig 11-1). In cases with mutations in *ANGPT1* or *TEK*, the etiology is thought to be due to maldevelopment of Schlemm canal.

Clinical Features

In infants, PCG presents with the classic triad of epiphora, photophobia, and blepharospasm. Until about 4 years of age, elevated IOP causes the cornea to stretch, leading to increased corneal diameter and enlargement of the globe (buphthalmos; Fig 11-2A), along with stretching of the scleral canal housing the optic nerve. The corneal stretching produces *Haab striae,* or breaks in Descemet membrane, and may lead to corneal edema and corneal opacification (Fig 11-2B; also see Figs 21-2 and 21-3 in BCSC Section 6, *Pediatric Ophthalmology and Strabismus*). As the cornea swells, the child may become irritable and photophobic. After age

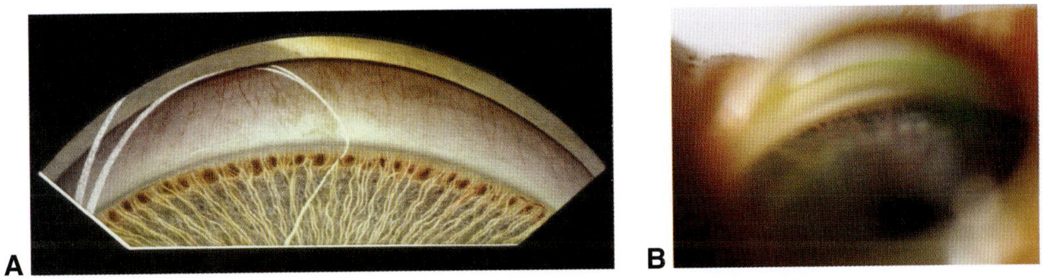

Figure 11-1 Anterior chamber angle in primary congenital glaucoma (PCG). **A,** Illustration of a gonioscopic view of the anterior chamber angle in primary congenital glaucoma reveals a deep angle with no angle recess; the iris appears as a scalloped line with less density of the iris fibers (rarefaction). **B,** Goniophotograph of the angle showing a similar view. Iris blood vessels are more prominently visible in eyes with PCG. *(Part A courtesy of Lee Allen and Wallace L.M. Alward, MD; part B courtesy of Robert Honkanen, MD.)*

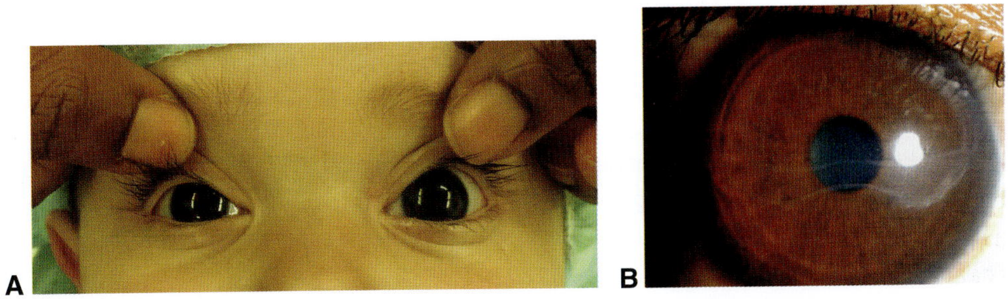

Figure 11-2 Primary congenital glaucoma. **A,** Photograph of a child with unilateral buphthalmos resulting from uncontrolled elevated intraocular pressure (IOP) in the left eye prior to surgery. **B,** Photograph of Haab striae, or breaks in Descemet membrane, which are visible after corneal edema clears. The striae are both horizontal and circumferential. *(Part A courtesy of JoAnn A. Giaconi, MD; part B courtesy of Deepak Edward, MD.)*

Table 11-8 Differential Diagnosis for Symptoms and Signs of Primary Congenital Glaucoma

Conditions associated with epiphora
Nasolacrimal duct obstruction
Corneal epithelial defect or abrasion
Conjunctivitis
Keratitis
Ocular inflammation (uveitis, trauma)
Conditions associated with corneal enlargement or apparent enlargement
X-linked megalocornea
Exophthalmos
Shallow orbits (eg, craniofacial dysostoses)
Axial myopia
Conditions associated with corneal clouding
Birth trauma with breaks in Descemet membrane
Keratitis: maternal rubella, herpes, phlyctenules
Corneal dystrophies: congenital hereditary endothelial dystrophies, posterior polymorphous corneal dystrophy
Corneal malformations: dermoid tumors, sclerocornea, choristomas, Peters anomaly
Keratomalacia
Metabolic disorders with associated corneal abnormalities: mucopolysaccharidoses, sphingolipidoses, cystinoses
Skin disorders affecting the cornea: congenital ichthyosis, congenital dyskeratosis
Conditions associated with optic nerve abnormalities
Optic nerve pit
Optic nerve coloboma
Optic nerve hypoplasia
Optic nerve malformation
Optic nerve atrophy
Physiologic cupping, particularly in a large optic nerve

3–4 years, the cornea ceases to enlarge further. Scleral stretching also ceases around this age. However, persistently elevated IOP may result in continued optic nerve damage.

Differential Diagnosis

The extensive differential diagnosis of PCG is presented in Table 11-8. PCG should be considered in the differential diagnosis of epiphora in children. PCG is a relatively rare disease and may go undetected or be misdiagnosed by primary care doctors and general ophthalmologists. Mild cases may be misdiagnosed as nasolacrimal duct obstruction, resulting in a delayed PCG diagnosis and irreversible damage. Physicians must be vigilant in their examination and urgently refer infants presenting with the classic triad of epiphora, photophobia, and blepharospasm to a specialist. Left untreated, almost all cases of PCG will progress to blindness.

Treatment and Prognosis

Treatment of PCG typically requires surgical intervention following a thorough examination with the patient under anesthesia (see the Surgical Management section later in this chapter). Medical therapy has limited long-term value but may be used to temporize or reduce corneal edema to improve visualization during surgery.

PCG generally has a better visual prognosis than do most secondary pediatric glaucomas. In US retrospective reviews, approximately two-thirds of patients with PCG have a visual acuity of 20/70 or better at final follow-up. However, in cases of newborn PCG, in cases of PCG diagnosed after age 1, or in patients with corneal diameters larger than 14 mm at diagnosis the prognoses may be very poor; severe dysgenesis can make IOP control difficult or there may be late-stage optic nerve damage at the time of diagnosis. More than 50% of patients with newborn PCG progress to legal blindness. The prognosis is best for patients whose glaucoma is diagnosed between the ages of 3 and 12 months, because most of these cases respond to angle surgery.

Ko F, Papadopoulos M, Khaw PT. Primary congenital glaucoma. *Prog Brain Res.* 2015; 221:177–189.

Juvenile Open-Angle Glaucoma

Juvenile open-angle glaucoma (JOAG) is a form of primary open-angle glaucoma that presents between the ages of 4 and 40 years with elevated IOP and usually normal-appearing angles. Because most cases of JOAG are inherited as an autosomal dominant trait, many families may be aware of their risk of developing this condition, leading to earlier screening and detection. Although the IOP is elevated, it does not cause corneal enlargement or Haab striae due to the later age of onset; however, progressive myopia may result and continue until 10 years of age. Medical therapy is used as first-line treatment, but many cases are refractory to maximal medical treatment and may require incisional glaucoma surgery. Angle procedures may be helpful in select cases.

Secondary Glaucomas due to Nonacquired Conditions

Pediatric glaucomas may be associated with various ocular and systemic abnormalities that are present at birth. The following sections discuss a few of the more common conditions associated with glaucoma. For more detailed information on each entity, please see BCSC Section 6, *Pediatric Ophthalmology and Strabismus,* and Section 8, *External Disease and Cornea.*

Axenfeld-Rieger Syndrome

Axenfeld-Rieger (A-R) syndrome is a spectrum of disorders characterized by anomalous development of the neural crest–derived anterior segment structures, including the anterior chamber angle, the iris, and the trabecular meshwork. Although this syndrome was initially separated into Axenfeld anomaly (posterior embryotoxon with multiple adherent peripheral iris strands), Rieger anomaly (Axenfeld anomaly plus iris hypoplasia and corectopia), and Rieger syndrome (Rieger anomaly plus developmental defects of the teeth or facial bones, including maxillary hypoplasia, redundant periumbilical skin, pituitary abnormalities, or hypospadias), these disorders are now considered variations of the same clinical entity and are combined under the name *Axenfeld-Rieger syndrome.*

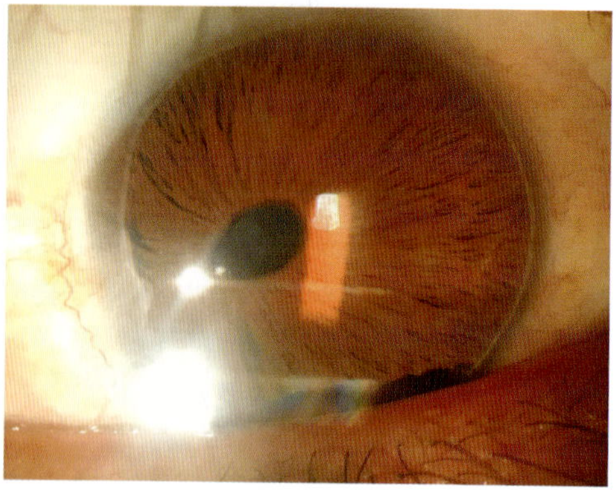

Figure 11-3 Photograph of an eye with Axenfeld-Rieger syndrome with prominent embryotoxon, iris hypoplasia, and corectopia. *(Courtesy of Jonathan Young, MD, PhD.)*

Most cases of A-R syndrome are of autosomal dominant inheritance, but sporadic cases can occur. The disorder is bilateral, with no sex predilection. Classic clinical manifestations of A-R syndrome include posterior embryotoxon of the cornea (a prominent and anteriorly displaced Schwalbe line; see BCSC Section 4, *Ophthalmic Pathology and Intraocular Tumors,* for details on the histology) (Fig 11-3; also see BCSC Section 8, *External Disease and Cornea,* Fig 6-4) and iris adhesions to the Schwalbe line that range from threadlike to broad bands. The iris may range from normal to markedly atrophic with corectopia, hole formation, and ectropion uveae (see Fig 11-3 and BCSC Section 8, *External Disease and Cornea,* Fig 6-5). Table 11-9 outlines the differential diagnosis of A-R syndrome to help distinguish it from other conditions that involve abnormalities of the iris, cornea, and anterior chamber.

Approximately 50% of cases of A-R syndrome are associated with glaucoma, typically occurring in middle or late childhood. Glaucoma is thought to develop as a result of abnormal formation of the trabecular meshwork or Schlemm canal. The development of glaucoma correlates to the height of the iris insertion in the angle, not to the number of iris processes or the degree of iris abnormality. Treatment is generally the same as for an open-angle glaucoma; however, angle surgery may not be possible if there are many iris processes. Possible treatments for glaucoma associated with A-R syndrome include medications, goniotomy, trabeculotomy, trabeculectomy, tube shunt surgery, and cyclodestructive procedures.

Peters Anomaly

Peters anomaly is a rare developmental condition presenting with an annular corneal opacity (leukoma) in the central visual axis (Fig 11-4), often accompanied by iris strands that originate at the iris collarette and adhere to the corneal opacity. The leukoma corresponds to a defect in the corneal endothelium and underlying Descemet membrane and posterior stroma. The lens may be in its normal position, with or without a cataract, or the lens may be adherent to the posterior layers of the cornea. Patients with corneolenticular adhesions have a higher likelihood of other ocular abnormalities, such as microcornea and angle anomalies, and of systemic abnormalities, including those of the heart, genitourinary tract, musculoskeletal system, ear, palate, and spine.

Table 11-9 Differential Diagnosis for Axenfeld-Rieger Syndrome

Condition	Differentiating Features
Iridocorneal endothelial syndrome	Unilateral Middle-age onset Corneal endothelial abnormalities Progressive changes
Isolated posterior embryotoxon	Lack of glaucoma-associated or iris changes
Aniridia	Iris hypoplasia Associated corneal and macular changes
Iridoschisis	Splitting of iris layers with atrophy of anterior layer
Peters anomaly	Corneal leukoma
Ectopia lentis et pupillae	Lens subluxation Pupillary displacement Axial myopia Retinal detachment Enlarged corneal diameters Cataract Prominent iris processes in the anterior chamber angle
Oculodentodigital dysplasia	Microphthalmia Microcornea Iris abnormalities Cataracts Glaucoma

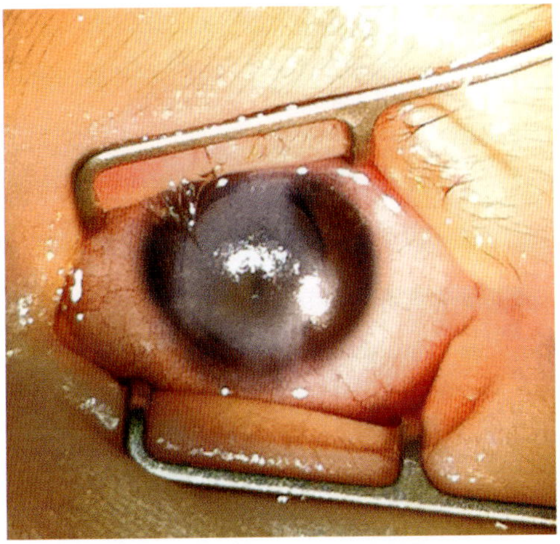

Figure 11-4 Photograph of an eye with Peters anomaly exhibiting central leukoma, which can be confused for corneal edema. *(Courtesy of JoAnn A. Giaconi, MD.)*

Peters anomaly is usually sporadic, although autosomal dominant and autosomal recessive forms have been reported. Most cases are bilateral, and angle abnormalities leading to glaucoma occur in approximately 50% of affected patients. As previously mentioned, glaucoma is thought to result from a malformed trabecular meshwork or Schlemm canal. Development of glaucoma is more common in patients with cataracts or corneolenticular adhesions. Elevated IOP typically presents in infancy but can also arise later in life.

Treatment of glaucoma associated with Peters anomaly can be difficult because of the iridocorneal dysgenesis. If possible, angle surgery is performed; alternative treatments include medications, trabeculectomy, tube shunt surgery, and cyclodestructive procedures.

Aniridia

Aniridia is a panocular, bilateral congenital disorder characterized by iris hypoplasia (Fig 11-5). Most patients with aniridia have only a rudimentary stump of iris; however, the iris appearance may vary greatly, with some patients having nearly complete but thin irides. Aniridia is associated with other ocular anomalies, including microcornea, anterior polar cataracts that may present at birth or develop later in life, and optic nerve and foveal hypoplasia resulting in pendular nystagmus and reduced visual acuity.

It had been thought that patients with aniridia develop glaucoma after the rudimentary iris stump rotates anteriorly to progressively cover the trabecular meshwork, resulting in synechial angle closure. A recent study, however, showed that aniridia patients without previous intraocular surgery did not have angle closure even when they had glaucoma. This suggests intraocular surgery, especially angle surgery, may trigger the formation of angle closure. IOP elevation in aniridia may not occur until the second decade of life or later. Occasionally,

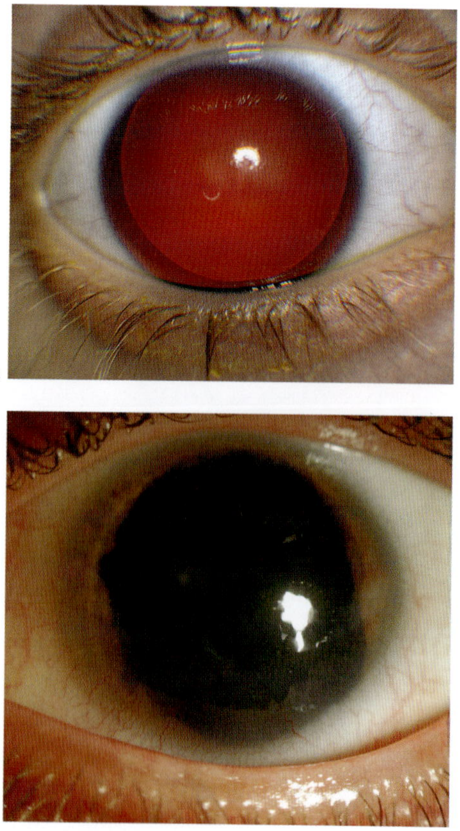

A

B

Figure 11-5 Iris morphology in aniridia in 2 patients with documented *PAX6* mutations. **A,** An eye with aniridia with no iris visible on slit-lamp biomicroscopy, exposing zonules and lens edge. **B,** An eye with aniridia in which remnants of rudimentary, hypoplastic iris tissue are present. Peripheral aniridic keratopathy, a classic finding in aniridia, is also present. *(Courtesy of Peter A. Netland, MD, PhD.)*

however, aniridia is associated with congenital glaucoma; primary maldevelopment of the drainage angle may result in elevated IOP at a younger age.

Patients with aniridia may have limbal stem cell abnormalities that eventually result in a corneal pannus, which begins in the peripheral cornea and slowly extends centrally. If corneal opacification threatens visual acuity, keratolimbal allograft stem cell transplantation can be performed. Implantation of an artificial iris can be performed for cosmesis; however, this implant is not recommended for children younger than 16 years.

Most cases of aniridia are familial and are transmitted with an autosomal dominant inheritance pattern; however, about one-third of cases result from isolated sporadic mutations in *PAX6*. Approximately 20% of sporadic cases are associated with a large chromosomal deletion that includes the adjacent Wilms tumor 1 gene *(WT1)*, a tumor suppressor gene, which results in an increased risk of Wilms tumor. Relatively few cases of Wilms tumor are seen in the familial form.

Two less-common forms of aniridia are associated with systemic abnormalities. *WAGR* (*W*ilms tumor, *a*niridia, *g*enitourinary anomalies, and mental *r*etardation) *syndrome* is an autosomal dominant form seen in 13% of patients with aniridia. *Gillespie syndrome* is an autosomal recessive form of aniridia associated with cerebellar ataxia and intellectual disability that occurs in 2% of those with aniridia.

Sturge-Weber Syndrome

Sturge-Weber syndrome (SWS; also known as *encephalofacial angiomatosis*) is a phakomatosis characterized by ipsilateral facial cutaneous hemangioma (port-wine stain), ipsilateral choroidal cavernous hemangioma, and ipsilateral leptomeningeal angioma associated with cerebral calcifications, seizures, focal neurologic deficits, and a variable degree of cognitive impairment. The condition is usually unilateral but can present bilaterally in rare instances. There is no race or sex predilection, and no inheritance pattern has been established. Glaucoma occurs in up to 70% of children with SWS and is more common when the cutaneous hemangioma involves the upper eyelid skin (Fig 11-6). Glaucoma is also more common in patients with choroidal hemangioma, iris heterochromia, and/or episcleral hemangioma. When glaucoma is seen in infants with this syndrome, congenital angle dysgenesis (similar to that seen in cases of PCG) is thought to be responsible. In these cases, treatment typically consists of angle surgery. However, these surgeries generally have a lower success rate in cases of SWS than in cases of PCG. Glaucoma that develops after the first decade of life may be caused by elevated episcleral venous pressure. Trabeculectomy, or preferably tube shunt surgery, should be performed with caution because of the increased risk of choroidal effusion and choroidal hemorrhage in these patients.

Neurofibromatosis

Neurofibromatosis (NF), the most common phakomatosis, has 2 recognizable forms. Neurofibromatosis 1 (NF1), also known as *von Recklinghausen disease* or *peripheral neurofibromatosis,* is the most common type, with a prevalence of 1 in 3000–5000 persons. NF1 is localized to band 11 of the long arm of chromosome 17 and is inherited in an autosomal

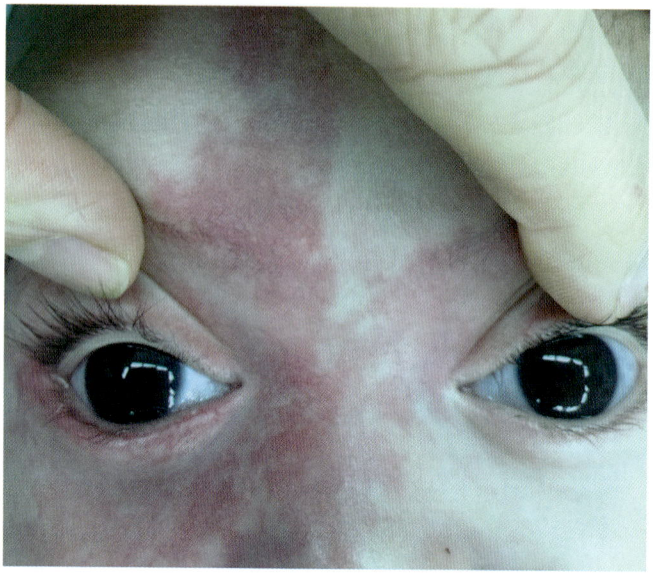

Figure 11-6 Photograph of a patient with Sturge-Weber syndrome; the facial hemangioma involves both upper eyelids. The patient also has glaucoma. *(Courtesy of JoAnn A. Giaconi, MD.)*

dominant pattern in approximately 50% of cases; the other 50% of cases are sporadic. In individuals with NF1, the neurofibromin gene is abnormal, and loss of tumor suppressor function leads to proliferation of neural tumors. The presence of ectropion uveae is a common ocular finding in this disease; its presence in a neonate warrants a workup for NF1. Other ocular findings associated with NF1 include Lisch nodules, choroidal lesions, optic nerve gliomas, eyelid neurofibromas, and glaucoma. Coexisting ptosis and glaucoma in a child should also prompt a workup for NF1; the ptosis may be due to an eyelid neurofibroma. Although the incidence of glaucoma in individuals with NF1 is low overall, the presence of an eyelid neurofibroma is strongly associated with glaucoma on the ipsilateral side. Systemic melanocytic lesions include cutaneous café-au-lait spots, cutaneous neurofibromas, and axillary or inguinal freckling. If glaucoma is present at birth it is thought to result from abnormal formation of angle structures. If it develops later in life, the mechanism is thought to be either infiltration of the angle with neurofibromatous tissue or angle closure caused by thickening of the ciliary body and choroid. Surgical treatment is often necessary, but success rates of surgical treatment in cases of NF1-associated glaucoma are lower than success rates for cases of PCG.

Neurofibromatosis 2 (also called *central neurofibromatosis*) is characterized by the presence of bilateral acoustic neuromas and is not associated with glaucoma.

Secondary Glaucomas due to Acquired Conditions

Many of the causes of secondary glaucoma in infants and children are similar to those in adults, including trauma, inflammation, steroid use, and topiramate-induced angle closure. The signs and symptoms at presentation will depend on the age of the child (whether the child is younger than or older than 3–4 years) and the extent of the IOP elevation and severity of vision loss. Lens-associated disorders that cause angle-closure glaucoma may occur in patients with Marfan syndrome, homocystinuria, Weill-Marchesani syndrome, and microspherophakia. Posterior segment disorders such as persistent fetal vasculature, retinopathy of prematurity, and familial exudative vitreoretinopathy, as well as tumors of the retina, iris, or ciliary body, can also result in glaucoma. The intraocular tumors known to lead to secondary glaucoma in infants and children include retinoblastoma, juvenile xanthogranuloma, and medulloepithelioma. Rubella and congenital cataract are also associated with secondary pediatric glaucoma.

Glaucoma Following Cataract Surgery

Glaucoma and suspicion of glaucoma develop in up to 50% or more of children who have undergone surgery for congenital cataract. The glaucoma is predominantly an open-angle type; however, angle closure may also occur as a late consequence of an enlarging Sommering ring that pushes the iris forward. The term "aphakic glaucoma" is commonly used to refer to this group of glaucomas; today, this term may be considered outdated because many of these young patients receive intraocular lens implants. Risk factors include cataract surgery in the first year of life (risk is greatest in individuals who have undergone surgery in first 6 weeks of life), postoperative complications, and small corneal diameter. The risk of developing glaucoma is the same whether patients are left aphakic or they receive an intraocular lens implant at the time of cataract extraction. Although most glaucoma following congenital cataract surgery develops in patients within 3 years of cataract surgery, these patients are always at risk for glaucoma and thus require lifelong follow-up. The underlying mechanism is unclear, but likely etiologies for open-angle cases include congenital anomalies of the outflow pathway, surgically induced inflammation, and altered intraocular anatomy postoperatively. Removing all residual cortex during cataract surgery may reduce the risk of IOP elevation.

Freedman SF, Lynn MJ, Beck AD, Bothun ED, Örge FH, Lambert SR; Infant Aphakia Treatment Study Group. Glaucoma-related adverse events in the first 5 years after unilateral cataract removal in the Infant Aphakia Treatment Study. *JAMA Ophthalmol.* 2015;133(8):907–914.

Evaluating the Pediatric Glaucoma Patient

Evaluation of a pediatric glaucoma patient differs from examination of an adult glaucoma patient. Ophthalmologists should proceed with an orderly system of examination and have the appropriate equipment for evaluating infants and young children in both the office and the operating room (Table 11-10). For examinations under anesthesia (EUAs), efficiency in measuring and recording data in the operating room is optimized by having all necessary equipment ready and gathered in a single place (Fig 11-7). Time under anesthesia should be minimized as much as possible. The effects of general anesthesia on the developing brain are unclear but are currently under study in a number of multicenter randomized studies.

Table 11-10 Supplies Needed for Examining Children Under Anesthesia

- Examination form/checklist
- Topical medications
  - Proparacaine or tetracaine
  - Mydriatics (do not use if proceeding with angle surgery)
  - Balanced salt solution for gonioscopy
  - Glycerol
  - Pilocarpine and apraclonidine if proceeding with angle surgery
- Tonometer: Tono-Pen, Perkins, or pneumatonometer. Measure IOP as soon as possible after induction.
- Calipers
- Koeppe or other gonioscopy lens
- Portable slit lamp
- Pachymeter
- A-scan ultrasonography system
- B-scan ultrasonography system
- Direct ophthalmoscope
- Retinoscope and lenses for refraction
- Indirect ophthalmoscope and lens
- Portable fundus camera

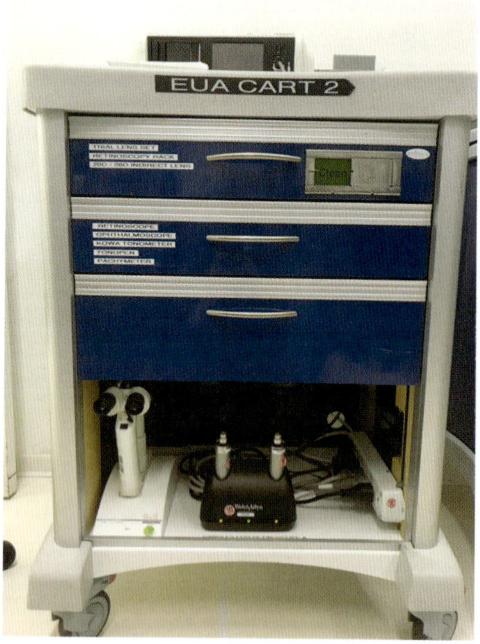

Figure 11-7 Photograph of a cart prepared for an examination under anesthesia (EUA) that contains all handheld instruments needed to perform a complete pediatric glaucoma examination in one place. *(Courtesy of JoAnn A. Giaconi, MD.)*

History

When evaluating an infant, the ophthalmologist should ask the caregiver whether the baby is fussy or irritable, whether the child is not feeding well or is losing weight, and whether the baby cries when taken outside into sunshine. It is important to elicit the caregiver's observations regarding any corneal clouding, specifically as to whether the clouding is intermittent or constant.

For evaluation of school-aged children, the ophthalmologist should inquire about the results of school vision screenings, changes in academic performance, and complaints about trouble seeing in the classroom. A complete record of the patient's history includes the names of any previous physicians who have been consulted; all prior ocular and systemic medical and surgical treatments; any family history of congenital glaucoma and other ocular and systemic disorders; medication use (with particular attention to all forms of steroids); and allergies.

Visual Acuity

Testing of visual acuity in infants and young children is discussed in BCSC Section 6, *Pediatric Ophthalmology and Strabismus*. Refraction should be performed to identify any myopia from axial enlargement and/or astigmatism from corneal irregularity. Decreased vision may be due to significant glaucomatous optic nerve damage, amblyopia, corneal scarring, or other associated ocular disorders (eg, retinal detachment, macular edema, cataract, lens dislocation).

External Examination

Before looking through a slit lamp, it is important to observe the child. Buphthalmos (see Fig 11-2A) and other signs and symptoms of PCG, including epiphora and blepharospasm, can be seen by observing a child from a distance. Systemic features that may be associated with primary and secondary glaucomas other than PCG should also be looked for, including those associated with chromosomal abnormalities, phakomatoses, connective tissue disorders, and A-R syndrome.

Anterior Segment Examination

As discussed previously, corneal enlargement and opacification are important signs associated with glaucoma in patients younger than 4 years. Corneal diameter can be measured with calipers or a ruler (Fig 11-8). The normal corneal diameter is approximately 9.5–10.5 mm in full-term newborns, increasing to 11–12 mm by 1 year of age. Table 11-11 compares normal pediatric measurements with adult measurements. A corneal diameter greater than 11.5 mm in a newborn and greater than 12.5 mm in children above the age of 1 year is suggestive of glaucoma. A difference in corneal diameter of 0.5 mm or greater between both eyes of the same patient may suggest glaucoma. Corneal edema may be due to elevated IOP or Haab striae and may range from a mild haze to dense opacification of the corneal stroma (Fig 11-9). Retroillumination after pupillary dilation may help make Haab striae visible. Evaluation for other anterior segment anomalies, such as aniridia, iridocorneal adhesions, and corectopia, may provide insight into the underlying diagnosis.

Tonometry

Accurate tonometry is important in the assessment of the pediatric glaucomas, but not always possible, especially in infants and very young children. A normal IOP measurement in

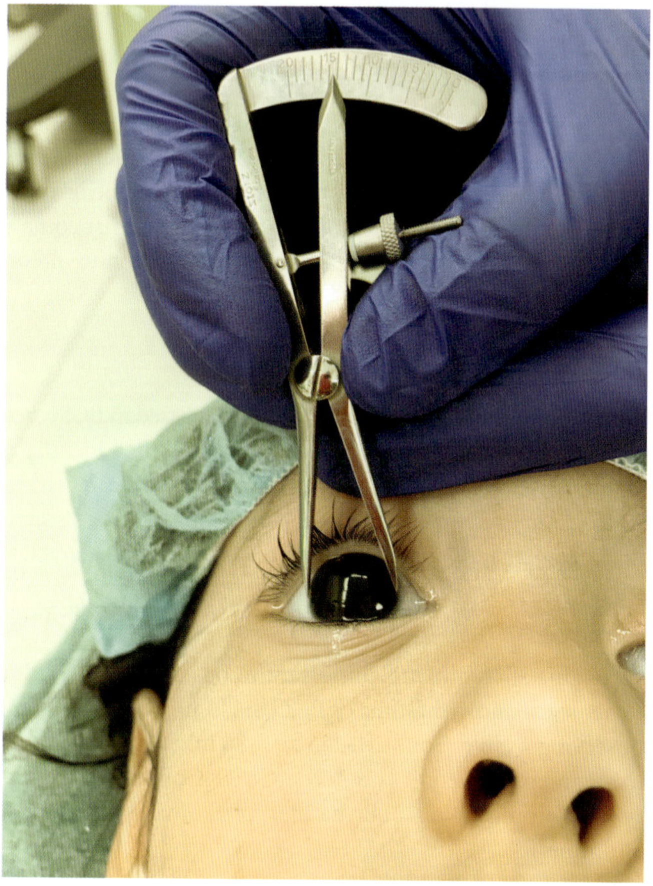

Figure 11-8 Photograph of corneal diameter measurement using calipers during an EUA. *(Courtesy of JoAnn A. Giaconi, MD.)*

Table 11-11 Comparisons of Normal Measurements in Pediatric and Adult Eyes

Age	Axial Length (mm)	Corneal Horizontal Diameter (mm)
Newborn	14.5–15.5	9.5–10.5
2-year-old	19.5–20.5	11.0–12.0
Adult	23.0–24.0	11.0–12.0

newborns ranges from 10 mm Hg to the low teens; by middle childhood, IOP increases to adult levels of 10–21 mm Hg. Glaucoma should be suspected if IOPs are elevated or asymmetric in a cooperative or anesthetized child; in an uncooperative or struggling child, IOP measurements may be falsely elevated.

The clinician may be able to successfully measure the IOP of an infant younger than 6 months by performing the measurement while the infant is feeding or immediately thereafter. In this group of patients, IOP can be measured with rebound tonometry (if the infant

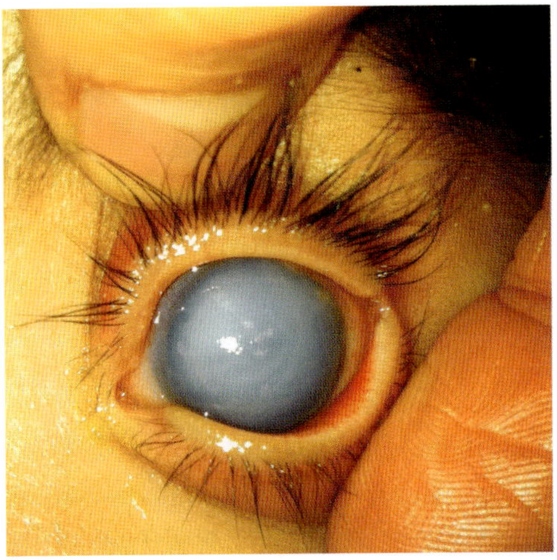

Figure 11-9 Photograph shows severe corneal edema from elevated IOP in newborn pediatric glaucoma. *(Courtesy of JoAnn A. Giaconi, MD.)*

can be held upright), the Tono-Pen (Reichert Ophthalmic Instruments), pneumotonometry, or a Perkins handheld applanation tonometer, if the palpebral fissure is sufficiently wide.

For children who are relatively cooperative in the clinic but too young for Goldmann tonometry, the rebound tonometer is very useful because it does not require topical anesthesia. This device has been shown to reduce the number of EUAs performed to obtain pressure measurements. However, despite these advantages, initial reports indicate that measurements in patients with congenital glaucoma were higher when taken with the rebound tonometer than when taken with the Perkins tonometer, especially at higher levels of IOP.

General anesthesia is usually required for accurate IOP assessment in older infants (≥6 months) and young children. However, most general anesthetic agents and sedatives unpredictably lower IOP. Exceptions include chloral hydrate, which does not affect IOP; ketamine, which may increase IOP; and midazolam, which has a negligible effect on IOP. In addition, the preparation for general anesthesia may cause infants to become dehydrated, which can reduce IOP. Increased IOP during general anesthesia may result from endotracheal intubation, upward drift of the eyes (Bell phenomenon), or possible induced laryngospasm. It is best to coordinate with the anesthesiologist before the child is brought to the operating room and arrange to take the IOP measurement immediately after induction of general anesthesia (preferably before intubation), which will ideally minimize the effects of anesthesia on IOP. It is also good practice to use the same general anesthetic for serial examinations.

Martinez-de-la-Casa JM, Garcia-Feijoo J, Saenz-Frances F, et al. Comparison of rebound tonometer and Goldmann handheld applanation tonometer in congenital glaucoma. *J Glaucoma.* 2009;18(1):49–52.

Pachymetry

The role of pachymetry in the diagnosis and management of pediatric glaucoma is unclear. The average central corneal thickness (CCT) is 540–560 μm in children without glaucoma.

CCT is lower than average in eyes with congenital glaucoma with buphthalmos and in children with Down syndrome; CCT is higher than average in eyes that have had surgery for congenital cataract and in individuals with aniridia. It is also slightly higher in premature infants but decreases as the infant ages. The effect of CCT on the accuracy of IOP measurements in these groups is unclear, and nomograms cannot accurately be used to "correct" IOP measurements for differences in CCT measurements.

Bradfield YS, Melia BM, Repka MX, et al; Pediatric Eye Disease Investigator Group. Central corneal thickness in children. *Arch Ophthalmol.* 2011;129(9):1132–1138.

Gonioscopy

Gonioscopy provides important information about the mechanism of the pediatric glaucoma as well as evidence of a patient's prior surgeries. An EUA is usually required for gonioscopic examination of younger children. A Koeppe lens allows direct visualization of the angle structures. In older children, indirect gonioscopy can be performed with a 4-mirror goniolens at the slit lamp.

The normal anterior chamber angle of an infant differs from the normal adult angle in several ways, including a less pigmented trabecular meshwork, a less prominent Schwalbe line, and a less distinct junction between the scleral spur and ciliary body band (Fig 11-10A). In PCG, the anterior chamber is deep, with a high anterior iris insertion. The angle recess is absent, and the iris root appears as a scalloped line of glistening tissue (Fig 11-10B). Although this tissue is not a true membrane, it has been referred to as the *Barkan membrane* and likely represents thickened and compacted trabecular meshwork (see Fig 11-1).

In eyes with JOAG, the angle usually appears normal. In patients with aniridia, gonioscopy reveals a rudimentary iris root.

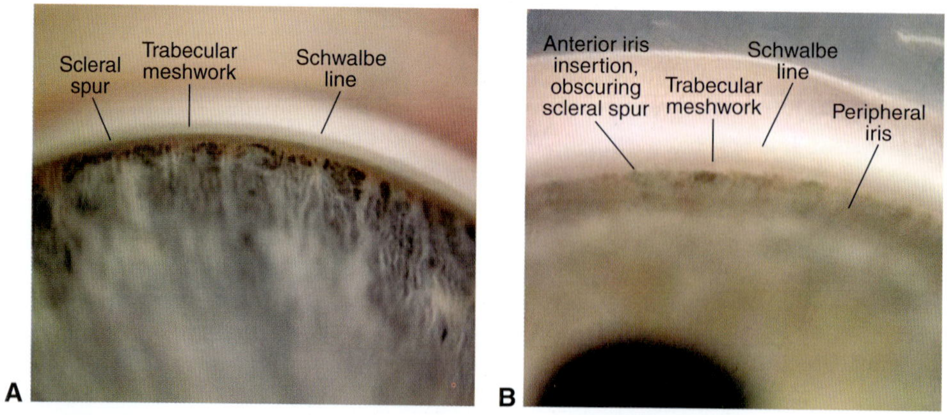

Figure 11-10 Gonioscopy of the anterior chamber angle. **A,** Anterior chamber angle of a nonglaucomatous infant eye, as seen by direct gonioscopy with a Koeppe lens. **B,** Typical appearance of the anterior chamber angle of an infant with primary congenital glaucoma. Note the scalloped appearance of the peripheral iris. The anterior iris insertion obscures the scleral spur. *(Courtesy of Ken K. Nischal, MD.)*

Optic Nerve and Fundus Evaluation

Visualization and documentation of the optic nerve are crucial in the evaluation and management of pediatric glaucomas. A highly magnified view of the nerve is ideal; this can often be achieved with direct ophthalmoscopy, which may be done in the office or operating room. In patients with small pupils, viewing through a direct ophthalmoscope can be enhanced through a Koeppe lens (Fig 11-11). Alternatively, a stereoscopic view can be achieved by viewing the nerve head through the central lens of a 4-mirror gonioprism with an operating microscope. Indirect ophthalmoscopy can be used, but this method may lead to underestimation of the cup–disc ratio (CDR). Slit-lamp biomicroscopy can be performed in older children with a dilated pupil. Photographs provide the best documentation and help the ophthalmologist evaluate changes over time.

Optic nerve imaging is possible on older, cooperative children and provides useful information that can be followed longitudinally. Normative databases for children do not yet exist in commercially available imaging platforms. However, it has been found that the

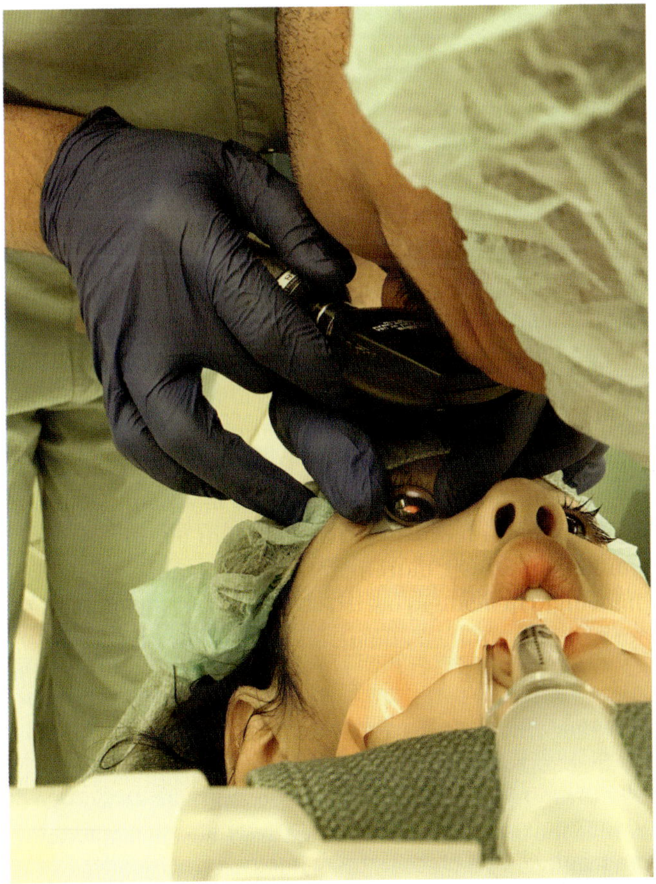

Figure 11-11 Photograph of an optic nerve examination with a direct ophthalmoscope using a Koeppe lens for an improved view. *(Courtesy of JoAnn A. Giaconi, MD.)*

retinal nerve fiber layer (RNFL) thickness of children over 5 years of age is similar to adult values; therefore, adult normative values can be used for comparison. Optical coherence tomography (OCT) parameters vary with age, axial length, and race, as they do for adults. OCT data for infants cannot be compared to data from adult normative databases. Another barrier to imaging in infants is the lack of commercially available portable handheld OCT machines.

A typical newborn without glaucoma has a small physiologic cup (CDR less than 0.3) with a pink rim. In individuals with PCG, the optic canal is stretched under high pressure and the lamina cribrosa is bowed backward, causing generalized enlargement of the cup. Enlarged or increasing CDR or CDR asymmetry greater than 0.2 between the 2 eyes is suggestive of glaucomatous cupping. Cupping may be reversible if the IOP is lowered before the child is 3 years old; however, lowering IOP does not reverse any existing atrophy of the optic nerve axons. Studies in which OCT is performed in children with PCG show diffuse RNFL loss rather than loss localized to the superior and inferior poles of the optic disc.

In children without glaucoma, CDR increases slightly from birth until approximately 10 years of age. The CDR of older children without glaucoma is similar to that seen in adults. Racial differences in CDR are present even at birth. Children of African, Middle Eastern, Hispanic, and East Asian descent have larger average CDRs than do children of European descent. Cupping in older children is similar to that seen in adult glaucomas; there are more focal defects and greater loss in the superior and inferior neural rim because their scleral canals do not stretch.

Allingham MJ, Cabrera MT, O'Connell RV, et al. Racial variation in optic nerve head parameters quantified in healthy newborns by handheld spectral domain optical coherence tomography. *J AAPOS.* 2013;17(5):501–506.

Samarawickrama C, Pai A, Tariq Y, Healey PR, Wong TY, Mitchell P. Characteristics and appearance of the normal optic nerve head in 6-year-old children. *Br J Ophthalmol.* 2012;96(1):68–72.

Visual Field Testing

Assessment of the visual field in children is useful, but the testing process can be challenging. Automated testing can begin at age 5 years; the results become more reliable as the child approaches 7–8 years of age. As for adults, abnormalities should be confirmed with repeat testing. Although there is no normative database for children, the age correction for mean deviation is small (0.7 dB/decade). Other indices, the pattern standard deviation, the glaucoma hemifield test, and glaucoma change probability are largely unaffected by age.

Patel DE, Cumberland PM, Walters BC, Russell-Eggitt I, Cortina-Borja M, Rahi JS; OPTIC Study Group. Study of optimal perimetric testing in children (OPTIC): normative visual field values in children. *Ophthalmology.* 2015;122(8):1711–1717.

A-Scan Ultrasonography

Serial measurements of axial length using A-scan ultrasonography can document progressive globe enlargement in patients under the age of 4 (Figs 11-12, 11-13). Axial length may

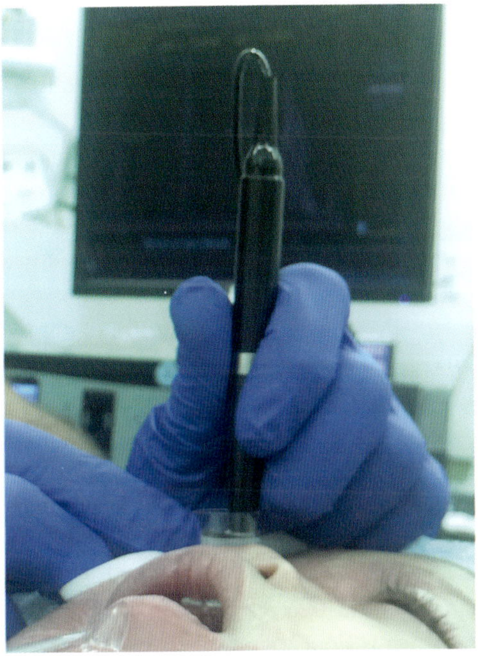

Figure 11-12 Photograph of axial length (AL) measurement obtained by A-scan ultrasonography, which is useful in detecting abnormally rapid globe elongation in eyes with uncontrolled IOP. *(Courtesy of JoAnn A. Giaconi, MD.)*

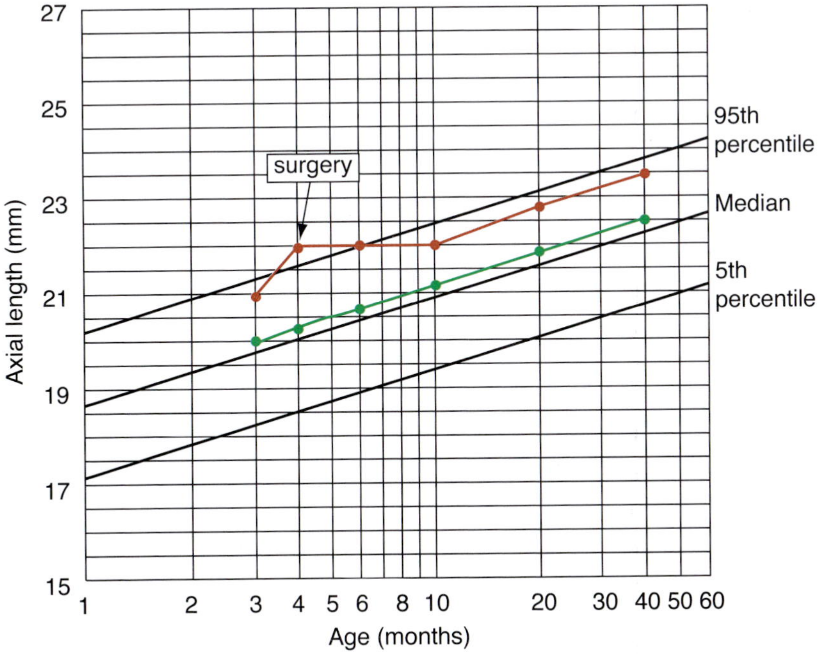

Figure 11-13 Graph of axial length showing normal pediatric growth with 95% confidence intervals. Charting AL on a graph helps identify abnormally long eyes or eyes that are growing at abnormal rates. *(Courtesy of JoAnn A. Giaconi, MD.)*

stabilize or decrease with control of IOP and thus serves as a critical marker for successful control of IOP.

Law SK, Bui D, Caprioli J. Serial axial length measurement in congenital glaucoma. *Am J Ophthalmol.* 2001;132(6):926–928.

Other Testing

B-scan ultrasonography can be performed if media opacities, particularly corneal edema, preclude fundus evaluation.

Treatment Overview

Surgical Management

Surgery is the preferred, definitive treatment of most cases of PCG; medications have limited long-term value. Although medication can better control IOP in other forms of pediatric glaucoma, a high percentage of these cases also eventually require surgery. Goniotomy and ab externo trabeculotomy are the procedures of choice for the treatment of PCG. Either procedure is appropriate if the cornea is clear. If the cornea is cloudy, poor visualization of the target structures makes goniotomy difficult to perform; trabeculotomy is preferred in these eyes because it is more easily performed. Angle surgery has a high success rate in children with PCG; the highest success rates have been observed in children diagnosed between 3 and 12 months of age.

Angle surgery may also be used to treat other forms of pediatric glaucoma, including glaucoma following congenital cataract surgery, glaucoma associated with aniridia, A-R syndrome, and SWS; however, the success rates are lower. Trabeculectomy and glaucoma tube shunt surgery should be reserved for congenital glaucoma cases in which goniotomy or trabeculotomy has failed or for cases in which angle surgery is not appropriate. Cyclodestruction is necessary in some intractable cases, but because of the risk of phthisis bulbi, it should be avoided if possible.

Glaucoma surgery in children poses unique difficulties. For example, in PCG, the anatomical landmarks are distorted in the buphthalmic eye, and the thin sclera presents additional difficulties during trabeculotomy and trabeculectomy. The surgeon performing glaucoma surgery in pediatric patients should be experienced in handling these challenges and able to provide the necessary environment for evaluating these patients postoperatively. Additional surgery is often required, so the surgeon should also develop a long-term plan in order to keep surgical options available for the future and to minimize the risk of visual compromise.

The decision to proceed with angle surgery is often made during an EUA; ideally, if glaucoma is diagnosed, angle surgery is performed during the same anesthesia session in order to minimize the number of general anesthesia exposures for the child. If both eyes have uncontrolled glaucoma it is the standard of care to perform bilateral surgery in the same session. If angle surgery is anticipated, it is best not to dilate the eye during the EUA in order to protect the lens during the surgical procedure.

Angle surgery

In a goniotomy, the angle is visualized with a surgical gonioscopic contact lens, a needle or appropriate blade is passed across the anterior chamber, and a superficial incision is made in the trabecular meshwork (Video 11-1, Fig 11-14). As mentioned, a clear cornea is required in order to visualize the angle.

VIDEO 11-1 Goniotomy.
Courtesy of Ken K. Nischal, MD.
Go to www.aao.org/bcscvideo_section10 to access all videos in Section 10.

In an ab externo trabeculotomy, Schlemm canal is cannulated from an external approach, and the trabecular meshwork is opened by breaking through Schlemm canal into the anterior chamber. The procedure begins with creation of a conjunctival flap, beneath which a partial-thickness scleral flap is created, similar to a trabeculectomy. Beneath that partial-thickness scleral flap, the surgeon identifies Schlemm canal, either by creating a radial incision into the scleral-corneal junction or by dissecting a deep scleral flap and noting the canal at the edges of this flap. Alternatively, the surgeon can identify the canal edges after unroofing the Schlemm canal by creating a single deep scleral flap. The surgeon inserts a rigid instrument (trabeculotome) into Schlemm canal and then rotates it into the anterior chamber (Fig 11-15), tearing the trabecular meshwork (Video 11-2). Alternatively, a 6-0 polypropylene suture or a fiber-optic microcatheter can be fed through Schlemm canal for its entire 360° circumference and pulled tautly into the anterior chamber (Video 11-3). There are other commercially available devices to perform an ab interno trabeculotomy. When performing a trabeculotomy, the surgeon must take care to avoid creating a false passage and entering the subretinal or suprachoroidal space.

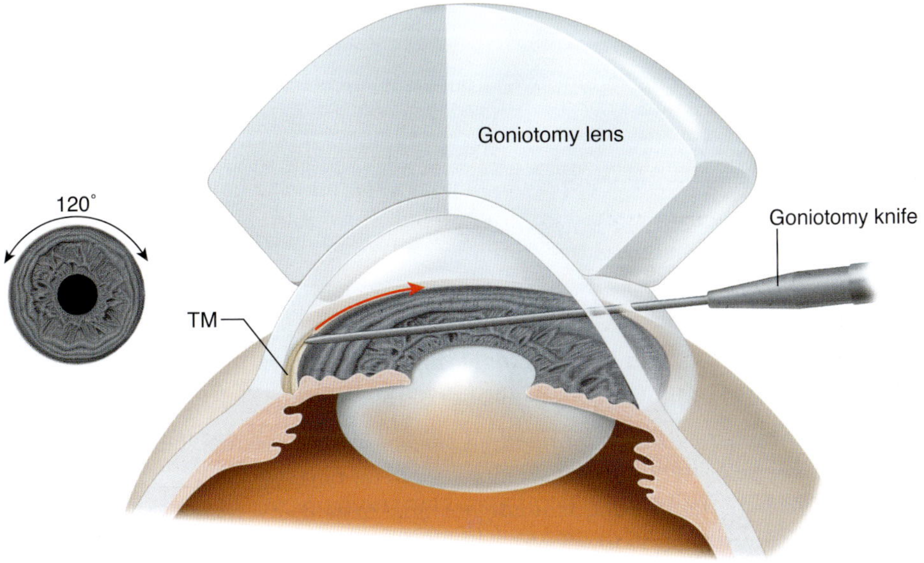

Figure 11-14 Illustration of a goniotomy incision as seen through a surgical contact lens. *(Illustration courtesy of Mark Miller.)*

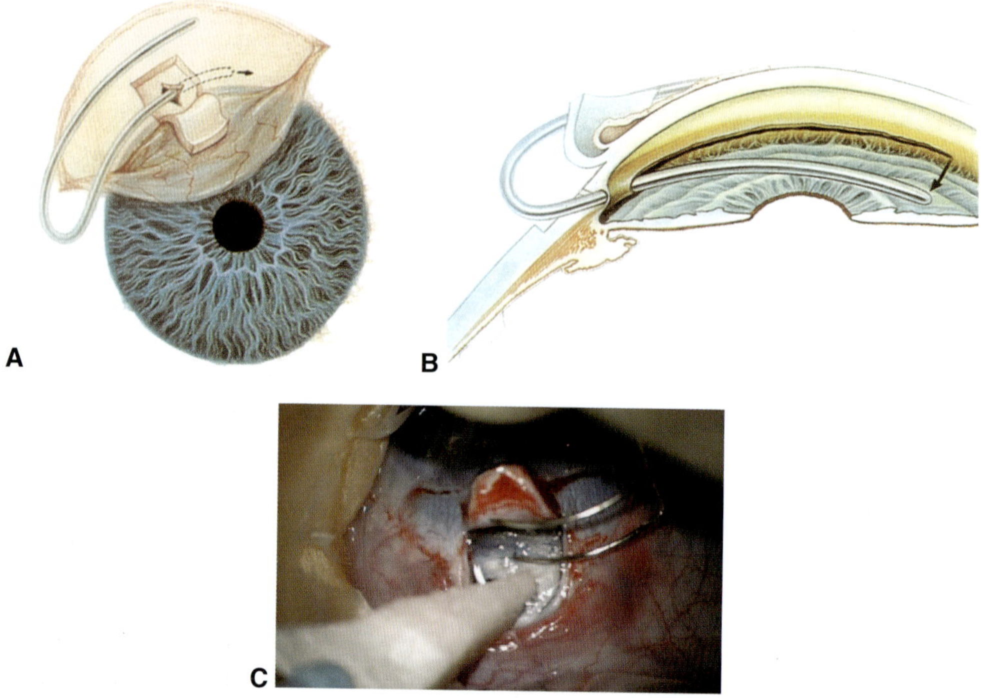

Figure 11-15 Trabeculotomy. **A,** Illustration of the probe as it is gently passed along Schlemm canal, with little resistance for 6–10 mm. **B,** By rotating the probe internally *(arrow),* the surgeon ruptures the trabecular meshwork and the probe appears in the anterior chamber with minimal bleeding. **C,** Photograph of the trabeculotome used in ab externo trabeculotomy allows the surgeon to open the angle over 1 quadrant. *(Parts A and B reproduced and modified with permission from Kolker AE, Hetherington J, eds.* Becker-Shaffer's Diagnosis and Therapy of the Glaucomas. *5th ed. Mosby; 1983. Part C courtesy of JoAnn A. Giaconi, MD.)*

VIDEO 11-2 Trabeculotomy over 1 quadrant.
Courtesy of Young Kwon, MD, PhD.

VIDEO 11-3 Trabeculotomy over 360°.
Courtesy of JoAnn A. Giaconi, MD.

Many surgeons inject viscoelastic into the anterior chamber at the start of goniotomy and trabeculotomy in order to prevent collapse of the chamber and to tamponade bleeding intraoperatively. To prevent a postoperative spike in IOP, thorough removal of the viscoelastic at the end of the procedure is necessary.

The success rates of these 2 angle surgeries are similar, but each procedure has its advantages (Table 11-12) and disadvantages. Complications associated with these procedures include hyphema, infection, iris damage, lens damage, and uveitis. Descemet membrane may be stripped during a trabeculotomy.

Table 11-12 Comparison of the Advantages of Goniotomy and Trabeculotomy

Goniotomy	Trabeculotomy
No postoperative conjunctival scarring	Ab externo approach more familiar to glaucoma surgeons who typically operate on adults
Faster procedure	Can be performed in opacified corneas
Less trauma to anterior segment tissues	Can be converted to a trabeculectomy if Schlemm canal cannot be cannulated

Angle surgery has a success rate of 70%–80% in infants presenting with PCG between 3 and 12 months of age; this success rate includes repeated angle procedures, which are common for this disease. Trabeculectomy or tube shunt surgery should be considered after 2 or more angle surgeries fail to control the IOP or when adjunctive medical therapy is inadequate.

Trabeculectomy and tube shunt surgery

If angle surgery is not successful, the surgeon must take several factors into account when deciding between trabeculectomy and tube shunt surgery as the next procedure. Trabeculectomy has a low success rate in children younger than 2 years and in aphakic eyes. Failure rates are high without the use of antifibrotics, but serious risks of bleb leaks and bleb infections are associated with the use of these agents. Due to the risk of blebitis and endophthalmitis, mitomycin C (MMC)–augmented trabeculectomy should be performed with caution in pediatric patients who are too young to understand good hygiene, which is necessary to minimize the risk of infection.

Tube shunt surgery is useful for lowering IOP, has higher success rates in children compared to trabeculectomy, and is associated with a lower risk of bleb-related infections. Success rates vary with different tube shunts, diagnoses, and patient ages. Complications include anterior migration of the tube with resultant corneal damage, tube blockage, tube erosion, infection, cataract, motility disturbances, bleb encapsulation with elevated IOP, and pupil distortion. In small eyes, the surgeon must ensure the posterior aspect of the drainage device plate does not compress the optic nerve. IOPs are usually higher after implantation of these devices than after successful trabeculectomy, and most children need to continue using topical ocular hypotensive medications, as is the case for adults.

Cyclodestruction

In children, cyclodestruction (discussed in Chapter 13) is reserved for cases refractory to other surgical and medical treatments. When these procedures are performed in pediatric patients, general anesthesia is required. The rate of complications is lower with cyclodestructive laser procedures than with cyclocryotherapy. A disadvantage of cyclodestructive procedures is the difficulty in titrating the results. Another disadvantage is the risk of serious complications—which include hypotony, uveitis, retinal detachment, phthisis bulbi, and blindness. The most common cyclodestructive modalities currently used are transscleral and endoscopic cyclophotocoagulation (ECP) with the diode laser. ECP is particularly useful in eyes with distorted anterior segment anatomy and in eyes with prior unsuccessful transscleral cyclophotocoagulation. Either procedure can be very useful for providing additional IOP lowering after tube shunt surgery.

Barkan O. Goniotomy for the relief of congenital glaucoma. *Br J Ophthalmol.* 1948;32(9): 701–728.

Medical Management

Although surgery is the mainstay of treatment for most pediatric glaucomas, medications are also frequently required. Medications can be used to lower IOP before surgery in order to reduce corneal edema and improve visualization during surgery. They may also be used after surgical procedures for additional IOP lowering. Primary medical therapy is used to treat most patients with JOAG, inflammatory glaucoma, glaucoma following cataract surgery, and other secondary glaucomas. The safety and efficacy of most of the glaucoma medications approved by the US Food and Drug Administration (FDA) have not been studied specifically in children in controlled clinical trials, although most clinicians are guided by extensive clinical experience. Topical β-blockers, topical carbonic anhydrase inhibitors (CAIs), and prostaglandin analogues are reasonable first-line agents in children. When the patient is a preadolescent or adolescent girl, clinicians must inquire about pregnancy before initiating any treatment that might affect a fetus. A full discussion of glaucoma medications and their mechanisms of action can be found in Chapter 12. See Table 21-4 in BCSC Section 6, *Pediatric Ophthalmology and Strabismus,* for a comparison of systemic and ocular adverse effects of glaucoma medications in children.

β-Adrenergic antagonists

Topical β-adrenergic antagonists, or β-blocker agents, must be used with caution in children. The systemic absorption of these agents is considerable—even with topical application—and can cause bronchospasm, bradycardia, and hypotension in susceptible children. β-Blockers should thus be avoided in children with asthma or significant cardiac disease. To decrease the risk of bronchospasm, the clinician may consider administering the cardioselective β-blocker betaxolol. The risk of adverse effects can also be diminished with occlusion of the nasolacrimal drainage system for 2 to 5 minutes after administration and use of the lowest effective dose (eg, timolol 0.25% or levobunolol 0.25% as opposed to 0.5%), particularly for young children. The clinician should teach parents how to occlude the nasolacrimal drainage system for administration at home. Patients with lighter irides may respond as well to timolol 0.25% or levobunolol 0.25% as they do to 0.5% of the same medication.

Carbonic anhydrase inhibitors

Topical use of dorzolamide or brinzolamide has a minimal risk of systemic adverse effects and is an excellent first-line therapy. Systemic CAIs (acetazolamide and methazolamide) provide slightly more IOP lowering than the topical preparations but are associated with numerous systemic adverse effects, including anorexia, diarrhea, weight loss, paresthesia, hypokalemia, risk of sickle cell crisis in patients with sickle cell anemia, and metabolic acidosis, which can affect bone growth. Children using other diuretics are particularly at risk for these adverse effects. Because of the risk of these adverse effects and of rare but life-threatening reactions such as Stevens-Johnson syndrome and aplastic anemia, systemic CAIs are reserved for patients at great risk of vision loss due to highly elevated IOP. The pediatric dosage of oral acetazolamide is 10–20 mg/kg/day.

α-Adrenergic agonists

The α_2-adrenergic agonist brimonidine, which crosses the blood–brain barrier, may have significant effects on the central nervous system, including apnea, hypotension, bradycardia, hypotonia, hypothermia, and somnolence. Infants and young children are particularly susceptible to brimonidine's adverse effects; thus α_2-adrenergic agonists are contraindicated in children younger than 2 years. Although brimonidine is FDA approved for use in children over the age of 2, there is some debate about the age at which children can safely use this drug. In general, it should be used with caution in children up to the teenage years. The lowest dose possible should be used and punctal occlusion employed to minimize systemic absorption.

The α_2-adrenergic agonist apraclonidine is better tolerated systemically in children, but the risk of follicular conjunctivitis increases with long-term use. Apraclonidine also acts as a vasoconstrictor and can be used to minimize bleeding during surgery.

Prostaglandin analogues

Prostaglandin analogues have minimal systemic side effects and are dosed once daily. They have been shown to effectively lower IOP in JOAG. Older children respond better to prostaglandin analogues than younger children and infants. These drugs have been shown to be well tolerated and effective in patients with uveitis; however, in some cases, they may cause or exacerbate uveitis.

Cholinergic agonists

Cholinergic agonists are seldom used for long-term glaucoma therapy, particularly in phakic eyes due to induced myopia. Echothiophate (Phospholine Iodide) is highly effective in many patients with aphakic glaucoma and can be dosed once daily; however, its use in children is associated with the development of iris cysts. Use of echothiophate also results in breakdown of the blood–aqueous barrier; therefore, it must be discontinued well in advance of any surgical procedure to prevent postsurgical inflammation. Cholinergic agents can be used intraoperatively to induce miosis, which facilitates angle surgery. They are sometimes used for a limited period of time after angle surgery to prevent peripheral anterior synechiae formation.

Rho kinase inhibitors

There are no published reports on the use of Rho kinase inhibitors in pediatric patients.

Chang L, Ong EL, Bunce C, Brookes J, Papadopoulos M, Khaw PT. A review of the medical treatment of pediatric glaucomas at Moorfields Eye Hospital. *J Glaucoma.* 2013;22(8):601–607.

Coppens G, Stalmans I, Zeyen T, Casteels I. The safety and efficacy of glaucoma medications in the pediatric population. *J Pediatr Ophthalmol Strabismus.* 2009;46(1):12–18.

Maeda-Chubachi T, Chi-Burris K, Simons BD, et al; A6111137 Study Group. Comparison of latanoprost and timolol in pediatric glaucoma: a phase 3, 12-week, randomized, double-masked multicenter study. *Ophthalmology.* 2011;118(10):2014–2021.

Prognosis and Follow-Up

The development of effective surgical techniques has greatly improved the long-term prognosis for pediatric glaucoma patients, particularly PCG patients asymptomatic at birth who present with onset of symptoms between 3 and 12 months of age. These patients typically have a good prognosis; many achieve visual acuity of at least 20/70 with 5-year follow up, although multiple surgeries may be required, and vision may still decline with longer follow-up. When symptoms are present at birth or when the disease is diagnosed after 12 months of age, the prognosis is poor, and the risk of blindness is high. Children with secondary pediatric glaucomas tend to have the worst prognosis; up to 50% lose light perception despite treatment. Early referral to vision rehabilitation may be helpful to patients and family.

Pediatric patients whose IOP is controlled by surgery may still experience morbidities related to previous IOP elevation, including amblyopia, corneal scarring, strabismus, anisometropia, cataract, lens subluxation, susceptibility to trauma due to scleral fragility, and recurrent IOP elevation in the affected or unaffected eye. These morbidities can cause serious long-term visual compromise and thus should be addressed promptly.

Amblyopia is a common cause of visual compromise, particularly in patients with unilateral glaucoma, corneal opacification, and/or anisometropia. It is important to treat amblyopia aggressively, addressing conditions contributing to its development, such as refractive error, strabismus, cataract, and corneal pathology. Haab striae and corneal scarring may cause astigmatism. Elevated IOP can lead to buphthalmos in patients with PCG and to progressive myopia and anisometropia in patients with JOAG. Refractive errors should be corrected with spectacles or contact lenses, and use of protective eyewear should be encouraged.

Strabismus may result from glaucoma tube shunt surgery or amblyopia. When performing surgery to correct strabismus, the surgeon should try to minimize conjunctival scarring in anticipation of future glaucoma surgeries and should be cognizant of the sites of prior trabeculectomies and tube shunt implants.

All cases of pediatric glaucoma require lifelong follow-up to monitor IOP, potential complications from prior surgeries, and secondary vision-threatening complications. Because IOP elevation may recur even years later, glaucoma and pediatric ophthalmologists should coordinate care. A team approach to care will involve low vision rehabilitation specialists, pediatricians, genetic counselors, educators, and parents or caregivers. Educating parents or caregivers about the need for lifelong care of a child with glaucoma and involving these children in their own care enhances the long-term management of this challenging disease (for more on low vision rehabilitation in pediatric patients, see BCSC Section 6, *Pediatric Ophthalmology and Strabismus*).

de Silva DJ, Khaw PT, Brookes JL. Long-term outcome of primary congenital glaucoma. *J AAPOS.* 2011;15(2):148–152.

Khitri MR, Mills MD, Ying GS, Davidson SL, Quinn GE. Visual acuity outcomes in pediatric glaucomas. *J AAPOS.* 2012;16(4):376–381.

CHAPTER 12

Medical Management of Glaucoma and Ocular Hypertension

Highlights

- Target pressure is an estimate of the intraocular pressure (IOP) level below which the rate of disease progression is expected to be sufficiently slow as to minimize the patient's risk of experiencing further symptomatic vision loss. Target pressure is determined based on an assessment of various clinical factors that influence the future risk of progression.
- There are 5 classes of topical ocular hypotensive medications that are prescribed for long-term use. They are frequently used in combination. Clinicians should tailor their selection among these agents for each patient based on their efficacy, contraindications, adverse effect profile, and cost.
- Prostaglandin analogues are the most commonly used IOP-lowering agents. They lower IOP by increasing uveoscleral outflow.

Introduction

The goal of currently available glaucoma therapy is to preserve visual function by lowering intraocular pressure (IOP). The treatment regimen chosen should achieve this goal with the lowest risk, the fewest adverse effects, and the least disruption to the patient's life, taking into account the cost of treatment. Although the long-term efficacy of treatment is judged by stability of the visual field, optic nerve, and other structural parameters, it is also regularly assessed by ensuring adequate IOP reduction.

The term *target pressure* refers to an IOP below which the clinician estimates the rate of disease progression to be sufficiently slow as to minimize the patient's risk of experiencing further symptomatic vision loss in his or her lifetime. The value of establishing a target pressure after an initial evaluation period of a patient with glaucoma or ocular hypertension is that it encourages thoughtful appraisal of various clinical factors that influence the future risk of progression and allows for an efficient assessment of the patient's IOP level at each subsequent visit. Even if the target pressure is achieved, the clinician must continue to evaluate the stability of structural and functional measures important in glaucoma.

Target pressure should be individualized for each eye, based on the IOP level at which damage is thought to have occurred and the severity of that damage. It can be adjusted on the basis of several factors, including the previously observed rate of progression (if known); life expectancy of the patient; and risk factors such as a history of disc hemorrhages, a thinner cornea, or a family history of severe vision loss in the setting of glaucoma (risk factors are discussed in more detail in Chapter 7 in this volume).

Evidence suggests that the severity of optic nerve injury may increase the likelihood of continued disease progression. Therefore, the more advanced the disease is on initial presentation, the lower the target pressure required to minimize the risk of further symptomatic vision loss will be. Furthermore, if severe vision loss is already present, further damage (loss of retinal ganglion cells) is likely to have a disproportionately greater impact on visual function and quality of life. Establishing a target IOP is part of the art of glaucoma management, because many different approaches can be used. Clinical trials to evaluate different approaches of determining the target pressure, or even the value of establishing a target pressure at all, are impractical to conduct; differences among groups would likely be small and would take a long period of time to detect because disease progression usually occurs slowly. In addition, simply establishing a target pressure does not guarantee it will be achieved, and it often takes a long time and many treatment adjustments to reach the target pressure.

Disease progression occurs in some patients despite reduction of IOP below the target pressure. If progression does occur at an unacceptable rate, downward revision of the target pressure may be required. Conversely, once a target pressure is established, it does not become a mandate; the risks of each sequential medical or surgical intervention thought to be required to achieve a given target pressure must be weighed against the potential benefit of further IOP reduction. Table 12-1 summarizes a general framework for estimating an appropriate target pressure; however, there is no system that would garner universal agreement.

After determining the target pressure, the clinician must decide whether to achieve this goal medically or surgically. For either approach, the anticipated benefits of any therapeutic intervention should justify the risks; regimens associated with substantial adverse effects should be reserved for patients with a high probability of progressive vision loss. In some cases, it may be necessary to accept an IOP level above the established target pressure because the adverse effects or risks of intensified therapy may be unacceptable. Both the risks and adverse events associated with specific treatment options and the risks of disease progression on the patient's overall quality of life must be considered.

Initial treatment of ocular hypertension and most glaucomas typically involves the use of medications or laser trabeculoplasty. When starting a patient on a medication, some clinicians favor using a unilateral treatment trial in order to assess the medication's efficacy; however, evidence suggests that this may be of limited value because of the occurrence of asymmetric IOP fluctuation between fellow eyes.

Ocular hypotensive agents are divided into several classes based on chemical structure and pharmacologic action. The classes in common clinical use include

- prostaglandin analogues, including 1 agent with a nitric oxide–donating moiety
- adrenergic drugs

Table 12-1 Estimating Target Pressure

Initial target pressure
Ocular hypertension (normal visual field and optic disc)
<25 mm Hg and 20% below baseline (if there is a decision to treat)
Mild glaucoma damage (optic disc damage with normal visual field)
<21 mm Hg and 25% below baseline
Moderate glaucoma damage (visual field damage in one hemifield outside the central 10°)
<18 mm Hg and 30% below baseline
Severe glaucoma damage (visual field damage in both hemifields and/or affecting the central 10°)
<15 mm Hg and 30% below baseline
Risk factors that may necessitate downward adjustment of target pressure
History of optic disc hemorrhage
Thinner central cornea
History of rapid progression or severe vision loss in the fellow eye
Family history of blindness due to glaucoma
Early age of onset of glaucoma damage
Factors that may allow upward adjustment of target pressure
Decreased life expectancy or other comorbidities
Prior history of stable or slowly progressive damage
High central corneal thickness

  - β-adrenergic antagonists (nonselective and β_1-selective)
  - adrenergic agonists (nonselective and α_2-selective)
- carbonic anhydrase inhibitors (topical and systemic)
- parasympathomimetic (miotic) agents
  - direct-acting cholinergic agonists
  - indirect-acting anticholinesterase agents
- Rho kinase inhibitors
- combination medications
- hyperosmotic agents

Table 12-2 lists the actions and adverse effects of the various glaucoma medications. See also BCSC Section 2, *Fundamentals and Principles of Ophthalmology,* for additional discussion of the mechanisms of action of these medications.

Netland PA, Tanna AP, eds. *Glaucoma Medical Therapy: Principles and Management.* 3rd ed. Kugler; 2020.

Prostaglandin Analogues

Mechanism of Action

Ocular hypotensive prostaglandin analogues are prodrugs that penetrate the cornea and become biologically active after being hydrolyzed by corneal esterase. They lower IOP by

Table 12-2 Glaucoma Medications

Class/Compound	Concentration	Dosing	Mechanism of Action	IOP Reduction	Adverse Effects: Ocular	Adverse Effects: Systemic	Comments, Including Time to Peak Effect and Washout
Prostaglandin analogues							
Latanoprost	0.005%	Once daily	Increases uveoscleral outflow primarily; also increases conventional outflow	25%–32%	Increased pigmentation of iris and lashes, hypertrichosis, trichiasis, distichiasis, blurred vision, keratitis, anterior uveitis, conjunctival hyperemia, exacerbation of herpes keratitis, CME, prostaglandin-associated periorbitopathy	Flulike symptoms, joint/muscle pain, headache	±IOP-lowering effect with miotic Peak: 10–14 hours Washout: 4–6 weeks Maximum IOP-lowering effect may take up to 6 weeks to occur
Travoprost	0.004%	Once daily	Same as above	25%–32%	Same as above	Same as above	Same as above
Bimatoprost	0.03%, 0.01%	Once daily	Same as above	27%–33%	Same as above	Same as above	Same as above
Bimatoprost sustained-release	10 µg sustained-release implant	FDA-approved for one-time use	Same as above	~30%	Conjunctival hyperemia, pain, irritation, corneal endothelial cell loss, photophobia, iritis	None	Intracameral implant composed of bimatoprost in a poly(D,L-lactide-co-glycolide) polymer matrix
Tafluprost	0.0015%	Once daily	Increases uveoscleral outflow	27%–31%	Same as above	Same as above	Same as above
Latanoprostene bunod	0.024%	Once daily	Increases uveoscleral outflow; nitric oxide may also increase conventional outflow	~32%	Same as above	Same as above	Same as above
β-Adrenergic antagonists (β-blockers)							
Nonselective							
Timolol maleate	0.25%, 0.50% solution or gel 0.1% gel	Solutions: 1–2 times daily Gels: once daily	Decreases aqueous humor production	20%–30%	Blurred vision, irritation, corneal anesthesia, punctate keratitis, allergy; aggravation of myasthenia gravis	Bradycardia, heart block, bronchospasm, lowered blood pressure, decreased libido, CNS depression, mood swings, reduced exercise tolerance, masked symptoms of hypoglycemia, exacerbation of myasthenia gravis	May be less effective if patient is taking systemic β-blockers; short-term escape, long-term drift; diabetic patients may experience reduced glucose tolerance and masking of hypoglycemic signs/symptoms Peak: 2–3 hours Washout: 1 month
Timolol hemihydrate	0.5%	Same as above	Same as above	20%–30%	Same as above	Same as above	—
Levobunolol	0.25%, 0.5%	Same as above	Same as above	20%–30%	Same as above	Same as above	Peak: 2–6 hours
Metipranolol	0.3%	2 times daily	Same as above	20%–30%	Same as above	Same as above	Report of iritis Peak: 2 hours

Class/Com[illegible]	[illegible]	[illegible]	[illegible]	[illegible]	[illegible]	[illegible]	[illegible]
Carteolo[illegible] hydroc[illegible]	[illegible]	[illegible]	[illegible]	[illegible]	[illegible]	[illegible]	[illegible]
Selective							
Betaxolol	[illegible]	[illegible]	[illegible]	[illegible]	[illegible]	[illegible]	[illegible] month
α_2-Adrener[illegible]							
Selective							
Apraclonid[illegible] hydrochlo[illegible]	[illegible]	[illegible] times daily	Decreases aqueous humor production	20%–30%	Irritation, ischemia, allergy, eyelid retraction, conjunctival blanching, follicular conjunctivitis, pruritus, dermatitis, ocular ache, photopsia, mydriasis	Hypotension, vasovagal attack, dry mouth and nose, fatigue	Useful in pre- or postlaser or cataract surgery Tachyphylaxis may limit long-term use Peak: <1–2 hours Washout: 7–14 days
Brimonidine tartrate preserved with benzalkonium chloride	0.15%, 0.2%	2–3 times daily	Decreases aqueous humor production, may increase uveoscleral outflow	20%–30%	Blurred vision, foreign-body sensation, eyelid edema, dryness, less ocular sensitivity/allergy than with apraclonidine, miosis	Headache, fatigue, hypotension, insomnia, depression, syncope, dizziness, anxiety, dry mouth	Highly selective for α_2-receptor Brimonidine should not be used in infants and young children Peak: 2 hours Washout: 7–14 days
Brimonidine tartrate preserved with Purite	0.1%, 0.15%	2–3 times daily	Same as above	Same as above	Same as above, except less allergy than with brimonidine 0.2%	Same as above, except less fatigue and depression than with brimonidine 0.2%	Same as above
Carbonic anhydrase inhibitors							
Oral							
Acetazolamide	125 mg	Seldom used for IOP-lowering therapy in adults	Decreases aqueous humor production	15%–20%	None	Poor tolerance of carbonated beverages, acidosis, depression, malaise, hirsutism, flatulence, paresthesias, numbness, lethargy, blood dyscrasias, diarrhea, weight loss, renal stones, loss of libido, impotence, bone marrow depression, hypokalemia, cramps, anorexia, taste disturbance, increased serum urate, enuresis	Use with caution in patients susceptible to ketoacidosis Contraindicated in patients with hepatic cirrhosis Adjust dose for chronic renal insufficiency Caution for using an oral CAI with other drugs that cause potassium loss Peak: 3–6 hours (sustained release) 2–4 hours (oral) Indicated for long-term therapy only in rare cases
	250 mg	2–4 times daily					
	500 mg (sustained release)	2 times daily					

(Continued)

Class/Compound	Concentration	Dosing	Mechanism of Action	IOP Reduction	Adverse Effects: Ocular	Adverse Effects: Systemic	Comments, Including Time to Peak Effect and Washout
Acetazolamide (parenteral)	500 mg 5–10 mg/kg	Usually every 6–8 hours	Same as above	Same as above	Same as above	Same as above	Same as above
Methazolamide	25 mg, 50 mg	2–3 times daily	Same as above	Same as above	Same as above	Same as above	Same as above
Topical							
Dorzolamide	2%	2–3 times daily	Same as above	15%–20%	Induced myopia, blurred vision, stinging, keratitis, punctate keratopathy, conjunctivitis, dermatitis	Less likely to induce systemic effects of CAI, but may occur; taste disturbance	Peak: 2–3 hours Washout: 48 hours
Brinzolamide	1%	2–3 times daily	Same as above	Same as above	Same as above, except less stinging when compared with dorzolamide	Same as above	Same as above
Parasympathomimetic agents (miotics)							
Cholinergic agonist (direct acting)							
Pilocarpine HCl	0.5%, 1.0%, 2.0%, 3.0%, 4.0%, 6.0%	2–4 times daily	Increases trabecular outflow	15%–25%	Posterior synechiae, keratitis, miosis, brow ache, cataract growth, angle-closure potential, myopia, retinal tear/detachment, dermatitis, change in retinal sensitivity, color vision changes, epiphora	Increased salivation, increased secretion (gastric), abdominal cramps	Exacerbation of cataract effect; more effective in lighter irides Peak: 1½–2 hours Washout: 48 hours
Anticholinesterase agent (indirect acting)							
Echothiophate iodide	0.125%	1–2 times daily	Same as above	15%–25%	Intense miosis, iris pigment cyst, myopia, cataract, retinal detachment, angle closure, punctal stenosis, pseudopemphigoid, epiphora	Same as pilocarpine; more gastrointestinal difficulties	Increased inflammation with ocular surgery; may be helpful in aphakia, anesthesia risks (prolonged recovery); useful in eyelid-lash lice, cataract surgery postoperatively
Rho kinase inhibitor							
Netarsudil	0.02%	Once daily	Increases conventional (trabecular) outflow, also decreases episcleral venous pressure	~20%–25%	Conjunctival hyperemia, subconjunctival hemorrhage, cornea verticillata, pain, blurred vision, increased lacrimation	None	—
Fixed combinations							
Timolol/ brinzolamide	0.5%/1%	2 times daily	Decreases aqueous humor production	25%–30%	Same as those of nonselective β-adrenergic antagonist, topical CAI	Same as those of nonselective β-adrenergic antagonist, topical CAI	—

Class/Compound	Concentration	Dosing	Mechanism of Action	IOP Reduction	Adverse Effects: Ocular	Adverse Effects: Systemic	Comments, Including Time to Peak Effect and Washout
Timolol/dorzolamide	0.5%/2%	2 times daily	Decreases aqueous humor production	25%–30%	Same as those of nonselective β-blocker, topical CAI	Same as those of nonselective β-blocker, topical CAI	Peak: 2–3 hours Washout: 1 month
Timolol/latanoprost	0.5%/0.005%	Once daily (nighttime)	Same as nonselective β-blocker and latanoprost	Greater than monotherapy with each individually	Same as those of nonselective β-blocker and latanoprost	Same as those of nonselective β-blocker and latanoprost	Not currently available in the United States
Timolol/travoprost	0.5%/0.004%	Once daily (nighttime)	Same as nonselective β-blocker and travoprost	25%–30%	Same as those of nonselective β-blocker and travoprost	Same as those of nonselective β-blocker and travoprost	Same as above
Timolol/bimatoprost	0.5%/0.03%	Once daily (nighttime)	Same as nonselective β-blocker and bimatoprost	Same as above	Same as those of nonselective β-blocker and bimatoprost	Same as those of nonselective β-blocker and bimatoprost	Same as above
Timolol/brimonidine tartrate	0.5%/0.2%	2 times daily	Same as nonselective β-blocker and α-agonist	Same as above	Same as those of nonselective β-blocker and α-agonist	Same as those of nonselective β-blocker and α-agonist	—
Brimonidine/brinzolamide	0.2%/1%	3 times daily	Decreases aqueous humor production; may increase uveoscleral outflow	26%–36%	Same as those of the individual components	Same as those of the individual components	—
Latanoprost/netarsudil	0.005%/0.02%	Once daily (nighttime)	Same as those of the individual components	31%–37%	Same as those of the individual components	Same as those of the individual components	—
Hyperosmotic agents							
Mannitol (parenteral)	20%	0.5–2.0 g/kg body weight	Creates osmotic gradient; dehydrates vitreous	—	IOP rebound, increased aqueous flare	Urinary retention, headache, congestive heart failure, diabetic complications, nausea, vomiting, diarrhea, electrolyte disturbance, confusion, backache, myocardial infarction	Contraindicated in patients in renal failure or on dialysis; caution in heart failure; useful in acute increased IOP
Glycerol (oral)	50%	1–1.5 g/kg body weight	Same as above	—	Similar to above	Similar to above; can cause problems in diabetic patients	Similar to above; may precipitate diabetic ketoacidosis

CAI = carbonic anhydrase inhibitor; CME = cystoid macular edema; CNS = central nervous system; IOP = intraocular pressure.

increasing aqueous humor outflow via the uveoscleral pathway and decreasing outflow resistance. The precise mechanism by which these changes occur has not been fully determined. It is thought that the ocular hypotensive prostaglandin analogues bind to various prostaglandin receptors, most importantly prostaglandin $F_{2\alpha}$ ($PGF_{2\alpha}$), triggering a cascade of events that lead to activation of matrix metalloproteinases. This in turn leads to remodeling of the ciliary body, trabecular meshwork, and possibly scleral extracellular matrix, so the flow rate of aqueous humor through these tissues is increased. Topical prostaglandin analogue therapy results in increased space between the muscle fascicles within the ciliary body, which is thought to be the primary location of uveoscleral outflow.

Available Agents and Dosing Frequency

Currently, 5 prostaglandin analogues are in widespread clinical use: latanoprost, travoprost, bimatoprost, tafluprost, and latanoprostene bunod. (See the section 2021 Update: Sustained-Release Bimatoprost Implant at the end of this chapter for information on an implant approved by the FDA in 2020.) These agents reduce IOP by 25%–33%. Tafluprost appears to be slightly less efficacious than latanoprost (see Table 12-2; see also the section General Approach to Medical Treatment in this chapter for discussion of preservatives). Latanoprostene bunod lowers mean diurnal IOP by 32% and is unique in that it is a *nitric oxide–donating* $PGF_{2\alpha}$ analogue. Nitric oxide is thought to increase trabecular outflow facility with a resultant 1 mm Hg IOP-lowering advantage over latanoprost in 1 clinical trial. See also BCSC Section 2, *Fundamentals and Principles of Ophthalmology.*

Prostaglandin analogues are used once daily and are less effective when used twice daily. Because some patients may respond better to 1 agent in this class than to another, switching drugs after a trial of 4–6 weeks may sometimes prove helpful.

Adverse Effects

An adverse effect unique to this class of drugs is the darkening of the iris and periocular skin as a result of an increased number of melanosomes within the melanocytes, without melanocyte proliferation. Increased iris pigmentation is permanent, and the frequency of this effect depends on the baseline iris color. Most published data relate to latanoprost and suggest a risk of up to 33% after 5 years of use. In particular, up to 79% of persons with green-brown irides and up to 85% of persons with hazel (yellow-brown) irides may be affected, compared with 8% of persons with blue irides. There is no evidence to suggest that increased iris or periocular skin pigmentation is associated with any risk to the patient such as an increased risk of melanoma.

Other adverse effects reported in association with the use of a topical prostaglandin analogue include conjunctival hyperemia (a result of vasodilation, more common with bimatoprost and travoprost), hypertrichosis (Figs 12-1, 12-2), trichiasis, and distichiasis. These effects are reversible upon drug discontinuation.

Use of prostaglandin analogue eyedrops has also been associated with the development of *prostaglandin-associated periorbitopathy* (see Fig 12-2), a complex of abnormalities that includes deepening of the upper eyelid sulcus, upper eyelid ptosis, enophthalmos, inferior scleral show, and possibly a tight orbit. These abnormalities appear to be the result of periorbital fat atrophy. It is not clear whether this periorbitopathy is reversible.

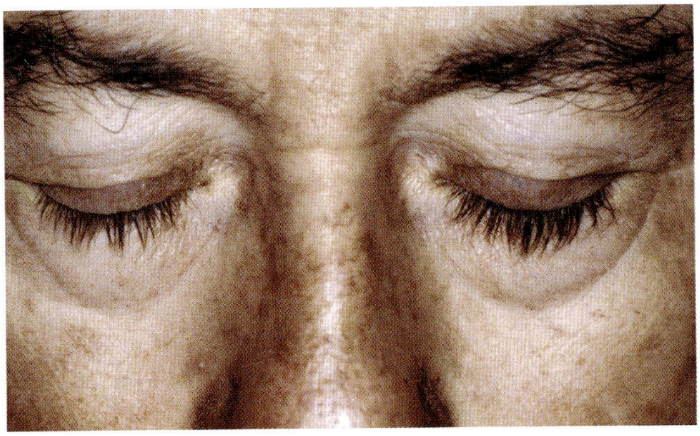

Figure 12-1 Hypertrichosis following use of latanoprost (left eye). *(Courtesy of F. Jane Durcan, MD.)*

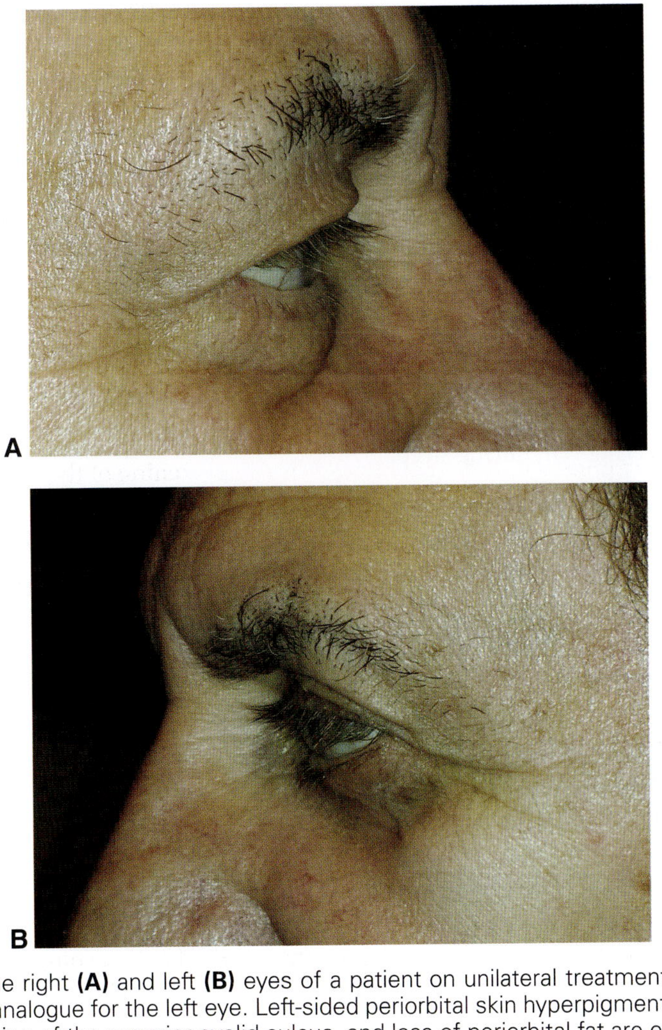

Figure 12-2 The right **(A)** and left **(B)** eyes of a patient on unilateral treatment with a topical prostaglandin analogue for the left eye. Left-sided periorbital skin hyperpigmentation, hypertrichosis, deepening of the superior eyelid sulcus, and loss of periorbital fat are evident. *(Courtesy of Chandrasekharan Krishnan, MD.)*

The development or exacerbation of preexisting cystoid macular edema (CME) can occur in certain predisposed eyes (ie, aphakic eyes, pseudophakic eyes with open posterior capsules, and eyes with uveitis). Reactivation of herpetic keratitis has been reported. Nongranulomatous anterior uveitis may occur as an idiosyncratic reaction in approximately 1% of patients.

Camras CB, Alm A, Watson P, Stjernschantz J. Latanoprost, a prostaglandin analog, for glaucoma therapy. Efficacy and safety after 1 year of treatment in 198 patients. Latanoprost Study Groups. *Ophthalmology.* 1996;103(11):1916–1924.

Weinreb RN, Ong T, Scassellati Sforzolini B, et al. A randomised, controlled comparison of latanoprostene bunod and latanoprost 0.005% in the treatment of ocular hypertension and open angle glaucoma: the VOYAGER study. *Br J Ophthalmol.* 2015;99(6):738–745.

Adrenergic Drugs

β-Adrenergic Antagonists

Mechanism of action

Topical β-adrenergic antagonists, or *β-blockers,* lower IOP by inhibiting cyclic adenosine monophosphate (cAMP) production in the ciliary epithelium, thereby reducing aqueous humor secretion by 20%–50%, with a corresponding IOP reduction of 20%–30%. In healthy eyes, β-blocker administration reduces aqueous secretion and lowers IOP; interestingly, however, there is a compensatory reduction in aqueous outflow facility that dampens the magnitude of IOP reduction. The effect on aqueous production occurs within 1 hour of instillation and can last for up to 4 weeks after discontinuation of the medication. Because systemic absorption occurs, an IOP-lowering effect may also be observed in the untreated contralateral eye. β-Blockers have much less effect on aqueous production during sleep, as aqueous production is already reduced during the nocturnal period; thus, they are ineffective in lowering IOP during sleep.

Available agents and dosing frequency

In the United States and Europe, 5 topical β-adrenergic antagonists are approved for the treatment of glaucoma: (1) betaxolol, (2) carteolol, (3) levobunolol, (4) metipranolol, and (5) timolol. Betaxolol, the only topical β_1-selective antagonist, is less effective in lowering IOP than the others, which are nonselective β-adrenergic antagonists. Most β-blockers are approved for twice-daily therapy. In many cases, the nonselective agents can be used once daily. Generally, dosing first thing in the morning is preferred in order to effectively blunt an early-morning pressure rise while minimizing the risk of systemic hypotension during sleep. Many nonselective β-blockers are available in more than 1 concentration. Clinical experience has shown that in many patients, timolol maleate 0.25% is as effective as timolol maleate 0.5% in lowering IOP.

In approximately 10%–20% of patients treated with topical β-blockers, IOP is not significantly lowered. Patients already taking a moderate or high dose of a systemic β-blocker may experience little additional IOP lowering from the addition of a topical ophthalmic β-blocker. Extended use of β-blockers may result in tachyphylaxis due to receptor upregulation. Physiologic changes in the trabecular meshwork may occur in response to decreased IOP and aqueous humor flow rate, resulting in decreased outflow facility. The underlying disease process responsible for decreased outflow facility and IOP elevation may also worsen during the course of therapy.

Adverse effects

Topical β-blockers are generally very well tolerated when administered to individuals without specific contraindications. The ocular and systemic adverse effects of β-adrenergic antagonists are listed in Table 12-2. Plasma drug levels from topical medications can approach those achieved with systemic administration because of their absorption in the nasolacrimal drainage system and lack of first-pass hepatic metabolism. However, administering topical medications in a gel vehicle results in reduced systemic absorption and decreased plasma concentrations of β-blockers compared with the equivalent solution. Punctal occlusion also reduces systemic absorption.

Systemic adverse effects of β-adrenergic antagonists include bronchospasm, bradycardia, increased heart block, systemic hypotension, reduced exercise tolerance, and central nervous system (CNS) depression. Patients with diabetes mellitus may experience reduced glucose tolerance and masking of hypoglycemic signs and symptoms. In addition, abrupt withdrawal of ophthalmic β-blockers can exacerbate symptoms of hyperthyroidism.

Before a β-blocker is prescribed, the clinician should ask whether the patient has a history of asthma, because β-blockers may induce severe, life-threatening bronchospasm in susceptible patients. β_2-Receptors are present in bronchial smooth muscle cells, and their inhibition results in bronchospasm in susceptible individuals. Because betaxolol is a β_1-selective antagonist, it is safer than the nonselective β-blockers for use in patients with asthma. In addition, betaxolol may be less likely to cause depression. However, β-blocker–related adverse effects can still occur with its use.

Prior to initiation of therapy with a topical β-blocker, the patient's pulse should be measured; the β-blocker should be withheld if the pulse rate is slow or if more than first-degree heart block is present. Administration of topical β-blockers has been associated with the development of signs and symptoms of myasthenia gravis in patients without a preexisting diagnosis and can exacerbate the condition in patients already known to have the disease. The mechanism by which this occurs is unclear.

Other adverse effects of β-blockers include lethargy, mood changes, depression, altered mentation, light-headedness, syncope, visual disturbance, corneal anesthesia, punctate keratitis, allergy, impotence, reduced libido, and alteration of serum lipids (reduction in high-density lipoprotein). In children, β-blockers should be used with caution, because of the relatively high systemic levels achieved.

Adrenergic Agonists

Nonselective adrenergic agonists

The nonselective adrenergic agonists epinephrine (adrenaline) and dipivefrin (a prodrug of epinephrine) reduce aqueous humor production, increase uveoscleral outflow, and improve conventional outflow facility. Both have largely been superseded by other classes of drugs and are now used in the management of glaucoma only in rare cases due to the frequent occurrence of local adverse effects. Neither is available in the United States.

α_2-Selective adrenergic agonists

Mechanism of action α_2-Selective agonists lower IOP primarily by reducing aqueous humor production. The α_2-adrenoceptor found on the ciliary epithelium is coupled to an inhibitory G protein. It is thought that when this adrenoceptor is bound by catecholamines or pharmacologically active α_2-agonists, an intracellular cascade results in reduction in the activity of adenylate cyclase and the intracellular concentration of cAMP, with a resultant reduction in the rate of aqueous humor production. An alternate or possibly complementary mechanism by which aqueous humor production is reduced may be anterior segment vasoconstriction and reduced blood flow to the ciliary body. After a longer period of therapy, increased uveoscleral outflow was observed with the selective α_2-adrenergic agonist brimonidine, but not with apraclonidine. How uveoscleral outflow may be increased with brimonidine is unclear, but evidence points to relaxation of ciliary smooth muscle cells. As with β-blockers, systemic absorption of α_2-selective agonists may lead to a crossover effect, although it appears to be small.

Available agents and dosing frequency Brimonidine tartrate is the most commonly used α_2-adrenergic agonist. Apraclonidine hydrochloride (*para*-aminoclonidine), an α_2-adrenergic agonist and clonidine derivative, is used for long-term therapy only in rare instances because of the frequent occurrence of tachyphylaxis and a hypersensitivity reaction that can cause blepharoconjunctivitis. Use of apraclonidine is mostly limited to perioperative administration to blunt acute IOP spikes that may occur after laser iridotomy, laser trabeculoplasty, Nd:YAG laser capsulotomy, and cataract extraction. Brimonidine is similarly effective when used perioperatively.

Tachyphylaxis is less profound with brimonidine than with apraclonidine. Brimonidine's peak IOP reduction is approximately 26% (2 hours post dose), which is comparable to the reduction achieved by a nonselective β-blocker and superior to that of the selective β-blocker betaxolol. At trough (12 hours post dose), the IOP reduction is only 14%–15%, or less than the reduction achieved with nonselective β-blockers. Studies have shown that brimonidine does not lower nocturnal IOP. Though approved for therapy 3 times daily in the United States, brimonidine is commonly used twice daily, particularly when used in combination with at least 1 other agent.

Adverse effects The incidence of ocular allergic reactions (eg, follicular conjunctivitis and contact blepharodermatitis; Fig 12-3) is lower with brimonidine than with apraclonidine. This is a delayed-type hypersensitivity reaction that is dose dependent, with a 1-year incidence of approximately 15% for brimonidine tartrate 0.2% preserved with benzalkonium chloride (BAK) and 10% for brimonidine tartrate 0.15% preserved with sodium chlorite (Purite). The incidence of allergy continues to increase beyond 1 year. Cross-sensitivity to brimonidine in patients with known hypersensitivity to apraclonidine is minimal. The incidence of long-term intolerance to brimonidine due to local adverse effects, however, is high (>20%). Granulomatous anterior uveitis is rare but has been reported in association with the use of brimonidine.

α_2-Selective agonists have some α_1-binding activity. The ocular effects of α_1-adrenergic agonists include conjunctival vasoconstriction, pupillary dilation, and eyelid retraction. Apraclonidine has a much greater affinity for α_1-receptors than does brimonidine and

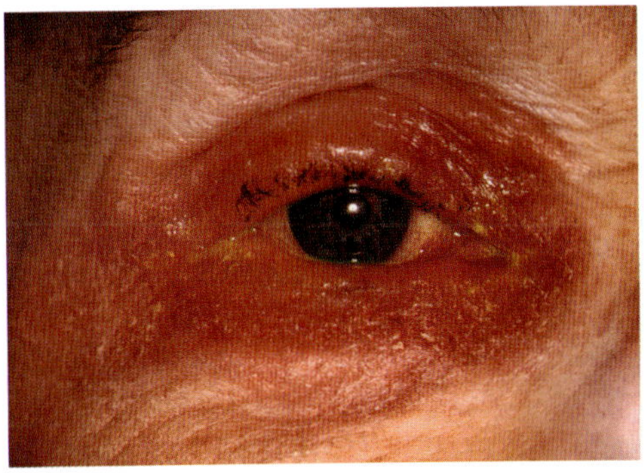

Figure 12-3 Contact blepharodermatitis following α-adrenergic agonist use. *(Courtesy of F. Jane Durcan, MD.)*

is therefore more likely to produce these effects. In some patients, apraclonidine causes mydriasis, whereas brimonidine commonly causes miosis.

Systemic adverse effects of α_2-selective agonists include xerostomia (dry mouth) and lethargy, both mediated by their clonidine-like CNS activity. Patients taking these medications should be advised to perform punctal occlusion. Brimonidine should not be used in infants and young children because of the risk of CNS depression, apnea, bradycardia, and hypotension, due to a combination of the lower volume of distribution and presumed increased CNS penetration of the drug.

Monoamine oxidase inhibitors and tricyclic antidepressants may interfere with metabolism of apraclonidine and brimonidine, resulting in toxicity.

Carbonic Anhydrase Inhibitors

Mechanism of Action

Carbonic anhydrase inhibitors (CAIs) decrease aqueous humor production by inhibiting the activity of ciliary epithelial carbonic anhydrase. Systemic CAI therapy may further decrease aqueous humor formation because of the resultant renal metabolic acidosis, which may reduce the activity of the Na^+,K^+-ATPase in the ciliary epithelium. The enzyme carbonic anhydrase is present in many tissues, including corneal endothelium, iris, retinal pigment epithelium, red blood cells, epithelial cells lining the choroid plexus of the brain, and kidney. More than 90% of the ciliary epithelial enzyme activity must be inhibited to decrease aqueous production and lower IOP.

Available Agents and Dosing Frequency

The topical CAI agents, dorzolamide and brinzolamide, are available for long-term treatment of elevated IOP and are associated with fewer systemic adverse effects than are the systemic CAIs. In the United States, these agents are currently approved for use 3 times daily, but most clinicians prescribe them for twice-daily use in many patients. Dosing 3 times per day dosing results in slightly greater IOP reduction. For patients taking an oral CAI at a full dose and the appropriate dosing frequency, there is no advantage to adding a topical CAI.

Systemic CAIs can be given orally or intravenously and are most useful in patients who present with severely elevated IOP or as a temporizing measure until surgery can be performed. Oral CAIs begin to act within 1 hour of administration, with maximal effect within 2–4 hours, whereas intravenous CAIs begin to act within 15 minutes. Sustained-release acetazolamide can reach peak effect within 3–6 hours of administration. Because of the adverse effects of systemic CAIs, however, long-term therapy should be reserved for patients whose IOP is not controlled with topical therapy and who have refused surgery or in whom surgery would be inappropriate.

The most commonly used oral CAIs are acetazolamide and methazolamide. Methazolamide has a longer duration of action and is less bound to serum protein than is acetazolamide; however, it is also less effective than acetazolamide. Methazolamide and sustained-release acetazolamide are the best tolerated of the systemic CAIs. Methazolamide is metabolized by the liver. Acetazolamide, which is not metabolized, is excreted by the kidney; it must be used with caution and at an adjusted dose in patients with renal insufficiency.

Because oral CAIs are potent medications that are associated with significant adverse effects, the lowest dose that reduces the IOP to an acceptable range should be used. Methazolamide is often effective in doses as low as 25–50 mg, given 2 or 3 times daily. Sustained-release formulations of acetazolamide may have fewer adverse effects than its standard formulation. The typical adult dosage of acetazolamide is 250 mg 4 times daily for the standard formulations or 500 mg twice daily for the sustained-release formulation.

Adverse Effects and Contraindications

Common adverse effects of topical CAIs include taste disturbance, blurred vision, burning upon instillation, and punctate keratopathy. Although many topical medications cause burning upon instillation, this is particularly common and more intense with dorzolamide, a solution formulated at a low pH due to the low solubility of the molecule at physiologic pH levels. Use of brinzolamide, a suspension, results in white deposits in the tear film. Eyes with compromised endothelial cell function may also be at risk of corneal decompensation with use of either of these drugs.

Adverse effects of systemic CAI therapy are usually dose related and are driven primarily by the resultant metabolic acidosis. Many patients experience paresthesias of the fingers or toes and report loss of energy and anorexia. Weight loss is common. Severe mental depression, abdominal discomfort, diarrhea, loss of libido, impotence, and taste disturbance, especially with carbonated beverages, may also occur. Patients with sickle cell anemia are at risk of sickle cell crisis. There is an increased risk of formation of calcium oxalate and calcium phosphate renal calculi. Because methazolamide causes less acidosis, it may be less likely than acetazolamide to cause nephrolithiasis.

As the urine becomes more alkaline, ammonia excretion is reduced. Systemic CAIs are contraindicated in patients with hepatic cirrhosis, because either systemic agent can precipitate hepatic encephalopathy due to increased serum ammonia levels.

CAIs are sulfonamides and thus are often thought to cause allergic reactions in individuals with known sulfonamide antibiotic allergies. Only about 10% of patients with hypersensitivity to sulfonamide antibiotics experience allergic reactions when exposed to sulfonamide nonantibiotics such as CAIs. Such a response is thought to represent a predisposition to allergic reactions rather than true cross-reactivity. It is prudent, however, to avoid prescribing CAIs to patients with a history of a severe allergic reaction to any sulfonamide. Aplastic anemia and other blood dyscrasias, Stevens-Johnson syndrome, and hepatic necrosis are very rare but potentially fatal idiosyncratic reactions to CAIs. Although routine complete blood counts have been suggested, they are not predictive of blood dyscrasias and are not routinely recommended. Hypokalemia is a potentially serious complication that is especially likely to occur when an oral CAI is used concurrently with another drug that causes potassium loss (eg, a thiazide diuretic). Serum potassium should be monitored regularly in such patients.

Fraunfelder FT, Fraunfelder FW, Chambers WA. *Drug-Induced Ocular Side Effects.* 7th ed. Butterworth-Heinemann; 2014.

Parasympathomimetic Agents

Parasympathomimetic agents, or *miotics,* have been used in the treatment of glaucoma for more than 100 years. Traditionally, they are divided into direct-acting cholinergic agonists and indirect-acting anticholinesterase agents.

The direct-acting agent pilocarpine continues to be used in certain circumstances, although it is not commonly prescribed for long-term use. In patients with pigmentary glaucoma, pilocarpine is effective in blunting the IOP spike that can occur with jarring physical activities such as running. This drug is also useful in the management of elevated IOP in aphakic eyes and in patients whose drainage angles are persistently occludable despite laser iridotomy (plateau iris syndrome). It has been associated with poor patient adherence to the treatment regimen because of its adverse effect profile and because of its 3- or 4-times-daily dosing schedule; therefore, it is infrequently used. Lower concentrations and dosing frequencies may be acceptable for management of angles with persistent iridotrabecular contact with a patent peripheral iridotomy.

Indirect-acting agents fell out of favor because of their ocular and systemic adverse effects. They can, however, be very effective and well tolerated in aphakic eyes with glaucoma, but they are rarely used.

Mechanism of Action

Parasympathomimetic agents reduce IOP by causing the longitudinal ciliary muscle fibers that insert into the scleral spur, trabecular meshwork, and inner wall of Schlemm canal to contract, thereby improving outflow facility by causing an unfolding of the trabecular meshwork and widening of the Schlemm canal. Direct-acting agents affect the motor end plates in the same way as acetylcholine, which is transmitted at postganglionic parasympathetic junctions, as well as at other autonomic, somatic, and central synapses. Pilocarpine can reduce IOP by 15%–25%. Indirect-acting agents inhibit the enzyme acetylcholinesterase, thereby prolonging and enhancing the action of naturally secreted acetylcholine.

Adverse Effects

Miotic agents have been associated with numerous ocular adverse effects. Induced myopia resulting from ciliary muscle contraction is an adverse effect of all cholinergic agents; brow ache may accompany the ciliary spasm. The miosis interferes with vision in dim light conditions; in patients with significant lens opacities, vision is adversely affected in all ambient lighting conditions. Because miotic agents have been associated with retinal detachment, a peripheral retinal evaluation is suggested before the initiation of therapy. Miotics, particularly the indirect-acting agents, may be cataractogenic. In addition, the indirect-acting agents may induce formation of iris pigment epithelial cysts, may cause epiphora by both direct lacrimal stimulation and punctal stenosis, and may cause ocular surface changes that result in drug-induced ocular pseudopemphigoid.

Other potential ocular adverse effects include increased bleeding during surgery and increased inflammation and severe fibrinous iridocyclitis postoperatively. Because miotics can break down the blood–aqueous barrier, they should be avoided, if possible, in patients with uveitic glaucoma. Use of miotics occasionally induces paradoxical angle closure, particularly in eyes with phacomorphic narrow angles; contraction of the ciliary muscle leads to forward movement of the lens–iris interface and increased anteroposterior lens diameter, which may cause or exacerbate pupillary block in an eye with a large lens.

Systemic adverse effects, seen mainly with indirect-acting medications, include diarrhea, abdominal cramps, increased salivation, bronchospasm, and even enuresis. Depolarizing muscle relaxants such as succinylcholine cannot be used for up to 6 weeks after stopping indirect-acting agents.

Rho Kinase Inhibitors

Mechanism of Action

The Rho family of G proteins are activated by various cytokines and regulate various aspects of cell structure, including cell stiffness, cell morphology, cell adhesion, apoptosis, and smooth muscle contraction. The effectors of these G proteins are the Rho kinases (ROCK1 and ROCK2). Activated Rho kinase phosphorylates various downstream proteins, including myosin light chain (MLC) phosphatase.

The net result of Rho kinase activity is increased phosphorylation and activation of MLC. Phosphorylated MLC interacts with actin, altering the physical characteristics of the cytoskeleton and thereby leading to increased cell stiffness and smooth muscle cell contraction. Rho kinase inhibitors lower IOP primarily by relaxing the cytoskeleton of outflow cells in the trabecular meshwork and Schlemm canal, increasing conventional (trabecular) outflow facility.

Available Agents and Dosing Frequency

Ripasudil, a mixed ROCK1 and ROCK2 inhibitor, was the first Rho kinase inhibitor available for clinical use to lower IOP and has been approved in Japan. The only Rho kinase inhibitor approved for use in the United States is netarsudil, which was approved by the US Food and Drug Administration (FDA) in 2017. Like ripasudil, netarsudil is a mixed

ROCK1 and ROCK2 inhibitor; however, it also is a norepinephrine transporter (NET) inhibitor. The NET inhibitor activity is thought to result in a reduction of episcleral venous pressure and may also decrease aqueous humor secretion, though the latter has not been demonstrated in humans. In clinical trials, its IOP-lowering efficacy was similar to or slightly lower than that of timolol. Some clinical trials were focused on eyes with fairly low baseline IOP because it was thought the drug might be particularly effective in such eyes. In 2 clinical trials in which the mean baseline diurnal IOP was approximately 22 mm Hg, the IOP reduction achieved with once-daily netarsudil 0.02% was approximately 20%. The drug lowers IOP by an additional 1.3–2.5 mm Hg when combined with latanoprost. Although mean IOP lowering with netarsudil used as monotherapy or in combination with latanoprost in clinical trials appears to be modest, some patients respond very well, experiencing substantial IOP lowering.

Netarsudil is used once daily. The hyperemia that commonly occurs with this class of agents is most intense during the first few hours after instillation; therefore, nighttime dosing is preferable.

Kahook MY, Serle JB, Mah FS, et al. Long-term safety and ocular hypotensive efficacy evaluation of netarsudil ophthalmic solution: Rho Kinase Elevated IOP Treatment Trial (ROCKET-2). *Am J Ophthalmol.* 2019;200:130–137.

Tanna AP, Johnson M. Rho kinase inhibitors as a novel treatment for glaucoma and ocular hypertension. *Ophthalmology.* 2018;125(11):1741–1756.

Adverse Effects

The most common adverse event associated with the use of Rho kinase inhibitors is conjunctival hyperemia, which occurs in more than 50%–60% of patients and is thought to be a result of conjunctival vascular smooth muscle cell relaxation. With netarsudil, subconjunctival hemorrhages occur in approximately 15%–20% of patients; eye pruritis, punctate keratitis, increased lacrimation, blepharitis, and decreased visual acuity were each reported in about 5%–10% of patients. Cornea verticillata was observed in approximately 15%–25% of patients after 1 year of use; it is similar in appearance to that observed after long-term use of amiodarone (Fig 12-4). Cornea verticillata does not seem to adversely affect visual function

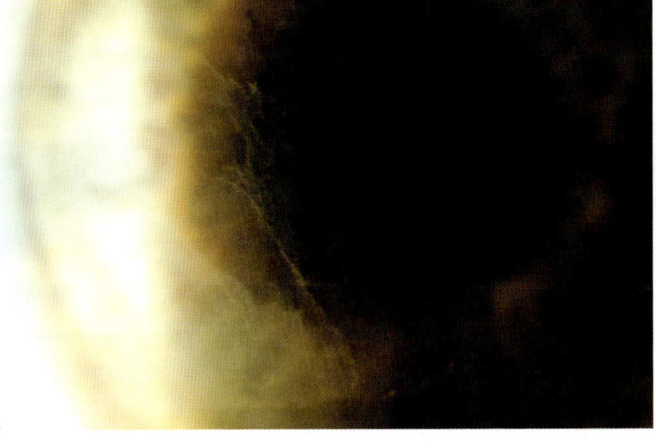

Figure 12-4 Cornea verticillata after use of netarsudil for 3 months. *(Courtesy of Angelo P. Tanna, MD.)*

and resolves after a mean of about 1 year after discontinuation of the drug. It is thought to occur as a result of lysosomal accumulation of phospholipids within corneal epithelial cells.

Combined Medications

Medications combined in a single bottle have the potential benefits of improved convenience and patient adherence. Fixed combinations consisting of timolol and another agent—a CAI (dorzolamide or brinzolamide), an α_2-adrenergic agonist (brimonidine), or a prostaglandin analogue (latanoprost, travoprost, or bimatoprost)—are available in many countries (see Table 12-2). In addition, fixed combinations of (1) brimonidine and brinzolamide and (2) latanoprost and netarsudil are available.

In general, the efficacy of fixed-combination formulations is similar to that of each of the components instilled separately. In the case of fixed-combination agents that include timolol and are administered twice daily, the total amount of the β-blocker may actually be more than necessary, because nearly the full effect of a β-blocker can be achieved with once-daily dosing. The ocular adverse effects are the same as for both drugs given individually. In general, except in the setting of an acutely elevated or dangerously high IOP, the clinician should make sure each component of the fixed combination is effective in further lowering the IOP by adding the individual components sequentially.

Hyperosmotic Agents

Hyperosmotic agents are used to control acute episodes of severely elevated IOP. Common hyperosmotic agents include oral glycerol and intravenous mannitol.

When given systemically, hyperosmotic agents increase blood osmolality, creating an osmotic gradient between the blood and the vitreous humor that draws water from the vitreous cavity and reduces IOP. Because of the increased gradient, the higher the dose administered and the more rapid the administration, the greater the subsequent IOP reduction will be. A substance distributed only in extracellular water (eg, mannitol) is more effective than a drug distributed in total body water (eg, urea). The osmotic agent enters the eye more rapidly when the blood–aqueous barrier is disrupted than when it is intact, reducing the effectiveness of the drug and its duration of action.

Hyperosmotic agents are rarely administered for longer than a few hours because their effects are transient (a result of the rapid reequilibration of the osmotic gradient). They become less effective over time, and a rebound elevation in IOP may occur if the agent penetrates the eye and reverses the osmotic gradient.

Adverse effects of these drugs include headache, confusion, backache, acute congestive heart failure, and myocardial infarction. The rapid increase in extracellular volume and cardiac preload caused by hyperosmotic agents may precipitate or aggravate congestive heart failure. Intravenous administration is more likely to cause this problem than oral administration. In addition, subdural and subarachnoid hemorrhages have been reported after treatment with hyperosmotic agents. Glycerol can precipitate hyperglycemia or even ketoacidosis in patients with diabetes mellitus, because it is metabolized into glucose and ketone bodies. Hyperosmotic agents are contraindicated in patients with renal failure.

General Approach to Medical Treatment

Long-Term Therapy

The ophthalmologist should tailor ocular hypotensive therapy to the individual needs of the patient, including establishing a target IOP. Though important, IOP is only one of several factors to monitor. The effectiveness of the therapy can be determined only by careful, repeated scrutiny of the patient's optic nerve, retinal nerve fiber layer, and visual field status (see Chapters 5 and 6).

Characteristics of the medical agents available for the treatment of glaucoma are summarized in Table 12-2. When making management decisions, ophthalmologists should consider the efficacy, adverse effect profile, and cost of the drug, as well as the likelihood of patient adherence to the drug regimen. Treatment is usually initiated with a single topical medication, unless the baseline IOP is extremely high, in which case 2 or more medications may be indicated. A discussion with the patient regarding treatment options can be beneficial for determining the optimal choice.

Prostaglandin analogues and β-blockers are reasonable choices as first-line therapy for open-angle glaucoma, as is laser trabeculoplasty in most cases. Prostaglandin analogues are the most commonly used first-line agents because of their superior efficacy, once-daily dosing, and favorable safety profile. Although the local adverse effects of β-blockers are minimal, these drugs have a greater potential for systemic adverse effects, and they lack nocturnal IOP-lowering efficacy. If prostaglandin analogues and β-blockers are contraindicated or ineffective, netarsudil (Rho kinase inhibitor), brimonidine (α_2-adrenergic agonist), or a topical CAI are all reasonable options.

If 1 agent is not adequate to reduce the IOP to the desired range, the initial agent may be discontinued and another tried, or another agent can be added. Laser trabeculoplasty, if appropriate, can be considered at any point during the stepwise process of intensifying treatment, or as the initial treatment (see Chapter 13 for more information on this procedure).

For patients on a prostaglandin analogue, if a second agent is required, it is reasonable to add a β-blocker, α_2-adrenergic agonist, topical CAI, or Rho kinase inhibitor. All have similar additive mean diurnal IOP-lowering efficacies, although CAIs may have better nocturnal efficacy. The decision as to which of these to select should be based on each drug's adverse effect profile, dosing frequency, possible contraindications, and patient preference.

Again, customizing the choice of agent to the patient's needs is helpful when selecting additional medication(s). In some circumstances, this might include parasympathomimetic agents for aphakic eyes. Clearly, when 3 or more medications are required, patient adherence to the medication regimen becomes more difficult, and the potential for local and systemic adverse effects increases. The use of fixed-combination agents can be very helpful for adherence but does not alter the adverse effect profile. Further, patients may not be able to tolerate multiple topical agents because of preservative toxicity. BAK, the agent most commonly used as a preservative, is present in most of the currently available topical ophthalmic eyedrops. If a reaction is suspected, an ocular hypotensive agent with an alternative preservative or preservative-free formulation can be used (Table 12-3).

For rehabilitation of the ocular surface, it may be beneficial to stop all topical medications—if the level of glaucomatous damage permits—and have the patient use preservative-free artificial tears frequently. During this period, the temporary use of oral CAIs may be helpful to lower IOP, if clinically warranted.

Patients sometimes fail to associate systemic adverse effects with topical drugs and, consequently, seldom volunteer symptoms. The ophthalmologist must make sure to inquire about these symptoms. In addition, communicating with the primary care physician is important not only to provide information about the potential adverse effects of glaucoma medication but also to discuss the effects that other currently prescribed medications for systemic disease might have on the glaucomatous process. Modification of oral β-blocker therapy for hypertension, for example, may affect IOP.

Therapy for Acute Intraocular Pressure Elevation

The goals of medical treatment of acute IOP elevation are to prevent further damage to the optic nerve; to clear corneal edema, if present; and to reduce intraocular inflammation. Hyperosmotic agents and systemic CAIs may be required in order to lower IOP in eyes with severe IOP elevation in preparation for definitive treatment. When the IOP is severely elevated, ischemia of the pupillary constrictor muscle can interfere with the miotic action of pilocarpine and other parasympathomimetic agents. Therefore, in patients with acute primary angle closure, lowering the IOP also allows pupillary constriction before an iridotomy is performed (see Chapter 9). Severely elevated IOP may cause collapse of Schlemm canal and closure of the collector channels; reduction of IOP may help restore conventional outflow.

Table 12-3 Preservative-Free and Alternatively Preserved Ocular Hypotensive Agents

Medication	Preservative
Brimonidine 0.1%, 0.15% (Alphagan P)	Sodium chlorite (Purite)
Dorzolamide/timolol (Cosopt PF)	Preservative-free unit dose vials
Latanoprost 0.005% (Xelpros)	Potassium sorbate, borate, propylene glycol
Tafluprost 0.0015%	Preservative-free unit dose vials
Timolol 0.25%, 0.5% (Timoptic in Ocudose)	Preservative-free unit dose vials
Timolol gel-forming solution 0.25%, 0.5% (Timoptic XE)	Benzododecinium bromide (a detergent closely related to BAK)
Travoprost 0.004% (Travatan Z)	Borate, sorbitol, propylene glycol, and zinc (Sofzia)

BAK = benzalkonium chloride.

Administration of Ocular Medications

Patients should be shown how to instill eyedrops properly and should be given instruction on nasolacrimal occlusion, which can be used to reduce the systemic absorption of topical ocular medications and to prolong their ocular contact time. Directing the patient to close their eyes for 1–3 minutes after instillation of the eyedrop will also promote corneal penetration and reduce systemic absorption of the drug by reducing the flow of medication-containing tears into the nasolacrimal drainage system.

Proper instillation procedures are especially important with the use of β-blockers, α_2-adrenergic agonists, and topical CAIs (to minimize the likelihood of taste disturbance). In addition, these procedures ensure that there is a sufficient amount of time between the instillation of different medications; eyedrops that need to be administered at the same time should be separated by 5 minutes to prevent washout of the first drug by the second. Patients should be taught how to space their medications, and instructional charts should be given. A dosing aid device may also be considered, especially for patients who live alone or who are unable to successfully instill eyedrops.

Use of Glaucoma Medications During Pregnancy or by Breastfeeding Mothers

Often, IOP decreases during pregnancy, both in healthy subjects and in patients with glaucoma. However, glaucoma patients who are pregnant frequently continue to require ocular hypotensive medical therapy throughout the pregnancy. As mentioned previously, topical ocular hypotensive medications are systemically absorbed; they subsequently cross the placenta and enter the fetal circulation or can be secreted into breast milk. Unfortunately, there is little definitive information concerning the safety of glaucoma medication use in pregnant women or breastfeeding mothers.

The decision as to whether to continue ocular hypotensive therapy during pregnancy, and what agents to use, should be made in collaboration with the patient and her obstetrician. Ideally, these plans should be formulated and implemented prior to conception, if possible. The theoretical risk of teratogenicity and other adverse outcomes necessitates an assessment of the potential benefits of treatment and a careful evaluation of the treatment regimen.

With all topical ocular hypotensive medications, pregnant and breastfeeding patients should be advised to perform nasolacrimal occlusion during eyedrop instillation. In general, it is prudent to minimize the use of medications in pregnant women whenever possible. The lowest effective dose should be given. The clinician may want to consider laser trabeculoplasty or other surgical intervention in cases in which the benefits outweigh the potential risks. Antifibrotic agents, however, should be avoided since there is evidence of human fetal risk based on adverse reaction data.

Mathew S, Harris A, Ridenour CM, et al. Management of glaucoma in pregnancy. *J Glaucoma.* 2019;28(10):937–944.

Pellegrino M, D'Oria L, De Luca C, et al. Glaucoma drug therapy in pregnancy: literature review and Teratology Information Service (TIS) case series. *Curr Drug Saf.* 2018;13(1):3–11.

Prostaglandin analogues

Previously listed in Pregnancy Category C (a classification system that has been abandoned by the FDA; Category C included drugs for which animal studies showed an adverse effect on the fetus but there were no adequate studies in humans), $PGF_{2\alpha}$ analogues have been shown to be embryocidal in rodent studies when administered at extremely high doses (15–97 times the human dose). Travoprost is teratogenic in rats at intravenous doses that correspond to exposure levels up to 250 times the human exposure at the maximum recommended human ocular dose. $PGF_{2\alpha}$ exerts abortifacient activity by increasing uterine contractility and may induce labor, albeit at much higher doses than those used in topical therapy. It is unlikely that topically administered prostaglandin analogues place the fetus at significant risk during pregnancy.

β-Blockers

β-Blockers (formerly listed in Pregnancy Category C) are often used for the treatment of systemic hypertension during pregnancy. There have been reports of growth retardation, arrhythmia, bradycardia, and lethargy affecting the fetus or newborn exposed to systemically or topically administered β-adrenergic antagonists. These agents are concentrated in breast milk and are relatively contraindicated in breastfeeding mothers because of their potential adverse effects on infants.

α_2-Agonists

Previously listed in Pregnancy Category B (Category B included drugs for which animal studies failed to demonstrate a risk to the fetus, but there were no adequate and well-controlled studies in pregnant women), brimonidine is a preferred agent for use during pregnancy. Because brimonidine has been linked to apnea in infants, its use should be discontinued in pregnant women prior to delivery to minimize the risk of this complication in the newborn. Brimonidine should also be avoided in breastfeeding mothers. For more information about brimonidine use in infants and children, see Chapter 11.

Carbonic anhydrase inhibitors

The CAIs (Pregnancy Category C) are teratogenic in rodents, and there are case reports of forelimb deformities in infants whose mothers were on systemic CAIs during pregnancy. Systemic CAIs should be avoided for the treatment of glaucoma in pregnant women. It may be preferable to also avoid the use of topical CAIs in pregnant women if possible, particularly during the first trimester.

Use of Glaucoma Medications in Elderly Patients

There are specific considerations regarding the use of glaucoma medications in elderly patients. First, elderly patients generally have greater difficulty instilling their medications than do younger patients; consequently, their adherence to the treatment regimen may be affected. Instillation difficulties may be due to tremor, poor coordination, or a comorbidity such as arthritis. Adherence may also be affected in elderly patients with reduced mental capacity or poor memory and a complicated drug regimen, especially because such individuals are often already taking multiple systemic medications for other ailments. Second, elderly persons have a greater susceptibility to systemic adverse effects of glaucoma medications. The incidence and severity of systemic adverse effects may be higher with β-blockers and α_2-adrenergic agonists in these patients. For example, a significant proportion of asymptomatic elderly patients suffer a significant, but reversible, reduction in pulmonary function with the use of β-blockers.

Generic Medications

Many glaucoma medications are available as generic drugs. Although the generic agents are required to be chemically or biologically equivalent to the brand-name product, in some cases there may be differences in formulation that could potentially alter a drug's effect. Brimonidine and bimatoprost, for example, are available in generic formulations that differ in concentration of the active ingredients from the brand-name products (see Table 12-2). The use of lower-cost generic medications has been shown to improve patient adherence to medication regimens.

Patient Adherence to a Medication Regimen

Glaucoma medications are effective only if patients use them. The first step toward improving patient adherence to a medication regimen is patient education. If patients understand the disease and the nature and benefits of treatment, adherence is increased; it is also enhanced when patients are aware of the possible adverse effects of a medication. Patient education should include a discussion of treatment alternatives.

The ophthalmologist must make sure that the patient understands the treatment regimen. Simpler medication regimens can improve patient adherence. The fewest number of medications, instilled with the lowest necessary frequency, is optimal. If the patient requires multiple medications and doses, it may be helpful to coordinate administration with daily events, such as meals or brushing teeth. A written schedule for medications can also be very helpful. Finally, as mentioned previously, proper instillation of eyedrops, by the patient or someone else, is essential and should be confirmed by the ophthalmologist.

2021 Update: Sustained-Release Bimatoprost Implant

In 2020, the US FDA approved an intracameral sustained-release biodegradable bimatoprost implant for 1-time use. The bimatoprost sustained-release implant is composed of 10 µg bimatoprost in a poly(D,L-lactide-co-glycolide) polymer matrix that slowly degrades after implantation in the anterior chamber.

The efficacy and safety of this implant (10 µg or 15 µg) compared to twice-daily topical timolol were evaluated in a 20-month phase 3 clinical trial in which there was a 52-week active treatment period and an additional 8 months of extended follow-up. Subjects in the bimatoprost implant groups underwent 3 administrations of the implant at 16-week intervals. Mean diurnal IOP lowering was similar with both the 10-µg and 15-µg implants, and neither was inferior to timolol. There was evidence of sustained IOP lowering with the bimatoprost implant; most subjects (69.2%) in the 10-µg bimatoprost implant group required no additional IOP-lowering treatment through month 20, a full year after the administration of the third implant.

The most concerning adverse effect observed in the clinical trial was a decrease in corneal endothelial cell density (CECD). At 20-month follow-up, a ≥20% decrease in CECD from baseline was seen in 10.2% and 21.8% of study eyes that received the 10-μg and 15-μg implants, respectively.

CHAPTER 13

Surgical Therapy for Glaucoma

This chapter includes related videos. Go to www.aao.org/bcscvideo_section10 or scan the QR codes in the text to access this content.

Highlights

- Laser trabeculoplasty is an effective primary or adjunctive treatment for open-angle glaucoma and ocular hypertension.
- The number of surgical options for glaucoma patients has expanded greatly in the past decade.
- Tube shunt surgery and trabeculectomy have an important role in the management of glaucoma.
- Cataract surgery can be effective in the management of angle-closure disease.

Introduction

Surgical treatments for glaucoma are designed to lower intraocular pressure (IOP) by reducing resistance to aqueous humor outflow or, in the case of cyclodestructive procedures, by reducing aqueous production. Aqueous outflow can be improved by enhancing the physiologic aqueous outflow pathways or by creating alternate paths. *Incisional surgery* is usually undertaken when there is either documented progressive glaucomatous damage or a high risk of further damage despite maximally tolerated medical therapy. Other reasons for proceeding to surgery are situations in which medical treatment is not appropriate, not tolerated, or not properly used by a particular patient.

Incisional surgery is the first-line treatment for primary congenital glaucoma (see Chapter 11). For most other types of glaucoma, medication and/or laser surgery is tried as the initial therapy. The clinician must exercise caution when recommending incisional surgery because potential adverse effects (infections, hypotony, cataracts) can result in vision loss. Early studies of trabeculectomy as initial therapy for glaucoma, which were performed before the advent of many contemporary glaucoma medications, suggested that trabeculectomy might offer some advantages: better control of IOP, reduction in the number of patient visits to the physician, and possibly better preservation of the visual field, for example. The results of the Collaborative Initial Glaucoma Treatment Study (CIGTS; see Chapter 7) confirmed that initial surgical therapy achieves better IOP control compared with initial medical therapy; however, this did *not* translate to better visual field stabilization on average. In both the surgical and medication groups, there was a low incidence of visual field progression. The 9-year follow-up data suggested that initial surgery resulted in less visual field progression than did initial medical therapy in subjects with advanced visual field loss at baseline; in contrast, subjects with diabetes mellitus had more visual field loss over time if treated initially with surgery. Based on the results of this study and on current practice, most clinicians defer incisional surgery for open-angle glaucoma (OAG) unless medical and laser therapy fails. Surgical treatment can be considered earlier in patients with advanced visual field loss at presentation.

Although traditional surgeries (trabeculectomy and tube shunt surgery) are quite effective in lowering IOP, they are associated with significant risk. Thus, over the past several years, there has been a strong push to develop safer and reasonably effective alternatives. These "minimally invasive" procedures differ from traditional surgeries in that they make use of the physiologic aqueous outflow pathways. This is in contrast to trabeculectomy and tube shunt surgeries, in which a new pathway into the subconjunctival space is created.

When surgery is indicated, various factors guide the selection of the appropriate procedure. With the proliferation of minimally invasive glaucoma surgery (MIGS) devices and procedures, clinicians have a broad range of options. Each type of surgery has its own indications and contraindications; however, there is much overlap, few comparative studies are available, and the surgeon's personal preference is often the most important factor in the selection of a procedure. Table 13-1 presents the procedures discussed in this chapter according to their location and mechanism of action.

Musch DC, Gillespie BW, Lichter PR, Niziol LM, Janz NK; CIGTS Study Investigators. Visual field progression in the Collaborative Initial Glaucoma Treatment Study: the impact of treatment and other baseline factors. *Ophthalmology.* 2009;116(2):200–207.

Laser Trabeculoplasty

In *laser trabeculoplasty (LTP),* laser energy is applied to the trabecular meshwork in discrete spots, usually covering 180°–360° per treatment. The goal of LTP is to reduce IOP by increasing outflow facility. Different laser wavelengths and delivery systems can be used. In current clinical practice, the most commonly employed are selective laser trabeculoplasty (SLT), argon laser trabeculoplasty (ALT)*, and MicroPulse (Iridex) laser trabeculoplasty (MLT).

Mechanism of Action

When LTP was first attempted in the 1970s, the belief was that the application of thermal energy to the trabecular meshwork (TM) would create holes, thereby bypassing the primary site of resistance to aqueous outflow and reducing IOP. Subsequent electron microscopy studies showed that this hypothesized mechanism of action was incorrect. Although the actual mechanism of LTP remains unclear, several theories have been put forward. In ALT, thermal damage to the treated trabecular meshwork causes shrinkage of collagen fibers, stretching and widening adjacent areas of the uveoscleral TM. This may play a role

*Note: This term is based on the historical use of argon laser technology; most green lasers currently used in ophthalmology are diode-pumped solid-state (eg, frequency-doubled Nd:YAG or Nd:YLF) lasers.

Table 13-1 Locations and Mechanisms of Action for Intraocular Pressure Reduction

I. **Decrease Inflow**
   A. External cyclophotocoagulation
      1. Discrete
      2. Continuous
   B. Endocyclophotocoagulation
II. **Increase Outflow**
   A. Into subconjunctival space
      1. Trabeculectomy
      2. Plate-based tube implant
      3. EX-PRESS shunt
      4. Short aqueous stent (eg, XEN, PreserFlo)
      5. Nonpenetrating deep sclerotomy
   B. Through Schlemm canal
      1. Nonincisional: laser trabeculoplasty
      2. Trabecular disruption
         a. Goniotomy
         b. Trabeculotomy
         c. Trabectome
      3. Trabecular bypass
         a. iStent
         b. Hydrus
      4. Canal expansion/support
         a. Hydrus
      5. Canaloplasty (external or internal)

in improving aqueous outflow facility; however, other lasers are as effective despite causing little or no damage to the collagen fibers. In all forms of LTP, possible mechanisms of action include the following:

- stimulation of cell division
- release of cytokines from treated trabecular meshwork cells resulting in alterations of the extracellular matrix of the TM or biomechanical changes in the Schlemm canal endothelial cells
- recruitment of monocytes and macrophages in the TM
- increased phagocytic activity of cells in the TM

Alvarado JA, Alvarado RG, Yeh RF, Franse-Carman L, Marcellino GR, Brownstein MJ. A new insight into the cellular regulation of aqueous outflow: how trabecular meshwork endothelial cells drive a mechanism that regulates the permeability of Schlemm's canal endothelial cells. *Br J Ophthalmol.* 2005;89(11):1500–1505.

Indications and Contraindications

LTP is indicated to lower IOP in patients with open-angle glaucoma or ocular hypertension. Historically, LTP was reserved for patients failing maximally tolerated medical therapy. However, it has been shown to be more effective when done earlier and is cost-effective compared with medical therapy. Accordingly, many surgeons now use LTP as a first-line treatment option. Patients who have difficulty applying topical medications, who have poor adherence to treatment, or who have significant ocular surface disease are all good candidates for trabeculoplasty.

LTP should be performed only in patients with an open angle. In a patient with advanced glaucoma and significantly elevated IOP, other treatment options should be considered. Although it has not been well studied, LTP should generally be avoided in eyes with anterior uveitis because of the risk of increased inflammation and formation of peripheral anterior synechiae (PAS); however, the technique has been shown to have potential benefit when the inflammation is very well controlled and the etiology of the IOP elevation is thought to be steroid induced. LTP is not effective in eyes with iridocorneal endothelial (ICE) syndrome, angle neovascularization, or extensive PAS.

Technique

A topical hypotensive agent, most commonly brimonidine or apraclonidine, is given before the procedure to reduce the risk of a postoperative IOP spike. A gonioscope designed for laser treatment is placed on the eye with methylcellulose, allowing the surgeon to visualize anatomic landmarks, with the goal of recognizing the trabecular meshwork. Care must be taken to identify the Schwalbe line, as this line can be mistaken for pigmented trabecular meshwork in some patients. Individuals with a heavily pigmented trabecular meshwork have a higher risk of postoperative IOP spikes; thus, lower energy settings should be used for these patients.

Laser-specific techniques

Common laser settings are shown in Table 13-2. In *argon laser trabeculoplasty,* a beam is focused at the junction of the anterior nonpigmented and the posterior pigmented edge of the trabecular meshwork (Fig 13-1A). Care must be taken to avoid applying the laser too far posteriorly, as this will promote the formation of focal PAS. The power setting should be titrated to achieve blanching of the trabecular meshwork or small bubble formation. If

Table 13-2 Laser Trabeculoplasty Settings

	Selective Laser Trabeculoplasty	Argon Laser Trabeculoplasty	MicroPulse Laser Trabeculoplasty
Power	0.4–1.0 mJ (titrated to bubble formation)	300–1000 mW (titrated to small bubble formation)	1000–2000 mW
Spot size	400 µm (fixed)	50 µm	300 µm
Duration	3 nanoseconds (fixed)	0.1 seconds	0.3 seconds with a 15% duty cycle
Treatment area (in 1 session)	Up to 360°	Up to 180°	Up to 360°
Wavelength	532 nm	514 nm	532 or 577 nm

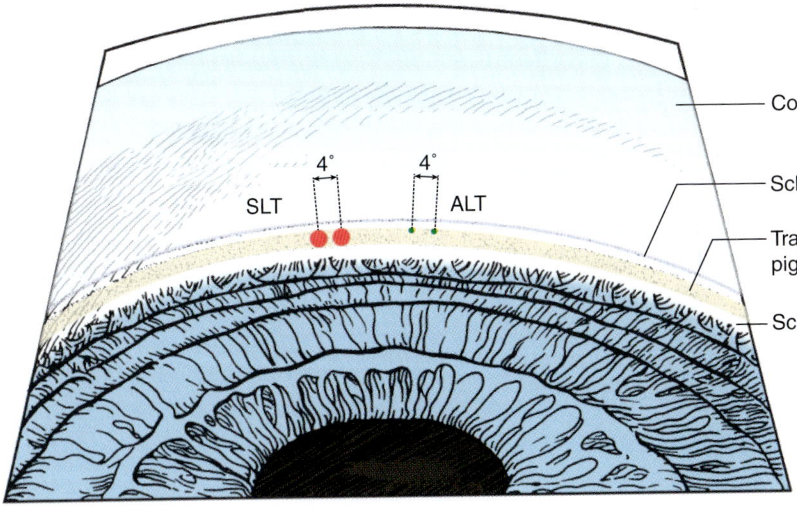

Figure 13-1 Illustration shows positioning of laser spots on the trabecular meshwork for argon laser trabeculoplasty (ALT) and selective laser trabeculoplasty (SLT).

a large bubble appears, the power is reduced and titrated to achieve the desired endpoint. Approximately 40–50 spots are applied over 180° of the TM. Usually, only half of the TM is treated to reduce the risk of postoperative IOP spikes and to allow for a second treatment if necessary in the future.

Selective laser trabeculoplasty targets intracellular melanin. A frequency-doubled (532-nm) Q-switched Nd:YAG laser with a fixed 400-µm spot size and 3-nanosecond pulse is applied to the TM (Fig 13-1B), with laser energy titrated to the appearance of cavitation bubbles or just below that. Treatment can be applied to 180°–360° of the TM, but most surgeons treat 360° in 1 session. Typically, 80–120 spots are applied over 360°.

MicroPulse laser trabeculoplasty applies energy to the trabecular meshwork at the same wavelength as in SLT. Unlike SLT, MLT uses a thermal laser application that is substantially longer but has a 15% duty cycle, meaning that energy is delivered in a sinusoidal pattern, "on" for 15% of the application time and "off" for 85%. This allows the tissue to cool during the application of each individual laser spot and may decrease the thermal injury to both the target and adjacent tissues. Approximately 120–140 confluent spots are applied over 360° of the TM.

Postoperative Care

For ALT, postoperative steroids or nonsteroidal anti-inflammatory drugs (NSAIDs) have been shown to improve patient comfort. One randomized controlled trial with SLT suggests that the use of steroids or NSAIDs may result in improved IOP outcomes. There are no studies on postoperative medications after MLT; however, none are specifically indicated. Patients are usually examined between 4 and 6 weeks after treatment to determine whether an adequate IOP response has occurred.

Complications

Complications from LTP include inflammation, IOP spike, and pain. IOP elevations are of particular concern in patients with advanced glaucoma. Such increases are usually evident by the first hour postoperatively. The adjunctive use of topical apraclonidine or brimonidine has been shown to blunt postoperative pressure elevation. Other medications that can reduce IOP spikes include β-blockers and pilocarpine. Hyperosmotic agents and oral carbonic anhydrase inhibitors may be helpful in eyes with IOP spikes not responsive to topical medications. In rare cases, patients have prolonged, intractable IOP elevation requiring incisional surgery. Treatment of 180° can decrease the risk of postoperative IOP spikes, especially with ALT.

With ALT, PAS can form if the laser is applied too posteriorly. Low-grade anterior segment inflammation can occur after treatment with any LTP method. Other complications include hyphema and reactivation of herpes simplex virus. In rare cases, patients can develop keratitis leading to irregular astigmatism.

Efficacy

SLT and ALT seem to have similar efficacy in lowering IOP. Approximately 80% of patients with medically uncontrolled OAG experience a drop in IOP for at least 6 months following LTP. Among patients who had an initial response, 50% maintain a significantly lower IOP level for 3–5 years after treatment. The success rate at 10 years is about 30%. Higher success rates are seen in older patients with primary open-angle glaucoma (POAG) and pseudoexfoliative glaucoma.

Treatment can be repeated with SLT and MLT, although success rates seem to decline with each subsequent treatment. Because the initial ALT treatment is usually applied to only 180° of the trabecular meshwork, the laser can be applied to the untreated half of the meshwork later, if needed. However, in previously treated areas, repeat ALT may be less effective and associated with an increased risk of IOP elevation. SLT can be used in areas of prior ALT treatment, with results similar to those in eyes undergoing repeat SLT. LTP is less effective in patients with angle-recession glaucoma, inflammatory glaucoma, or abnormal angle structure.

The Glaucoma Laser Trial (GLT) was a multicenter randomized clinical trial that assessed the efficacy and safety of ALT as an alternative to topical medical therapy in patients with newly diagnosed, previously untreated POAG. As initial therapy, ALT appeared to be at least as effective as medication in reducing IOP, preventing visual field loss, and slowing an increase in cup–disc ratio. The study was flawed in that 1 eye was assigned to ALT while the fellow eye was assigned to timolol treatment, which can have an IOP-lowering effect on the contralateral eye, potentially confounding the results. More than half of the eyes treated initially with laser required the addition of 1 or more medications to control IOP over the course of the study.

The Laser in Glaucoma and Ocular Hypertension (LiGHT) Trial was a prospective randomized study that compared SLT to medical treatment in the initial management of ocular hypertension and glaucoma. At 36 months, IOP control was similar between the 2 groups, while SLT was more cost-effective. Patients who had SLT scored similarly or better on quality-of-life measures compared with patients using medication.

Gazzard G, Konstantakopoulou E, Garway-Heath D, et al; LiGHT Trial Study Group. Selective laser trabeculoplasty versus eye drops for the first-line treatment of ocular hypertension and glaucoma (LiGHT): a multicentre randomised controlled trial. *Lancet.* 2019;393(10180):1505–1516.

Glaucoma Laser Trial Research Group. The Glaucoma Laser Trial (GLT) and Glaucoma Laser Trial Follow-up Study: 7. Results. *Am J Ophthalmol.* 1995;120(6):718–731.

Hutnik C, Crichton A, Ford B, et al. Selective laser trabeculoplasty versus argon laser trabeculoplasty in glaucoma patients treated previously with 360° selective laser trabeculoplasty: a randomized, single-blind, equivalence clinical trial. *Ophthalmology.* 2019;126(2):223–232.

Wang W, He M, Zhou M, Zhang X. Selective laser trabeculoplasty versus argon laser trabeculoplasty in patients with open-angle glaucoma: a systematic review and meta-analysis. *PLoS One.* 2013;8(12):E84270.

Cyclodestruction

Mechanism of Action

Cyclodestructive procedures aim to reduce aqueous production by damaging or destroying the nonpigmented ciliary epithelium. In addition, cyclodestructive procedures (specifically, external approaches) affect the ciliary muscle, which may increase uveoscleral outflow. Laser energy can be applied internally or externally. Internal delivery allows for a more targeted approach with less collateral tissue destruction, but it involves entry into the eye, which introduces a risk of infection and requires the use of an operating room. External delivery can be performed in the office in appropriate patients.

Pantcheva MB, Kahook MY, Schuman JS, Noecker RJ. Comparison of acute structural and histopathological changes in human autopsy eyes after endoscopic cyclophotocoagulation and trans-scleral cyclophotocoagulation. *Br J Ophthalmol.* 2007;91(2):248–252.

Indications and Contraindications

Historically, cyclodestructive procedures were reserved for patients with poor vision potential, as it was thought that those undergoing these procedures were at high risk of postoperative vision decline. However, experience has shown that patients who had cyclodestructive procedures often have acceptable visual outcomes. The procedure is useful in all types of glaucoma, especially for elderly patients when other glaucoma surgeries are refused or not appropriate because of poor health. It is also useful for patients who cannot stop antiplatelet and/or anticoagulation therapy and thus have a higher risk of suprachoroidal hemorrhage with incisional glaucoma surgery. In addition, cyclodestructive procedures can be used in painful eyes with poor vision potential in an attempt to provide comfort by lowering the IOP. However, there is a small risk of sympathetic ophthalmia with cyclodestructive procedures; thus, eyes without light perception should be treated with caution. The combination of corticosteroid and cycloplegic therapy can be very effective in controlling pain in such eyes.

Technique

Local anesthesia (retrobulbar, peribulbar, or sub-Tenon) is administered before the procedure. This can be done in the office if the patient can tolerate a periocular injection while awake.

External cyclodestruction (transscleral cyclophotocoagulation)

There are 2 ways (Video 13-1) to deliver the laser energy externally: by means of discrete treatment spots or broad, continuous application. Discrete delivery is easier to perform but may be associated with more collateral tissue damage. Sweeping application is technically more challenging in patients with tight orbits.

VIDEO 13-1 Transscleral cyclophotocoagulation.
Courtesy of Lauren Bierman, MD.
Scan the QR code or access the video at www.aao.org/bcscvideo_section10.

Discrete transscleral cyclophotocoagulation involves use of a fiber-optic probe to deliver 810-nm diode laser energy through the sclera to the ciliary processes. In this approach, 16–20 treatment spots are applied 360°. The probe is placed so that the energy is delivered posterior to the limbus, in order to target the ciliary processes (Fig 13-2). Care is taken to avoid the 3-o'clock and 9-o'clock positions to prevent damage to the long posterior ciliary nerves.

Continuous transscleral cyclophotocoagulation (MicroPulse; Iridex) also uses 810-nm diode laser energy delivered with a fiber-optic probe. However, the probe is moved in a continuous sweeping manner in applying the energy posterior to the limbus. The laser cycles on and off in a sinusoidal pattern with a duty cycle of 31.3%. A variety of settings are used for continuous transscleral cyclophotocoagulation.

Internal cyclodestruction (endocyclophotocoagulation)

To perform endocyclophotocoagulation (ECP), the surgeon views the ciliary epithelium with an endoscopic probe placed in the ciliary sulcus, posterior to the iris. Laser energy is

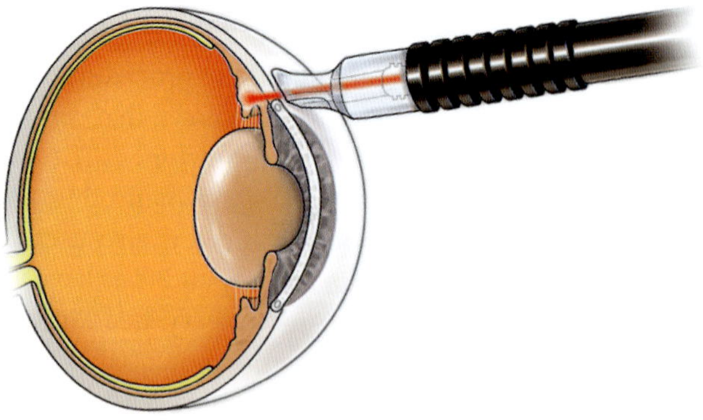

Figure 13-2 Cyclodestruction. The diode laser handpiece attachment (example of 1 manufacturer's device) is aligned with the limbus and ready to treat. *(Figure developed by Angelo P. Tanna, MD, and illustrated by Wendy Hiller Gee.)*

delivered directly to the target tissue. This procedure is performed in the operating room, often in combination with cataract surgery.

A clear corneal incision is created, and the eye is filled with viscoelastic, with particular attention paid to widening the sulcus. The probe is introduced into the eye, and 0.2–0.5 W of continuous-wave diode laser energy is initially applied to the ciliary processes. The energy is titrated to an endpoint of whitening and shrinking the ciliary processes without rupturing the tissue. The laser is applied in a continuous fashion, treating between 270° and 360° of ciliary processes (if treating 360°, a second incision is required). The effect of the treatment is related to both the amount of energy applied and the distance between the laser probe and the ciliary processes.

Postoperative Care

After surgery, topical and/or subconjunctival steroids are used to control inflammation. Cycloplegics mitigate postoperative pain by paralyzing the ciliary muscles, which are often inflamed after treatment. Medical ocular hypotensive therapy is continued in the immediate postoperative period and then tapered as appropriate. Oral analgesics, including narcotics, may be required for pain control.

Complications

Cyclodestructive procedures may result in prolonged hypotony, pain, inflammation, cystoid macular edema, hemorrhage, retinal detachment, and phthisis bulbi. Sympathetic ophthalmia is a rare but serious complication. Endophthalmitis is a risk with the endoscopic approach.

Ishida K. Update on results and complications of cyclophotocoagulation. *Curr Opin Ophthalmol.* 2013;24(2):102–110.

Efficacy

All forms of cyclophotocoagulation have been shown to lower IOP. A randomized study comparing continuous and discrete external cyclophotocoagulation showed a similar reduction in IOP, number of glaucoma medications, and retreatment rates at 18 months.

No prospective randomized study has shown that cataract surgery combined with ECP is more effective than cataract surgery alone, although a prospective nonrandomized study and a retrospective study have done so. These procedures often need to be repeated, as their IOP-lowering effect diminishes over time.

Aquino MC, Barton K, Tan AM, et al. Micropulse versus continuous wave transscleral diode cyclophotocoagulation in refractory glaucoma: a randomized exploratory study. *Clin Exp Ophthalmol.* 2015;43(1):40–46.

Francis BA, Berke SJ, Dustin L, Noecker R. Endoscopic cyclophotocoagulation combined with phacoemulsification versus phacoemulsification alone in medically controlled glaucoma. *J Cataract Refract Surg.* 2014;40(8):1313–1321.

Pérez Bartolomé F, Rodrigues IA, Goyal S, et al. Phacoemulsification plus endoscopic cyclophotocoagulation versus phacoemulsification alone in primary open-angle glaucoma. *Eur J Ophthalmol.* 2018;28(2):168–174.

Laser Peripheral Iridotomy

In laser peripheral iridotomy (LPI), laser energy is used to create a hole in the peripheral iris, providing an alternate pathway for aqueous to pass into the anterior chamber.

Mechanism of Action

As described in Chapter 9, primary angle closure occurs as a result of a relative increase in central iridolenticular contact. This creates greater resistance to aqueous flow through the pupil to the anterior chamber *(pupillary block),* increasing the pressure posterior to the iris, causing it to bow anteriorly. This, in turn, narrows the anterior chamber angle. An iridotomy provides an alternate pathway for aqueous to pass into the anterior chamber (Fig 13-3), thus relieving the pupillary block and allowing the iris to fall back and subsequently widen the angle.

Indications and Contraindications

LPI is performed when iridotrabecular contact is thought to be caused by relative pupillary block. Patients with acute primary angle closure (APAC), primary angle closure (PAC), and primary angle-closure glaucoma (PACG) all benefit from iridotomy. In addition, it is often performed in primary angle-closure suspects (PACS), although it is unclear whether LPI is beneficial for these patients (see later section on Efficacy for further discussion). Eyes with

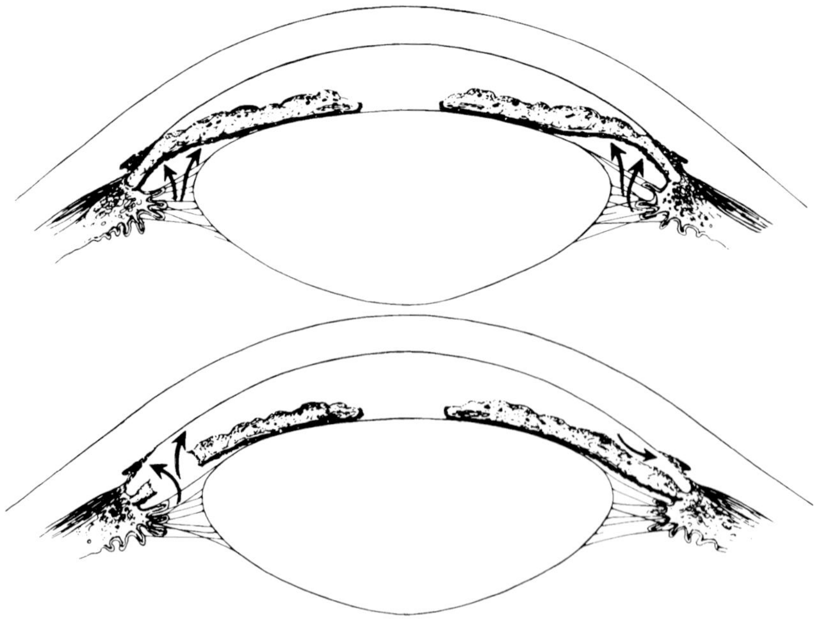

Figure 13-3 Illustration of eye with angle closure *(top).* Laser iridotomy or surgical iridectomy breaks the pupillary block and results in opening of the entire peripheral angle *(bottom)* if no permanent peripheral anterior synechiae are present. *(Reproduced and modified with permission from Kolker AE, Hetherington J, eds.* Becker-Shaffer's Diagnosis and Therapy of the Glaucomas. *5th ed. Mosby; 1983.)*

secondary angle closure due to pupillary block also benefit from iridotomy. Multiple and/or larger iridotomies may be indicated for patients with significant posterior synechiae.

In patients with a very shallow or flat peripheral anterior chamber, LPI can cause damage to the corneal endothelium. In patients who have angle closure without pupillary block (eg, neovascular glaucoma, ICE syndrome), iridotomy is ineffective. Eyes that have already developed 360° of synechial angle closure (due to chronic iridotrabecular contact) do not benefit from iridotomy.

Technique

A cooperative patient and an adequate view of the iris are necessary. Lowering the IOP before iridotomy is helpful in reducing corneal edema that may be present in acute angle closure and in allowing perfusion of the iris constrictor muscle. IOP reduction can also help to alleviate pain, which in turn improves patient cooperation. Topical, oral, and intravenous ocular hypotensive medications can all be used to lower IOP, and pain control can also be achieved with oral analgesics. IOP reduction can also be achieved by performing a careful paracentesis. Pretreatment of the iris with a green laser is useful in patients with a higher risk of bleeding (eg, in patients on anticoagulation or antiplatelet therapy).

A topical hypotensive agent is administered before the iridotomy to prevent postoperative IOP spikes. Pilocarpine is instilled to constrict the pupil, which in turn stretches the iris and allows for easier iris penetration by the laser. However, pilocarpine may be ineffective in patients with prolonged acute angle closure resulting in iris constrictor muscle ischemia.

An Abraham iridotomy lens with methylcellulose is used in this procedure. Prior to performing iridotomy, the surgeon should evaluate the iris to consider where to place the iridotomy, which should be located as far peripherally as possible. Making the iridotomy in an area where the iris is thinner (an iris crypt, for example) lessens the amount of energy needed. The Nd:YAG and green lasers can be used to create an iridotomy. In patients with thicker and darker irides, some surgeons advocate pretreatment with a green laser to thin the iris before using the Nd:YAG laser to penetrate the iris (Table 13-3). When the laser pierces through the iris, a release of fluid and pigment into the anterior chamber will usually be seen. Transillumination is useful in locating the iridotomy but does not signify patency. The iridotomy should be of sufficient size. There is evidence that creating a larger iridotomy in eyes with small iridotomies can help deepen the anterior chamber.

Table 13-3 Laser Settings for Peripheral Iridotomy and Iridoplasty

	Thermal Laser (Green) Pretreatment	Nd:YAG Laser Peripheral Iridotomy	Thermal Laser (Green) Peripheral Iridotomy	Laser Iridoplasty
Energy	200–400 mW	2–5 mJ per shot (can be in burst mode)	800–1000 mW	200–400 mW
Spot size	200–500 μm	N/A	50 μm	200–500 μm
Duration	0.2–0.5 seconds	N/A	0.1 seconds	0.5 seconds
Wavelength	514 nm	1064 nm	514 nm	514 nm

Postoperative Care

IOP is checked 30 minutes to 1 hour after the procedure to monitor for potential pressure spikes. Steroids are prescribed for approximately 1 week to treat postoperative inflammation associated with tissue disruption and bleeding. Topical hypotensive agents are also used when needed for IOP control. The patient is examined 1–6 weeks after LPI to confirm that the iridotomy is patent and the angle has deepened and to evaluate the fundus. Further evaluation can be considered if the angle remains narrow after iridotomy (see Chapter 9).

Lam DS, Chua JK, Tham CC, Lai JS. Efficacy and safety of immediate anterior chamber paracentesis in the treatment of acute primary angle-closure glaucoma: a pilot study. *Ophthalmology.* 2002;109(1):64–70.

Complications

Complications from iridotomy include bleeding, persistent postoperative inflammation, accelerated cataract formation, and lens damage. Retinal tear, postoperative IOP spike, and corneal endothelial damage can also occur. Visual dysphotopsias (glare, streaks, lines, halos) may be present and are thought to result from proximity of the iridotomy to the tear meniscus, which acts as a strong prism. Thus, some clinicians advocate temporal placement of the iridotomy, taking precautions to perform the iridotomy at a distance from the tear film. However, it is unclear whether the location of the iridotomy affects the likelihood of dysphotopsias, and a large prospective study suggests that it does not.

Srinivasan K, Zebardast N, Krishnamurthy P, et al. Comparison of new visual disturbances after superior versus nasal/temporal laser peripheral iridotomy. *Ophthalmology.* 2018;125(3):345–351.

Vera V, Naqi A, Belovay GW, Varma DK, Ahmed II. Dysphotopsia after temporal versus superior laser peripheral iridotomy: a prospective randomized paired eye trial. *Am J Ophthalmol.* 2014;157(5):929–935.

Efficacy

LPI is effective in deepening the angle recess in all forms of angle closure caused by pupillary block. However, some patients have persistent angle closure despite a patent iridotomy, and this requires further evaluation. LPI can be useful in controlling IOP in PAC patients, although approximately 40%–60% of PAC patients treated with LPI require long-term medical or surgical treatment as well. Iridotomy is also useful in the acute management of APAC. However, it is less effective than phacoemulsification for long-term IOP control. In 1 study, approximately 50% of patients who underwent LPI for APAC had IOP elevation above 21 mm Hg at 18 months, compared with 3% in the phacoemulsification group. Most PACG eyes will require additional IOP treatment despite iridotomy. The rate of conversion from PAC to PACG is low after iridotomy, though the rate of conversion from APAC to PACG is high despite iridotomy.

The Zhongshan Angle Closure Prevention (ZAP) trial prospectively enrolled 889 primary angle-closure suspects. Each patient had 1 eye treated with LPI, while the other eye was observed. At 6 years, control eyes were more likely to develop angle-closure disease (36 eyes vs 19 eyes; $P = .004$), most commonly on the basis of the formation of

PAS. However, there was a very low rate of conversion in both groups overall and no significant difference in acute angle-closure events or IOP elevation >24 mm Hg. (See also Chapter 9, Treatment Controversies sidebar.)

He M, Jiang Y, Huang S, et al. Laser peripheral iridotomy for the prevention of angle closure: a single-centre, randomised controlled trial. *Lancet.* 2019;393(10181):1609–1618.

Radhakrishnan S, Chen PP, Junk AK, Nouri-Mahdavi K, Chen TC. Laser peripheral iridotomy in primary angle closure: a report by the American Academy of Ophthalmology. *Ophthalmology.* 2018;125(7):1110–1120.

Peripheral Iridoplasty

Mechanism of Action

Peripheral iridoplasty (or *gonioplasty*) is performed by using a thermal laser (green or diode) to treat the peripheral iris stroma. This causes contraction of collagen fibers and thinning of the peripheral iris, pulling it away from the angle recess.

Indications and Contraindications

Peripheral iridoplasty is performed to prevent the development of primary angle closure and primary angle-closure glaucoma in eyes that have narrow angles despite a patent peripheral iridotomy. Occasionally, iridoplasty is used to break acute angle-closure attacks in eyes with an anterior chamber too shallow to allow iridotomy. Although there is controversy and a paucity of evidence, iridoplasty is thought to be beneficial in patients with plateau iris syndrome, phacomorphic angle closure, or nanophthalmos if iridotomy cannot adequately open the angle.

Technique

Pilocarpine is instilled to induce miosis and stretch the iris, and a topical aqueous suppressant is given to prevent postoperative IOP spikes. As with LPI, a cooperative patient and a good view to the iris are important for successful treatment.

About 16–20 evenly spaced laser burns are placed on the peripheral iris (see Table 13-3). A contact gonioscopy laser lens or Abraham iridotomy lens is used to enable peripheral placement of the spots. Long, slow burns are applied. The energy level and duration of laser treatment are adjusted based on iris color and tissue response. (See Chapter 9, Video 9-4.)

Postoperative Care

IOP is measured approximately 1 hour after treatment in order to detect IOP spikes. A corticosteroid is used to control postoperative inflammation and pain.

Complications

Complications include anisocoria, pupil distortion, persistent postoperative inflammation, PAS, and localized iris discoloration.

Efficacy

For patients with APAC, when iridotomy is not possible, iridoplasty is at least as effective as medical management in lowering IOP in the short term. The effectiveness of iridoplasty in preventing primary angle closure or primary angle-closure glaucoma is unclear. A randomized prospective trial comparing iridotomy alone to iridotomy and iridoplasty showed no difference in IOP reduction between the 2 groups at 1 year, but there was less PAS formation at 1 year in the iridoplasty plus iridotomy group. A randomized prospective study comparing peripheral iridoplasty to prostaglandin analogue therapy showed that prostaglandin analogue therapy was significantly more effective in IOP control at 1 year. A retrospective review of iridoplasty in plateau iris reported that the angle recess was wider at 6-year follow-up, which may help slow the development of PAC. (See also Chapter 9, Treatment Controversies sidebar.)

Narayanaswamy A, Baskaran M, Perera SA, et al. Argon laser peripheral iridoplasty for primary angle-closure glaucoma: a randomized controlled trial. *Ophthalmology.* 2016;123(3):514–521.

Sun X, Liang YB, Wang NL, et al. Laser peripheral iridotomy with and without iridoplasty for primary angle-closure glaucoma: 1-year results of a randomized pilot study. *Am J Ophthalmol.* 2010;150(1):68–73.

Trabeculectomy

Mechanism of Action

Trabeculectomy is an incisional procedure in which a fistula is created between the anterior chamber and the subconjunctival space, bypassing the normal aqueous outflow pathway. This procedure was initially performed as a full-thickness ("unguarded") procedure. High complication rates related to hypotony led to a major evolution in the surgical technique in that the fistula is now created under a partial-thickness flap of sclera ("guarding" the flow of aqueous) as a means of providing some resistance to aqueous flow through the fistula, thereby lowering the risk of postoperative hypotony.

Indications and Contraindications

Incisional glaucoma surgery is indicated when maximally tolerated medical therapy and laser treatments fail or are insufficient to prevent progressive damage. Failure of medical therapy may be the result of poor patient adherence. This can be an indication for surgery because further changes in medical therapy are unlikely to improve IOP control. Progression of visual field damage and uncontrolled IOP, even at low levels, are indications for surgery. Multiple visual field examinations may be required in order to confirm progression.

Because of the potential complications of incisional surgery, it is not reasonable to perform trabeculectomy in an eye with ocular hypertension and a low risk of developing functional loss. However, in less clear-cut situations—for example, when 1 eye has sustained significant glaucomatous damage, and the IOP is high in the fellow eye despite maximally tolerated medical therapy—some ophthalmologists recommend surgery prior to unequivocal evidence of damage. In eyes with severely elevated, medically uncontrollable IOP, surgery may be warranted in the absence of glaucomatous damage. In some cases without documented progression, the decision to proceed with surgery is based on clinical judgment that the IOP is too high for the stage of disease.

The absence of light perception is a contraindication for incisional glaucoma surgery. The risk of sympathetic ophthalmia should always be kept in mind when any procedure is considered in a blind eye or an eye with poor vision potential. Conditions that predispose to trabeculectomy failure, such as active anterior segment neovascularization or active anterior uveitis, are relative contraindications. The underlying problem should be addressed first, if possible, or a surgical alternative such as tube shunt surgery should be considered. It may be difficult to perform a successful trabeculectomy in an eye that has sustained extensive conjunctival injury (eg, from previous surgery or trauma). Patients with extremely thin or abnormal sclera (eg, from surgery, necrotizing scleritis, or degenerative myopia) have a higher likelihood of complications.

The success rate of trabeculectomy is lower in patients with diabetes; younger patients; patients with African, Asian, or Hispanic ancestry; and aphakic or pseudophakic patients who had prior cataract extraction through a scleral tunnel incision. However, with the advent of clear corneal incisions for cataract surgery and the use of antifibrotic agents during trabeculectomy, outcomes have improved in pseudophakic patients. Patients with certain types of secondary glaucoma, predisposition to an aggressive postoperative inflammatory response, or prior failed trabeculectomy have a higher risk of trabeculectomy failure. Use of topical fluorometholone for 1 month prior to surgery can reduce the need for postoperative interventions and the need for long-term postoperative glaucoma medications. Patients who are unwilling or unable to comply with postoperative care may not be good candidates for trabeculectomy.

Breusegem C, Spielberg L, Van Ginderdeuren R, et al. Preoperative nonsteroidal anti-inflammatory drug or steroid and outcomes after trabeculectomy: a randomized controlled trial. *Ophthalmology.* 2010;117(7):1324–1330.

Stiles MC. Update on glaucoma surgery. *Focal Points: Clinical Modules for Ophthalmologists.* American Academy of Ophthalmology; 2012, module 6.

Technique

Exposure

In order to obtain adequate exposure, a partial-thickness suture can be passed through the superior cornea to rotate the eye inferiorly (Fig 13-4A). Alternatively, a superior rectus bridle suture can be placed (Fig 13-4B); however, its use has been reported to increase the risk of trabeculectomy failure.

Conjunctival incision

The conjunctival incision can be made in 1 of 2 locations. A *fornix-based* trabeculectomy conjunctival flap is created by making an incision adjacent to or slightly posterior to the limbus (Fig 13-5; Video 13-2), while a *limbus-based* trabeculectomy flap is created by making an incision 8–10 mm posterior to the limbus (Fig 13-6). Fornix-based

A
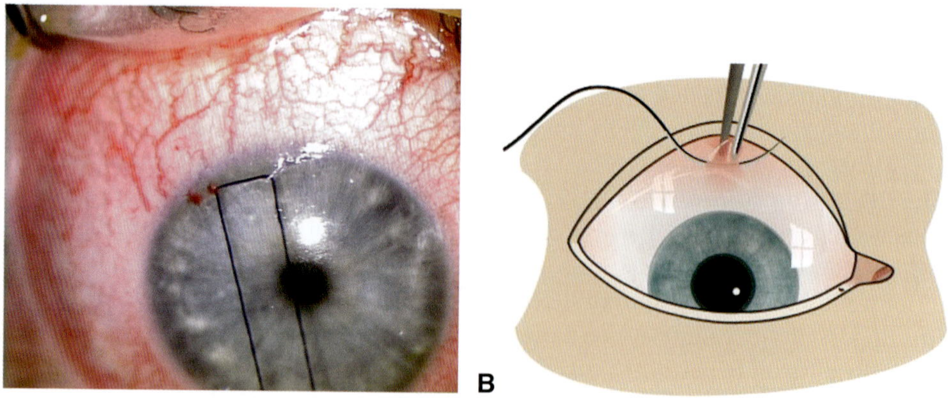
B

Figure 13-4 Options for trabeculectomy exposure. **A,** Corneal traction suture. **B,** Superior rectus bridle suture. *(Part A courtesy of Keith Barton, MD; part B courtesy of Alan Lacey. Both parts reproduced with permission of Moorfields Eye Hospital.)*

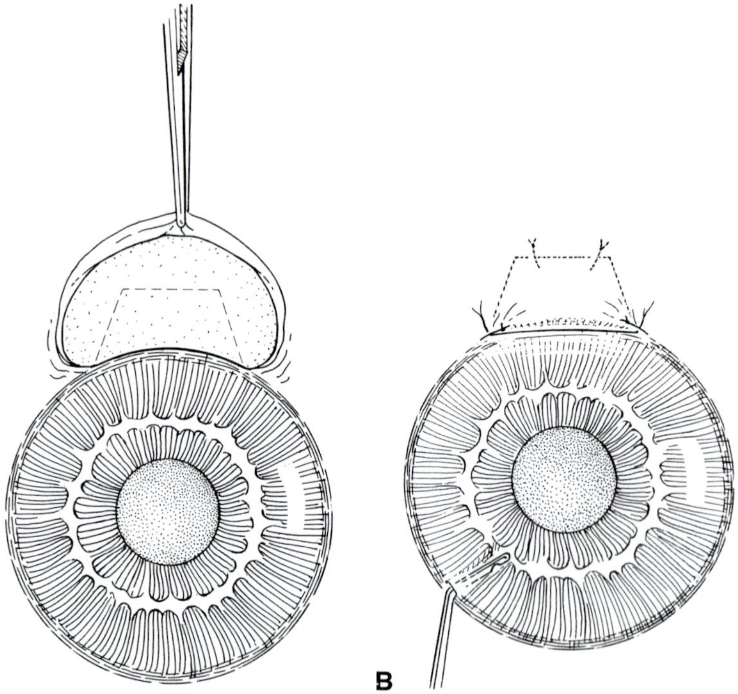
A B

Figure 13-5 Fornix-based conjunctival flap. **A,** Drawing shows the initial incision through conjunctiva at the limbus and the insertion of the Tenon capsule. The arc length of the initial incision is approximately 6–7 mm. Tissue adjacent to the incision is undermined with blunt scissors before the scleral flap is prepared. **B,** Incision is closed either at both ends with interrupted or purse-string sutures or with a running mattress suture. *(Modified with permission from Weinreb RN, Mills RP, eds.* Glaucoma Surgery: Principles and Techniques. *2nd ed. Ophthalmology Monograph 4. American Academy of Ophthalmology; 1998:43.)*

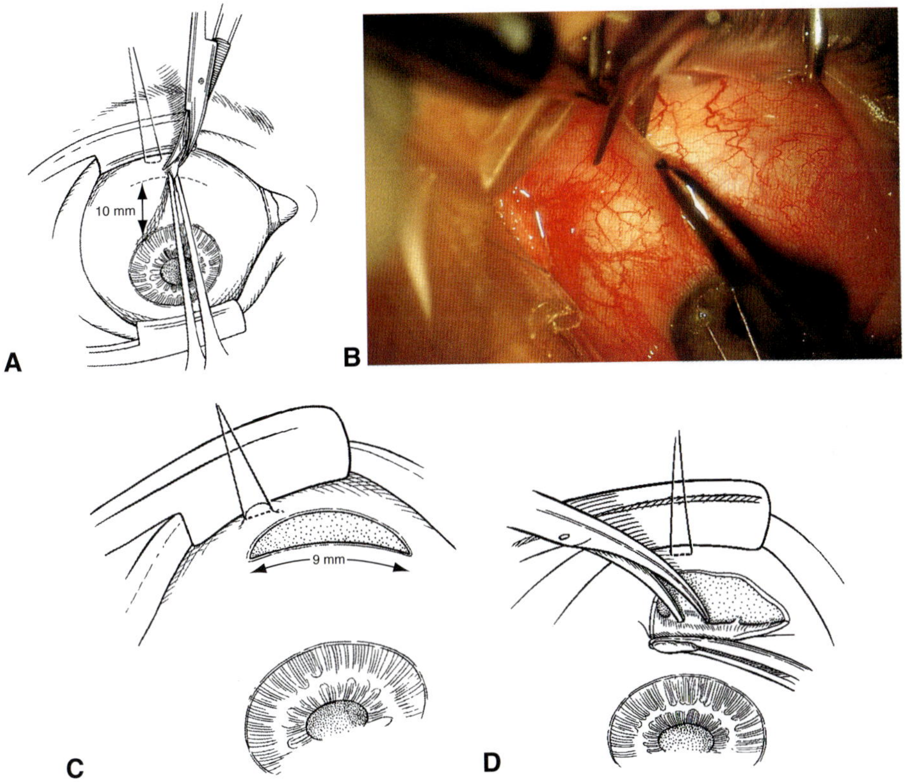

Figure 13-6 Limbus-based conjunctival flap. **A,** Drawing shows the initial incision through conjunctiva and Tenon capsule. **B,** Clinical photograph corresponding to part A shows the initial incision for creation of a limbus-based conjunctival flap. **C,** Completion of conjunctiva–Tenon incision 8–10 mm posterior to the limbus. **D,** Anterior dissection of conjunctiva–Tenon flap with excision of Tenon episcleral fibrous adhesions. *(Parts A, C, and D modified with permission from Weinreb RN, Mills RP, eds.* Glaucoma Surgery: Principles and Techniques. *2nd ed. Ophthalmology Monograph 4. American Academy of Ophthalmology; 1998:29–31. Part B courtesy of Robert D. Fechtner, MD.)*

trabeculectomies offer the advantages of better exposure, while limbus-based flaps reduce the risk of early wound leak because the incision is several millimeters away from the scleral flap. Fornix-based flaps are associated with more diffuse blebs.

VIDEO 13-2 Fornix-based trabeculectomy with running closure.
Courtesy of James A. Savage, MD.

Scleral flap

A partial-thickness scleral flap is created in the superior sclera, posterior to the limbus (Fig 13-7). This flap will ultimately cover the hole that allows aqueous to egress into the subconjunctival space. Whenever possible, the scleral flap is centered at 12 o'clock to help prevent postoperative bleb exposure and dysesthesia. Common flap shapes include triangular, rectangular, and trapezoidal.

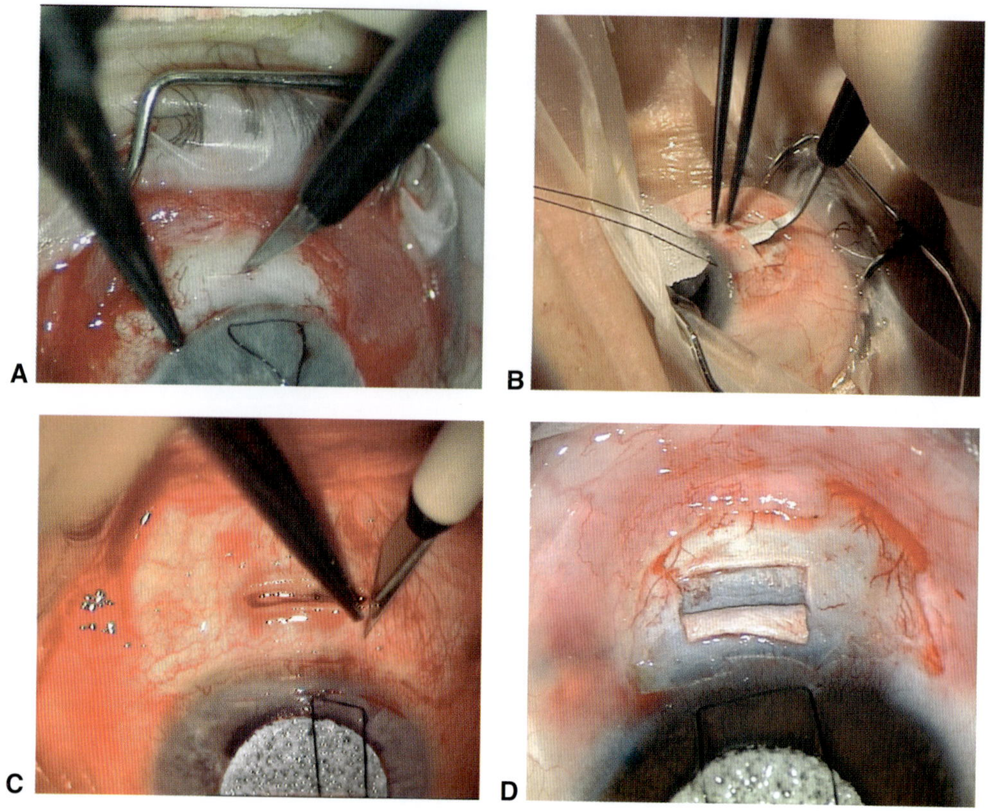

Figure 13-7 Clinical photographs showing creation of a scleral flap 4 mm wide and 2.0–2.5 mm from front to back at 50%–75% scleral depth. **A,** Posterior margin is dissected with a fine blade. **B,** Crescent knife is used to dissect a partial-thickness scleral tunnel. **C,** Sides of the tunnel are opened to create a flap. **D,** Final appearance. *(Courtesy of Keith Barton, MD. Reproduced with permission of Moorfields Eye Hospital.)*

Fistula creation

A paracentesis provides access to the anterior chamber to allow re-formation of the chamber with balanced salt solution or viscoelastic when needed. An incision into the anterior chamber is created under the scleral flap with a sharp blade. A corneoscleral block of tissue is removed (Fig 13-8), creating a fistula that allows aqueous to flow directly from the anterior chamber to the subconjunctival space. The fistula can be made freehand or with a trephining device such as a Kelly Descemet membrane punch. This fistula is typically centered underneath the scleral flap and is small enough so that the flap overlaps it on all sides.

Iridectomy

An iridectomy prevents iris from occluding the fistula (Fig 13-8D). Some surgeons do not perform an iridectomy in selected patients, as it is believed the risk of fistula occlusion is low in certain pseudophakic eyes. The risks of iridectomy (bleeding, inflammation) should be weighed against the risk of fistula obstruction.

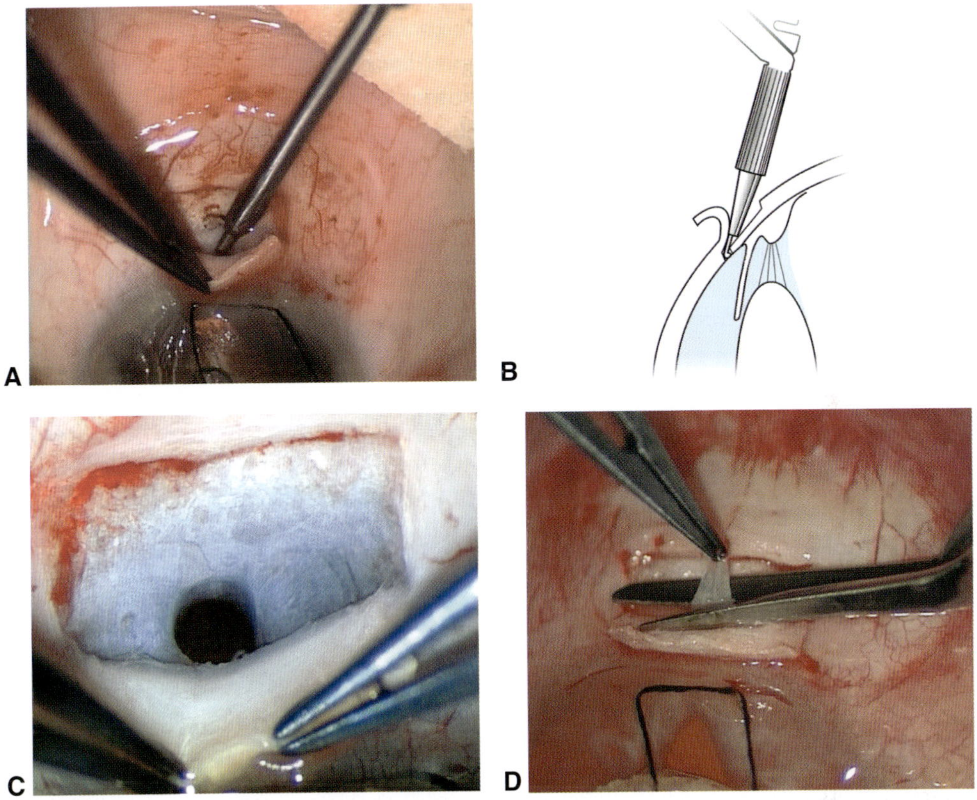

Figure 13-8 The surgeon can create a fistula by **(A)** inserting a punch under the scleral flap; **(B)** snaring the posterior lip of the anterior chamber entry site; and **(C)** removing a punch (0.75–1.0 mm) of peripheral posterior cornea. A peripheral iridectomy **(D)** is then made (shown here in an albino eye) with iridectomy scissors. *(Clinical photographs courtesy of Keith Barton, MD; illustration based on original drawing by Alan Lacey. All parts reproduced with permission of Moorfields Eye Hospital.)*

Closure of scleral flap and conjunctiva

The scleral flap is secured (Fig 13-9) with several nylon sutures (typically 10-0 or 9-0), which are tightened to provide appropriate resistance to aqueous flow. Some surgeons preplace these sutures before entering the anterior chamber to facilitate quick closure. Releasable sutures in the flap allow for suture removal postoperatively without a laser (Video 13-3). After the sutures are tied, the anterior chamber is re-formed with balanced salt solution, and scleral flap tension is titrated to achieve the desired rate of egress of aqueous humor.

VIDEO 13-3 Placement of a releasable suture for flap closure.
Courtesy of Marlene Moster, MD.

Conjunctival closure must be watertight to prevent postoperative complications and to maximize the success of the surgery. For a limbus-based flap, the Tenon capsule and conjunctiva are closed separately or in a single layer by means of a running suture on a

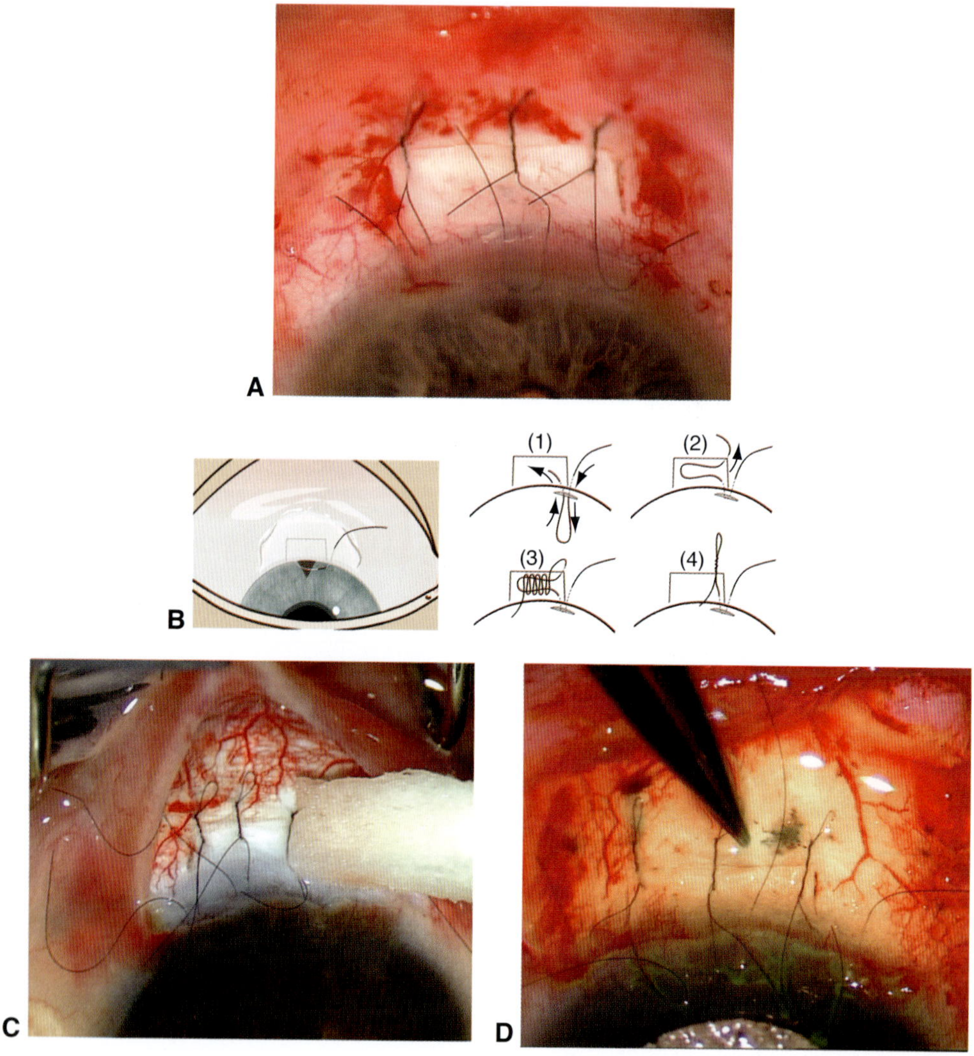

Figure 13-9 In a trabeculectomy with mitomycin C, the scleral flap is closed relatively tightly so that spontaneous drainage is minimal. Closure may be performed with releasable sutures **(A, B)** that can be removed later at the slit lamp in order to increase flow or with interrupted sutures that can be cut postoperatively by laser. Part B shows the sequence of movements for placing 1 type of releasable suture. The surgeon should check the flow at the end of scleral closure using a sponge **(C)** or fluorescein **(D).** *(Clinical photographs courtesy of Keith Barton, MD; drawing courtesy of Alan Lacey. All parts reproduced with permission of Moorfields Eye Hospital.)*

vascular needle. For a fornix-based trabeculectomy, the conjunctiva can be closed with 2 wing sutures or a running suture.

Antifibrotic Agents in Trabeculectomy

The increased use of mitomycin C and 5-fluorouracil has improved the rate of surgical success, especially in patients with risk factors for failure. Use of these antifibrotic agents has also led to higher rates of bleb leak, infection, and hypotony; but the increase is related to the longer survival of the trabeculectomy attained with these agents. Antifibrotic agents can be applied subconjunctivally by means of soaked sponges or injection.

5-Fluorouracil (5-FU) is a pyrimidine analogue that inhibits DNA synthesis through its action on thymidylate synthetase and thereby interferes with fibroblast proliferation. This agent can be used both intraoperatively (soaked on sponges) and postoperatively (injected subconjunctivally) to increase the success rate of trabeculectomy. 5-FU can be highly toxic to the corneal epithelium and thus should be used with caution in patients with ocular surface disease.

Mitomycin C (MMC) is a naturally occurring compound with antineoplastic and antibiotic activities. MMC is an alkylating agent that crosslinks DNA, thus inhibiting DNA replication and inducing apoptosis. It is cytotoxic to fibroblasts and vascular endothelial cells, thereby modulating the fibroproliferative and angiogenic steps of wound healing. It is administered by application of soaked sponges or subconjunctival injection. Both techniques lead to similar IOP outcomes, although injection may promote the formation of more diffuse blebs (Figs 13-10, 13-11). MMC is highly toxic, and intracameral exposure should be avoided.

A Cochrane review of the literature found that IOP was significantly lower with adjunctive MMC compared with 5-FU 1 year after trabeculectomy. Visual outcomes were similar between the groups.

Cabourne E, Clarke JC, Schlottmann PG, Evans JR. Mitomycin C versus 5-fluorouracil for wound healing in glaucoma surgery. *Cochrane Database Syst Rev.* 2015;11:CD006259. Epub 2015 Nov 6.

Esfandiari H, Pakravan M, Yazdani S, et al. Treatment outcomes of mitomycin C-augmented trabeculectomy, sub-Tenon injection versus soaked sponges, after 3 years of follow-up. *Ophthalmol Glaucoma.* 2018;1(1):66–74.

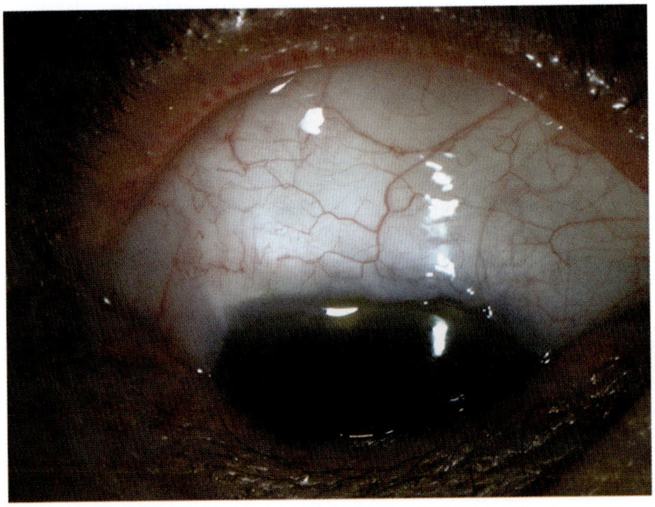

Figure 13-10 Clinical photograph shows a diffuse conjunctival bleb. Although it is difficult to see the bleb, the clues are the irregular conjunctival border at the limbus and scarring at the 10- and 2-o'clock positions, where sutures were placed during surgery. With careful slit-lamp examination, one will notice that the bleb is elevated off the sclera. *(Courtesy of JoAnn A. Giaconi, MD.)*

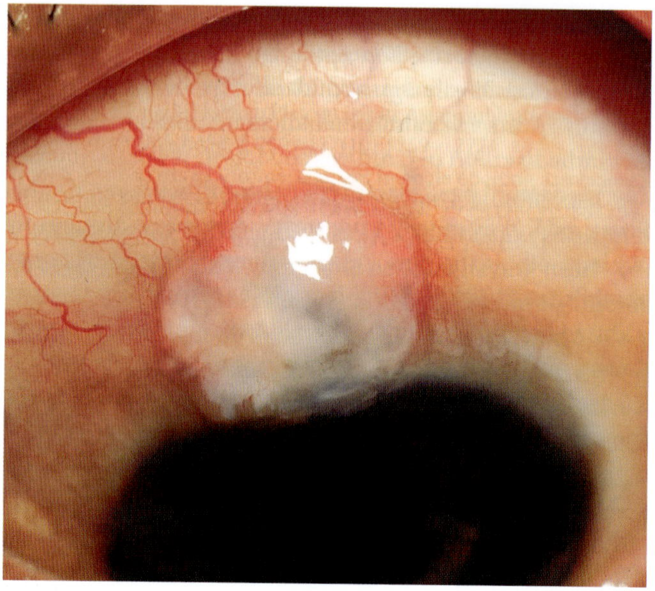

Figure 13-11 Clinical photograph of a localized conjunctival bleb. *(Courtesy of Jody Piltz-Seymour, MD.)*

Palanca-Capistrano AM, Hall J, Cantor LB, Morgan L, Hoop J, WuDunn D. Long-term outcomes of intraoperative 5-fluorouracil versus intraoperative mitomycin C in primary trabeculectomy surgery. *Ophthalmology.* 2009;116(2):185–190.

Postoperative Complications and Management

Although meticulous surgical technique is important, the success of an incisional glaucoma procedure depends to a great extent on careful postoperative management (Fig 13-12). Many complications can arise during the early and late postoperative period, compromising the success of the surgery, vision, and ocular health (Table 13-4). Thus, timely identification of potential complications is imperative.

Overfiltration occurs when there is too little resistance to aqueous flow from the anterior chamber into the subconjunctival space. It is usually caused by inadequately tightened scleral flap sutures. Other causes include intraoperative flap buttonhole and proximity of the fistula to the edge of the flap. Overfiltration may be associated with an exuberant bleb (in the absence of a bleb leak) and a shallow anterior chamber. Treatment options include reducing topical steroids (to allow the development of subconjunctival fibrosis) and placing additional scleral flap sutures (Video 13-4). The development of hypotony maculopathy (optic nerve and/or retinal edema and radial macular folds causing a decline or distortion in vision) is an indication for intervention.

VIDEO 13-4 Transconjunctival scleral flap suturing at slit lamp.
Courtesy of Susan Liang, MD.

Bleb leaks can occur at any point in the postoperative course. In the early postoperative period, leaks most commonly occur at the incision site. Unrecognized buttonholes

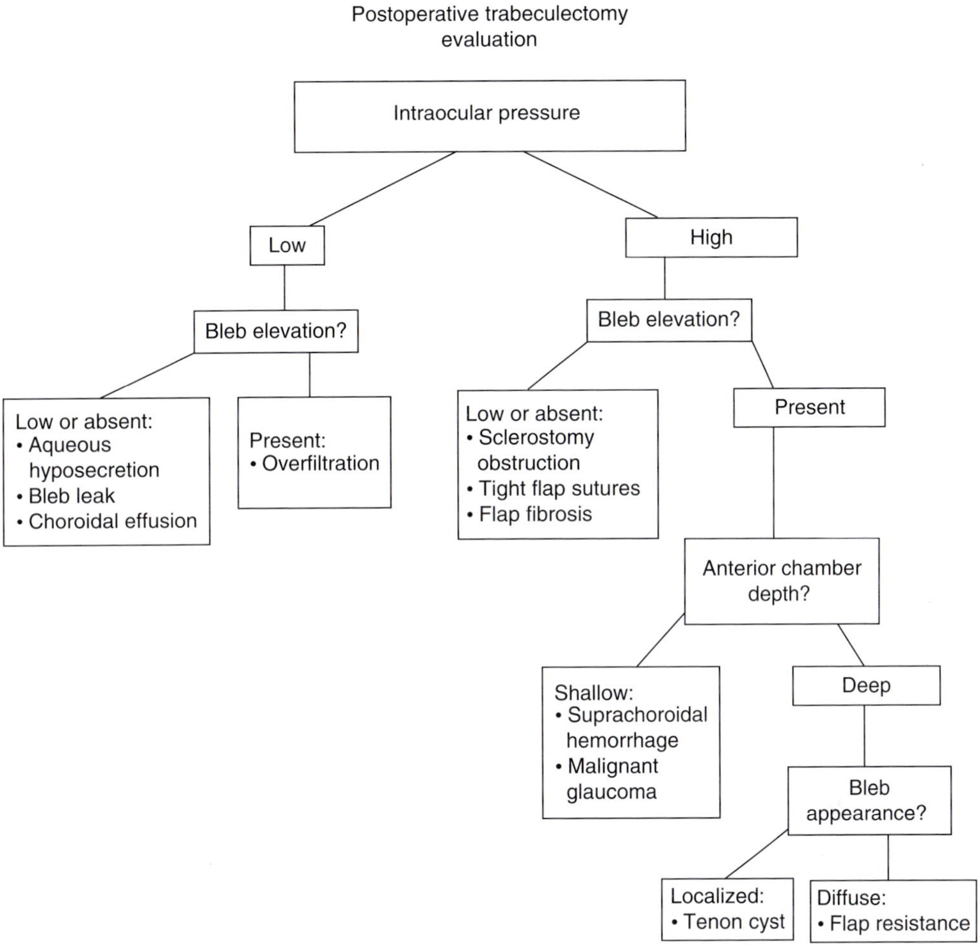

Figure 13-12 Algorithm depicts suggested evaluation approach after trabeculectomy. *(Courtesy of Chandrasekharan Krishnan, MD.)*

and flap suture erosion through the conjunctiva can also lead to leaks. They are often symptomatic (patients report experiencing excessive tearing) and can be found by performing a Seidel test (Video 13-5; see also Chapter 4). In addition to hypotony, patients with a leak may have a shallow or normal anterior chamber depth and a low-lying bleb. Untreated leaks can lead to early bleb fibrosis and infection.

VIDEO 13-5 Identifying a bleb leak.
Courtesy of Chandrasekharan Krishnan, MD.

There are several treatment options. Decreasing topical steroids can promote fibrosis and healing. Aqueous suppressants reduce the flow through the defect, allowing the leak to seal through epithelialization. Placement of an oversized contact lens can provide a scaffold for re-epithelialization and may also tamponade the leak. Suturing the site of the leak may be necessary if conservative measures fail.

Table 13-4 Complications of Trabeculectomy

Early Complications	Late Complications
Choroidal effusion	Cataract
Cystoid macular edema	Bleb migration
Dellen formation	Blebitis
Formation or acceleration of cataract	Endophthalmitis/bleb infection
Hyphema	Eyelid retraction
Hypotony	Hypotony
Hypotony maculopathy	Leakage or failure of the filtering bleb
Infection	Ptosis
Loss of vision	Symptomatic bleb (dysesthetic bleb)
Malignant glaucoma (aqueous misdirection)	
Persistent uveitis	
Shallow or flat anterior chamber	
Suprachoroidal hemorrhage	
Transient intraocular pressure elevation	
Wound leak	

Choroidal effusions can also occur at any time in the postoperative period when the IOP is low, with blebs of any size. Elderly patients with low IOP are more likely to develop choroidal effusions as compared to hypotony maculopathy (perhaps because of their greater scleral rigidity). The anterior chamber will be shallow, more so peripherally than centrally. Fundus examination discloses the classic grayish dome-shaped effusions, anchored in the region of the vortex veins.

Treatment includes use of cycloplegics to deepen the anterior chamber. If overfiltration or a bleb leak is the cause, decreasing steroids may be useful in promoting healing and fibrosis. If ciliary body inflammation (and aqueous hyposecretion) is the cause, increasing steroids is beneficial. Injecting viscoelastic into the anterior chamber can temporarily elevate the IOP and hasten recovery. If conservative management fails, the effusion can be drained in the operating room through posterior sclerotomies. The scleral flap is often reinforced at the same time to increase resistance to outflow (Video 13-6).

VIDEO 13-6 Scleral flap resuturing and choroidal drainage.
Courtesy of Lauren Blieden, MD.

Sclerostomy obstruction can occur at any point but is most frequent in the early postoperative phase (Fig 13-13). The condition is characterized by a low bleb, deep chamber, and elevated IOP. The sclerostomy may be blocked by a blood clot, fibrin, vitreous, or iris; gonioscopy is crucial to determine the cause of the obstruction. Laser iridoplasty or iridotomy can be used to manage iris tissue incarcerated in the sclerostomy. Tissue plasminogen activator can dissolve a blood clot quickly if needed.

Tight scleral flap sutures impair egress of aqueous humor, resulting in a low bleb, deep anterior chamber, and higher-than-desired IOP (Fig 13-14A). Moderate to firm digital ocular massage forces fluid through the flap, elevating the bleb and lowering the IOP. Determining the optimal time to cut 1 or more flap sutures can be a difficult balancing act (Fig 13-14B, C).

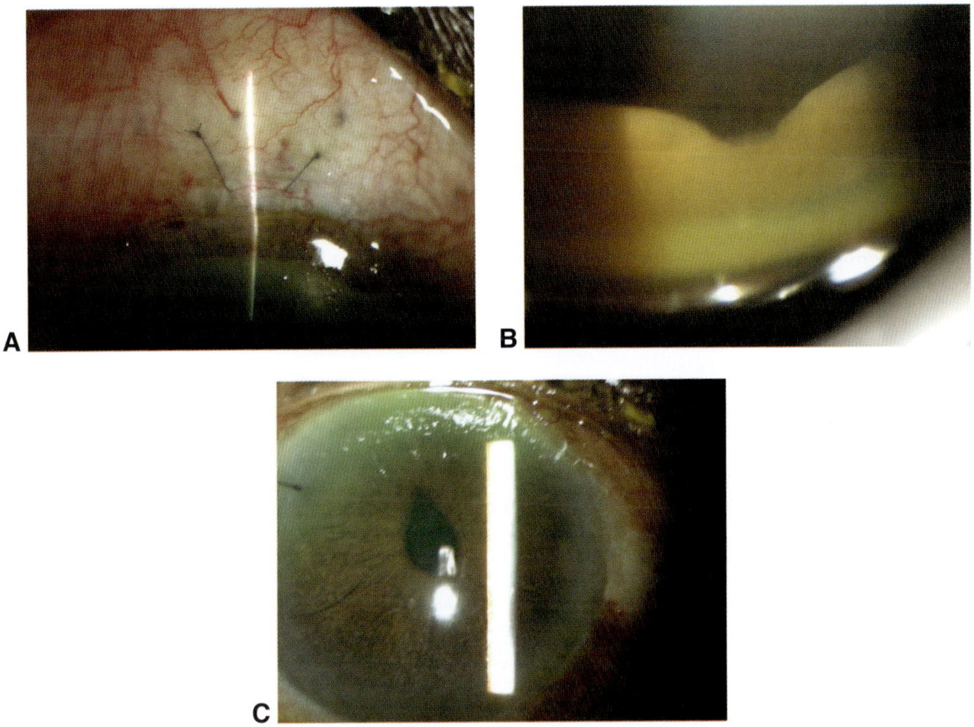

Figure 13-13 Sclerostomy obstruction. **A,** Patients with iris occlusion of the trabeculectomy fistula will have elevated intraocular pressure and a flat bleb. **B,** Gonioscopic photo reveals iris in the fistula. **C,** A peaked pupil should alert the physician to this possibility. *(Courtesy of Chandrasekharan Krishnan, MD.)*

If done too soon, overfiltration may occur; if done too late, the formation of fibrosis under the flap (from lack of flow) may result in inadequate long-term control of IOP.

Malignant glaucoma (also known as *aqueous misdirection*) and *suprachoroidal hemorrhage* can have very similar findings: shallow chamber, moderate to large bleb, and normal or high IOP (Fig 13-15). The chamber is very shallow centrally. Fundus evaluation (or B-scan ultrasonography if the view of the posterior segment is poor) is usually required to determine the cause of these findings. Treatment of suprachoroidal hemorrhage involves pain control and temporizing medical management of the IOP. Anticoagulant and antiplatelet therapy should be stopped if possible. Choroidal drainage should be delayed unless there is corneolenticular touch, intractable pain, or "kissing choroidals."

Malignant glaucoma is treated with cycloplegics and medical management of the IOP. Attempts can be made to break the vitreous face with the Nd:YAG laser (through the pupil in a pseudophakic patient or through a peripheral iridotomy in a phakic patient). If these approaches are unsuccessful, vitrectomy is warranted, with particular attention to disruption of the anterior hyaloid.

Fibrosis most commonly develops in the subconjunctival space but can occur at the level of the scleral flap as well. Adequate flow through the scleral flap and into the subconjunctival space in the early postoperative period is important for long-term surgical

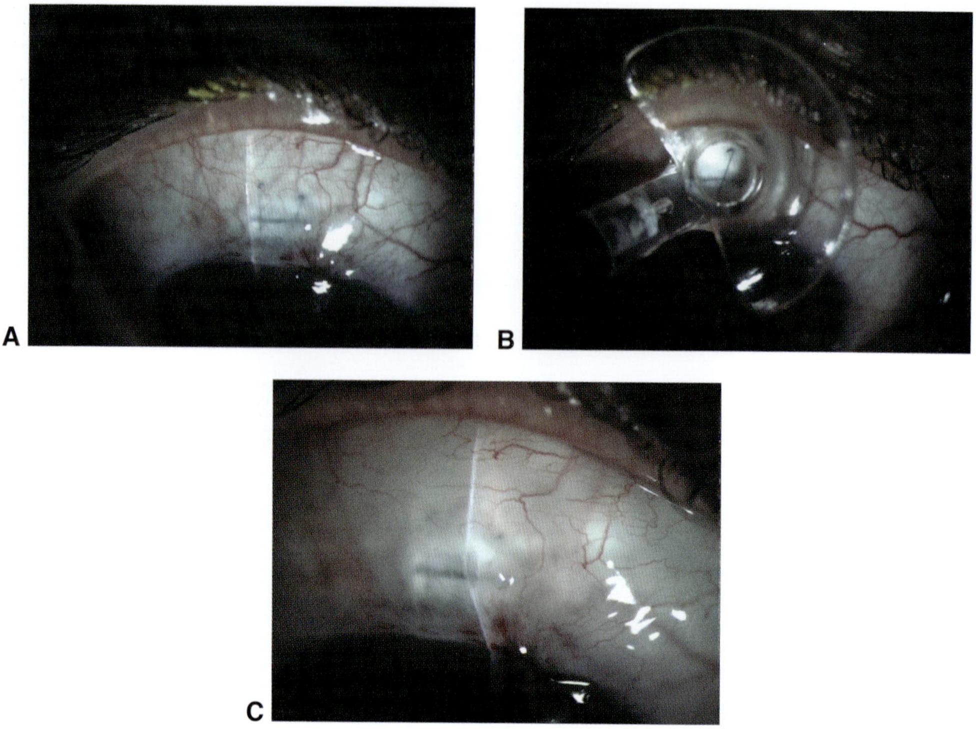

Figure 13-14 Tight scleral flap sutures. **A,** Tight flap sutures can cause a low bleb postoperatively. **B,** A laser goniolens can be used to visualize the suture. **C,** After the suture is cut with a green laser, the bleb should elevate quickly. *(Courtesy of Chandrasekharan Krishnan, MD.)*

success. Accordingly, control of fibrosis with topical steroids and subconjunctival antifibrotic agents (MMC, 5-FU) is of value. *Conjunctival hyperemia* in the postoperative period is a harbinger of subsequent fibrosis and necessitates the use of corticosteroid and/or antifibrotic therapy. Cutting or removing flap sutures increases flow and mitigates fibrosis. Transconjunctival needle revision (*bleb needling;* Video 13-7) can help disrupt fibrosis. A sharp-tipped instrument is introduced subconjunctivally to disrupt fibrotic tissue, allowing the formation of a more diffuse bleb.

VIDEO 13-7 Bleb needling.
Courtesy of Cynthia Mattox, MD.

Bleb-related infection (Fig 13-16) is a potentially vision-threatening complication after trabeculectomy, occurring in 1.5%–6.0% of patients. Patients typically present with tearing, irritation, pain, and/or blurry vision. Risk factors for infection include untreated blepharitis, presence of an inferior bleb, bleb leak, and thin-walled blebs (which tend to occur with localized blebs). The use of MMC and 5-FU is also a risk factor, as these agents are associated with a higher incidence of thin-walled blebs and bleb leaks. The formation

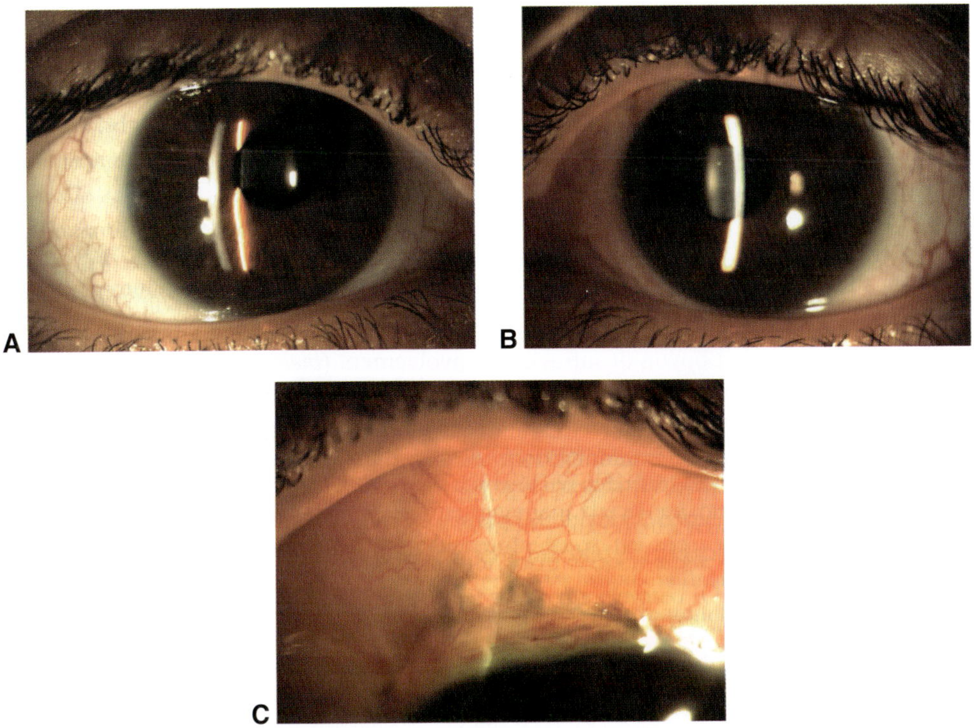

Figure 13-15 Malignant glaucoma after trabeculectomy. **A,** Early postoperative period. Note that the central chamber is flat. B-scan ultrasonography did not show any posterior abnormalities. **B,** The depth in the unaffected eye is shallow, which increases the risk for postoperative malignant glaucoma. **C,** The pressure in the surgical eye is not significantly elevated because the filtering bleb is functioning. *(Courtesy of Chandrasekharan Krishnan, MD.)*

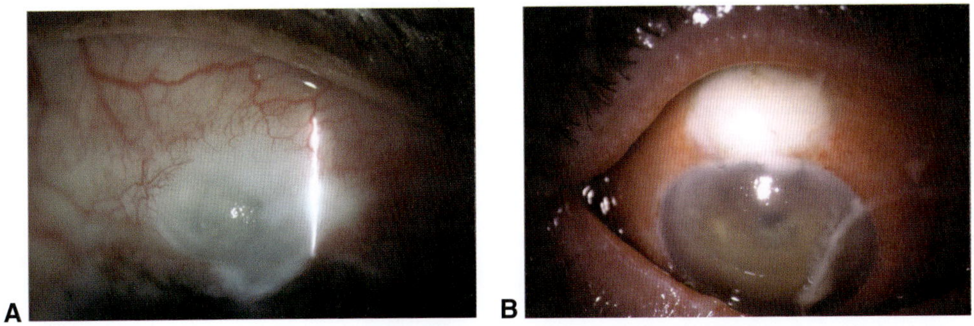

Figure 13-16 Bleb-related infection. **A,** Patients may present with blebitis, which is characterized by mucopurulent infiltrate within the bleb, localized conjunctival hyperemia, and minimal intraocular inflammation. **B,** Bleb-related endophthalmitis is characterized by diffuse bulbar conjunctival hyperemia, purulent material within the bleb, and anterior chamber cellular reaction; it is also sometimes characterized by hypopyon formation and marked vitritis. *(Part A courtesy of Chandrasekharan Krishnan, MD; part B courtesy of Keith Barton, MD. Part B is reproduced with permission of Moorfields Eye Hospital.)*

of thin-walled blebs and bleb leaks can be mitigated by fornix-based trabeculectomies and diffuse application of the antifibrotic agent.

One proposed classification scheme divides bleb-related infection into 3 stages, although these stages represent a continuum of infection:

- *stage 1:* erythema around the bleb, bleb infiltrate
- *stage 2:* anterior chamber inflammation
- *stage 3:* hypopyon and/or intravitreal involvement

Stage 1 and stage 2 bleb-related infection *(blebitis)* can be treated with topical fluoroquinolones or fortified topical and subconjunctival antibiotics as needed. Stage 3, indicated by the presence of a hypopyon or intravitreal involvement *(bleb-related endophthalmitis)*, warrants either a vitreous tap with injection of antibiotics or a vitrectomy. Patients with stage 1 and stage 2 bleb-related infection tend to fare well, while those with stage 3 tend to have poor visual outcomes.

Yassin SA. Bleb-related infection revisited: a literature review. *Acta Ophthalmol.* 2016;94(2):122–134.

EX-PRESS Shunt

The EX-PRESS Glaucoma Filtration Device (Alcon; Fig 13-17) is a shunt used in a variation on trabeculectomy. It was initially designed to be a stand-alone subconjunctival device inserted at the limbus. However, a high incidence of postoperative hypotony and erosion of the device through the conjunctiva necessitated a change in the surgical approach. The current technique for implantation follows steps similar to those used in trabeculectomy. The key difference is that the surgeon inserts the device underneath a partial-thickness scleral flap instead of removing a corneoscleral block of tissue. In addition, a peripheral iridectomy is not performed with the EX-PRESS shunt.

Several retrospective and prospective randomized trials comparing trabeculectomy with the EX-PRESS device to standard trabeculectomy have shown similar long-term IOP results, although vision recovery may be faster with the shunt than with trabeculectomy alone. Complications are similar, including hypotony, choroidal effusion, and infection. Device extrusion or migration is a rare complication that requires removal. EX-PRESS shunts are magnetic resonance imaging (MRI)-safe up to 3 Tesla.

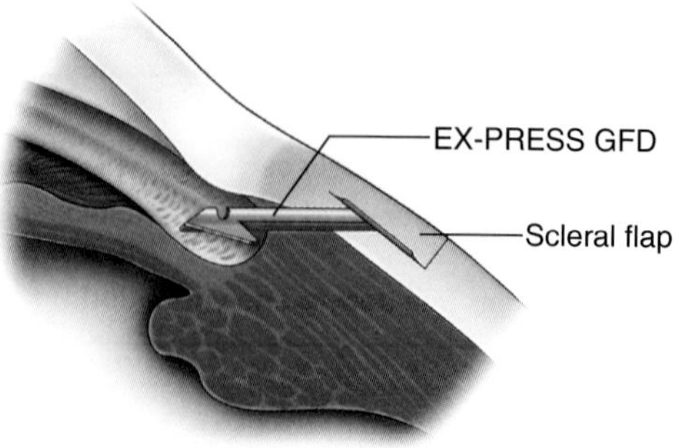

Figure 13-17 Schematic illustration of an EX-PRESS shunt placed under a scleral flap. GFD = glaucoma filtration device. *(© 2020 American Academy of Ophthalmology.)*

Gonzalez-Rodriguez JM, Trope GE, Drori-Wagschal L, Jinapriya D, Buys YM. Comparison of trabeculectomy vs Ex-PRESS: 3-year follow-up. *Br J Ophthalmol.* 2016;100(9):1269–1273.

Netland PA, Sarkisian SR Jr, Moster MR, et al. Randomized, prospective, comparative trial of EX-PRESS glaucoma filtration device versus trabeculectomy (XVT study). *Am J Ophthalmol.* 2014;157(2):433–440.

Plate-Based Tube Shunt Surgery

Mechanism of Action

Plate-based tube implants are designed to shunt aqueous from the anterior chamber to a space-maintaining plate in the equatorial subconjunctival space. Broadly speaking, plate-based tube implants can be divided into *valved* and *nonvalved* types. The *Ahmed Glaucoma Valve* (New World Medical; Video 13-8) has 2 leaflets in the plate that are designed to separate when the IOP is above a certain level (approximately 8–12 mm Hg). When the pressure is lower, the leaflets come together, preventing flow through the tube. The nonvalved *Baerveldt* (Johnson & Johnson Vision Care, Inc.; Video 13-9) and *Molteno* (Molteno Ophthalmic Limited) implants have no restriction to flow from the tube to the plate.

VIDEO 13-8 Ahmed valve implantation.
Courtesy of Simon K. Law, MD, PharmD.

VIDEO 13-9 Baerveldt tube shunt implantation.
Courtesy of JoAnn A. Giaconi, MD.

Indications and Contraindications

The indications and preoperative considerations for plate-based tube implants are similar to those for trabeculectomy. These implants were historically used in eyes that had failed multiple prior trabeculectomies, had active inflammation or neovascularization, or had severe conjunctival scarring. Over time, the indications for plate-based tube implants have expanded considerably. The Tube Versus Trabeculectomy Study (see Treatment Decisions and Data Sidebar) demonstrated superior success rates with tube shunt surgery in eyes with previous cataract surgery or trabeculectomy. The ongoing Primary Tube Versus Trabeculectomy Study is designed to evaluate outcomes of tube shunt surgery compared with trabeculectomy as the initial surgical intervention for eyes that failed medical therapy. These implants can cause corneal endothelial cell loss and corneal decompensation over time. Posterior placement of the tube may reduce the rate of corneal endothelial cell loss.

Technique

Exposure

Exposure is obtained by passing a partial-thickness traction suture through the cornea. Typically, the first implant is placed in the superotemporal quadrant. The placement of a second implant, if required, is dependent on surgeon preference.

Incision

A conjunctival incision can be made either at the limbus *(fornix-based flap)* or 5–6 mm posterior to the limbus *(limbus-based flap)*, depending on surgeon preference. Typically, about 90° of dissection is performed to provide ample space to implant the plate.

Placement of plate

The plate is then sutured onto the sclera about 8 mm posterior to the limbus. Prior to insertion, the muscles are identified to determine the appropriate location for the plate. For Baerveldt implants, the muscles must be isolated and lifted in order to place the wings of the plate underneath the rectus muscles. Nondissolving sutures are used to secure the plate. Care must be taken to avoid globe perforation, as the sclera is often relatively thin in this area.

Tube placement and management

The tube is cut to an appropriate length to ensure that it remains in the preferred location (pars plana, anterior chamber, or sulcus). If the tube is placed in the anterior chamber or the pars plana, the tube is cut bevel up. Alternatively, if the tube is placed in the sulcus, it is cut bevel down to prevent occlusion of the tube by the iris.

Valved devices must be primed to separate the leaflets of the valve. Nonvalved devices must be modified to prevent hypotony in the immediate postoperative period (Video 13-10). A dissolvable suture (or *ligature*) is tied around the tube near the tube–plate junction to restrict aqueous flow through the tube, thus allowing a capsule to form around the plate prior to dissolution of the suture. When the suture loosens (approximately 5–7 weeks postoperatively), resistance to flow from the capsule surrounding the plate prevents hypotony. A monofilament suture, called a *rip cord,* can be placed in or adjacent to the lumen of the tube and carried subconjunctivally. This rip cord can be pulled if necessary to lower the IOP within the first 6 weeks. Venting slits can be created between the ligature and the entry point of the tube into the eye to allow aqueous flow in the early postoperative period.

VIDEO 13-10 Intraoperative tube adjustments.
Courtesy of Chandrasekharan Krishnan, MD.

A 22- or 23-gauge needle is used to create an entry site for tube placement in the anterior chamber, ciliary sulcus, or pars plana (in a vitrectomized eye). When the tube is to be placed in the anterior chamber or sulcus, the needle is directed parallel to the iris in order to avoid tube–cornea touch. Some surgeons create a partial-thickness tunnel with the needle starting 3–6 mm posterior to the limbus.

Coverage of the tube can be reinforced with several different types of human donor materials (eg, cornea, pericardium, sclera), or the tube can be implanted through a long scleral tunnel or under a scleral flap (Video 13-11).

VIDEO 13-11 Tube coverage.
Courtesy of Chandrasekharan Krishnan, MD.

Closure

The conjunctiva is closed with dissolvable sutures. Fornix-based incisions can be closed with wing sutures, while limbus-based incisions can be closed with a running single- or 2-layer closure.

Postoperative Management

Plate-based tube implants tend to require fewer interventions in the postoperative period compared with trabeculectomy. However, complications can occur (Table 13-5).

Elevated IOP in the early postoperative period can have various causes. The *hypertensive phase* is marked by a sudden elevation of IOP after previously well-functioning surgery. Usually occurring between 3 weeks and 3 months after surgery, it is caused by decreased permeability of the capsule that forms around the end plate. Over time, the hypertensive phase may resolve as the capsule reorganizes and becomes more permeable to aqueous. Thus, management involves medical treatment to keep the pressure reasonably low while the capsule reorganizes. The incidence of this complication is higher with the Ahmed implant than with the Baerveldt implant, perhaps because the capsule is exposed to aqueous in the early postoperative period with the Ahmed device. Conversely, with Baerveldt implants, exposure of the capsule to aqueous is delayed by the ligature. The use of aqueous suppression early in postoperative management (when the IOP reaches approximately 10–12 mm Hg) is associated with a reduction in the incidence of the hypertensive phase and improved long-term outcomes. Evidence is mixed regarding the value of intraoperative or postoperative adjunctive MMC or 5-FU with tube shunt surgery; however, clinical trials are in progress.

Other causes of elevated IOP in the postoperative period include a defective valve mechanism and occlusion. Tubes can become occluded with fibrin, blood, vitreous, or iris tissue. A peripheral iridotomy can remedy iris occlusion, while fibrin and heme will usually clear over time without intervention. Elevated IOP in Baerveldt shunts that have been ligated can be managed by applying a green or diode laser to the ligature with settings similar to those used for nylon suture lysis. If a rip cord has been placed, it can be pulled. However, if these procedures are performed too early, hypotony may ensue. Fenestrations can also be created at the slit lamp to provide temporary IOP relief while waiting for the ligature to dissolve.

Shallow anterior chamber in the postoperative period occurs for reasons similar to those seen after trabeculectomy. *Choroidal effusions* and *malignant glaucoma* are managed in a similar fashion. *Overfiltration* may require a return to the operating room to either ligate the tube or place a suture in the lumen of the tube to restrict aqueous outflow.

Tube erosion occurs in 1%–8% of plate-based tube implant surgeries (Fig 13-18). The causes include mechanical factors, immune response, and fragile conjunctiva overlying the tube. Tube erosion requires surgical correction, as patients with this complication are at high risk for infection. Repair may involve placing a new allograft, moving the tube to a different location, or removing the tube (Video 13-12). The risk of endophthalmitis after tube shunt surgery is about 0.5% in 5 years. Management of endophthalmitis often requires tube removal.

Table 13-5 Complications of Tube Shunt Surgery and Options for Their Prevention and Management

Complication	Prevention or Management
Tube–cornea touch	Insert tube in anterior chamber parallel to the iris plane. Use a tube occlusion technique to avoid flat chambers with nonvalved shunts. Pars plana and ciliary sulcus insertion decrease this complication.
Flat chamber and hypotony	Valved devices can decrease overfiltration leading to these complications. With nonvalved devices, occlusion of tube by ligature or suture within tube can decrease early hypotony. Use viscoelastic agents if flat chamber develops. Ensure that entry site of tube is watertight around the tube (ie, carefully choose the needle size for creating the scleral track). Correct overdrainage early. Consider drainage of suprachoroidal effusions. Cycloplegics and corticosteroids can help deepen a shallow, but not a flat, chamber. A flat chamber resulting from a complication such as suprachoroidal hemorrhage must be managed based on the clinical setting.
Tube occlusion	Bevel the tube away from uveal tissue (iris) or vitreous. Generous vitrectomy should be performed if needed. Nd:YAG laser can be used to clear an occlusion; however, surgical intervention is often required.
Plate migration or tube retraction	Secure plate tightly to sclera with nonabsorbable sutures. If the plate migrates, the intraocular tube may become longer or retract. Plate migration toward the limbus requires repositioning of the plate in the equatorial subconjunctival space. Plate migration away from the limbus is rarely significant enough to warrant repositioning but may require a tube extender if the tube retracts from the anterior chamber.
Valve malfunction	Test valves for patency before insertion of the tube. Several techniques have been described to unclog a valve.
Tube or plate exposure or erosion	Tube or plate exposure can be repaired by removing any protruding sutures that have precipitated the erosion, securing tube tightly to sclera, covering tube with reinforcing material (eg, sclera, cornea, or pericardium), and mobilizing conjunctiva. Patch graft must be adequately covered with conjunctiva, or further erosion may occur. If adequate conjunctiva is not available, conjunctival autograft or amniotic membrane may be used. Exposure increases the risk of endophthalmitis. In some settings, the tube should be removed if adequate coverage cannot be achieved.
Diplopia	Prisms may resolve the diplopia. Strabismus surgery may be required for intractable diplopia.

VIDEO 13-12 Tube revision.
Courtesy of Chandrasekharan Krishnan, MD.

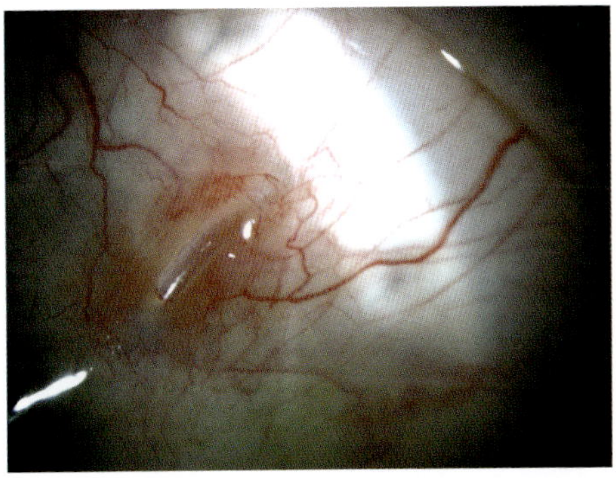

Figure 13-18 Tube exposures increase the risk of developing endophthalmitis and should be repaired urgently. *(Courtesy of Chandrasekharan Krishnan, MD.)*

Diplopia occurs in about 5% of patients. It is often due to displacement of the globe by a large bleb or injury or impingement of an extraocular muscle. Management with prisms is usually successful. If the deviation precludes prism use, strabismus surgery or tube removal may be indicated.

Bains U, Hoguet A. Aqueous drainage device erosion: a review of rates, risks, prevention, and repair. *Semin Ophthalmol.* 2018;33(1):1–10.

Cui QN, Hsia YC, Lin SC, et al. Effect of mitomycin C and 5-fluorouracil adjuvant therapy on the outcomes of Ahmed Glaucoma Valve implantation. *Clin Exp Ophthalmol.* 2017;45(2):128–134.

Pakravan M, Rad SS, Yazdani S, Ghahari E, Yaseri M. Effect of early treatment with aqueous suppressants on Ahmed Glaucoma Valve implantation outcomes. *Ophthalmology.* 2014;121(9):1693–1698.

Yazdini S, Doozandeh A, Pakravan M, Ownagh V, Yaseri M. Adjunctive triamcinolone acetonide for Ahmed Glaucoma Valve implantation: a randomized clinical trial. *Eur J Ophthalmol.* 2017;27(4):411–416.

Zheng CX, Moster MR, Khan MA, et al. Infectious endophthalmitis after glaucoma drainage implant surgery: clinical features, microbial spectrum, and outcomes. *Retina.* 2017;37(6):1160–1167.

TREATMENT DECISIONS AND DATA

Trabeculectomy or Tube Shunt Surgery?

In the Tube Versus Trabeculectomy (TVT) Study, 212 eyes with uncontrolled glaucoma that had previously undergone trabeculectomy or cataract surgery were randomized into 2 treatment groups. One group had trabeculectomy with MMC (0.4 mg/mL for 4 minutes), while the other underwent Baerveldt tube shunt surgery (350 mm^2).

At 5 years, mean IOP and number of glaucoma medications were similar between the groups. However, there was a significantly higher failure rate (defined as IOP >21, <20% reduction of IOP, persistent IOP <5, or loss of light perception) in the trabeculectomy group, and that group also required more reoperations. The "complete success" rate (achieving successful IOP control without medication) and quality-of-life

(Continued on next page)

(continued)

measures were similar between the 2 groups. The most common postoperative complications were shallow/flat anterior chamber, wound leak, and choroidal effusions in the trabeculectomy group. The most common postoperative complications in the tube group were shallow/flat anterior chamber, persistent corneal edema, and choroidal effusions. The trabeculectomy group required more postoperative clinic interventions. The rate of reoperation for complications was similar between the 2 groups. Importantly, over 40% of patients overall lost 2 or more lines of Snellen visual acuity over 5 years. This was not significantly different between the trabeculectomy and tube implant groups and was most commonly caused by cataract progression and persistent corneal edema.

The ongoing Primary Tube Versus Trabeculectomy Study is similar to the TVT Study, except that the participants had no prior intraocular surgery. At 3 years, both the mean IOP and number of glaucoma medications were significantly lower in the trabeculectomy group. In addition, more patients were able to achieve the target IOP without medical therapy with trabeculectomy (44%) than with tube shunt (13%). There were no significant differences in complication rates between the groups at 3 years.

Gedde SJ, Feuer WJ, Shi W, et al; Primary Tube Versus Trabeculectomy Study Group. Treatment outcomes in the Primary Tube Versus Trabeculectomy Study after 1 year of follow-up. *Ophthalmology.* 2018; 125(5):650–663.

Gedde SJ, Herndon LW, Brandt JD, Budenz DL, Feuer WJ, Schiffman JC; Tube Versus Trabeculectomy Study Group. Postoperative complications in the Tube Versus Trabeculectomy (TVT) Study during five years of follow-up. *Am J Ophthalmol.* 2012;153(5):804–814.

Gedde SJ, Schiffman JC, Feuer WJ, Herndon LW, Brandt JD, Budenz DL; Tube Versus Trabeculectomy Study Group. Treatment outcomes in the Tube Versus Trabeculectomy (TVT) Study after five years of follow-up. *Am J Ophthalmol.* 2012;153(5):789–803.

Kotecha A, Feuer WJ, Barton K, Gedde SJ; Tube Versus Trabeculectomy Study Group. Quality of life in the Tube Versus Trabeculectomy Study. *Am J Ophthalmol.* 2017;176:228–235.

Valved Versus Nonvalved Plate-Based Tube Implants

The Ahmed Baerveldt Comparison (ABC) Study and Ahmed Versus Baerveldt (AVB) Study compared the efficacy of the Ahmed FP7 and Baerveldt 350 implants over 5 years. A pooled data analysis showed that, at 5 years, the Baerveldt group had lower mean IOP (13.2 ± 4.8 mm Hg vs 15.8 ± 5.2 mm Hg) and were on fewer glaucoma medications (1.5 ± 1.4 vs 1.9 ± 1.5) than the Ahmed group. Visual acuity loss of 2 or more Snellen lines was similar between the groups (47% in the Ahmed group, 46% in the Baerveldt group). Failure rates (defined as IOP <6 or >18 mm Hg, IOP reduction <20% below baseline at 2 consecutive visits after 3 months, additional glaucoma procedures needed, or loss of light perception) were higher in the Ahmed group than in the Baerveldt group at 5 years (49% vs 37%). The most common reason for failure in both groups was elevated IOP.

More patients had serious complications (defined as a complication requiring reoperation or a loss of visual acuity of 2 or more lines) in the Baerveldt group than in the Ahmed group. Of note, 4% of patients in the Baerveldt group had failure due to hypotony.

Budenz DL, Feuer WJ, Barton K, et al; Ahmed Baerveldt Comparison Study Group. Postoperative complications in the Ahmed Baerveldt Comparison Study during five years of follow-up. *Am J Ophthalmol.* 2016;163:75–82.e3.

Christakis PG, Zhang D, Budenz DL, Barton K, Tsai JC, Ahmed IIK; ABC-AVB Study Groups. Five-year pooled data analysis of the Ahmed Baerveldt Comparison Study and the Ahmed Versus Baerveldt Study. *Am J Ophthalmol.* 2017;176:118–126.

Cataract Surgery in the Glaucoma Patient

After surgery for visually significant cataract, patients with ocular hypertension or glaucoma may have a reduction in IOP.

Ocular Hypertension

In the Ocular Hypertension Treatment Study (see Chapter 7), 42 patients underwent cataract surgery while enrolled in the control arm of the study. These patients were compared to patients in the control arm who did not undergo cataract surgery. At 36 months, the average IOP reduction in patients who had cataract surgery was 16.5%. Moreover, 40% of eyes that underwent cataract surgery had a ≥20% reduction in IOP at 36 months. Conversely, the mean IOP in eyes that did not undergo cataract surgery was unchanged at 36 months.

Mansberger SL, Gordon MO, Jampel H, et al; Ocular Hypertension Treatment Study Group. Reduction in intraocular pressure after cataract extraction: the Ocular Hypertension Treatment Study. *Ophthalmology*. 2012;119(9):1826–1831.

Primary Open-Angle Glaucoma

Many retrospective and prospective studies have shown that cataract surgery reduces IOP in patients with OAG. This reduction is thought to be the result of increased outflow facility. Hypothesized mechanisms for this effect include the following:

- anatomic changes in the eye from removal of the lens
- biochemical changes induced as a result of surgery
- irrigation of the TM

A meta-analysis found a mean IOP reduction of 3 mm Hg after cataract surgery in eyes with POAG, although the decrease in IOP seems to dissipate over time. However, in some patients, cataract surgery can be associated with acute and persistent IOP elevation. There is no evidence to support removal of cataracts that are *not* visually significant in the management of OAG.

Chen PP, Lin SC, Junk AK, Radhakrishnan S, Singh K, Chen TC. The effect of phacoemulsification on intraocular pressure in glaucoma patients: a report by the American Academy of Ophthalmology. *Ophthalmology.* 2015:122(7):1294–1307.

Masis M, Mineault PJ, Phan E, Lin SC. The role of phacoemulsification in glaucoma therapy: a systematic review and meta-analysis. *Surv Ophthalmol.* 2018;63(5):700–710.

Angle-Closure Glaucoma

With normal aging, the increase in the anteroposterior diameter of the lens leads to the development of relative pupillary block. This in turn can cause primary angle closure in predisposed eyes. Because an intraocular lens is substantially thinner than the crystalline lens, cataract surgery can be effective in the management of all stages of angle-closure disease by alleviating pupillary block.

The EAGLE study compared cataract surgery in eyes with clear lenses and non–visually significant cataracts to laser peripheral iridotomy combined with medical therapy in a prospective randomized controlled trial in patients with either primary angle closure (defined unconventionally in this study as the presence of ≥180° of synechial or appositional iridotrabecular contact with IOP ≥30 mmHg) or primary angle-closure glaucoma. At 3 years, the lensectomy group had lower IOP, were on fewer medications, and required fewer additional interventions to control IOP. (See also Chapter 9, Treatment Controversies sidebar.)

In patients with PAS, goniosynechialysis may lower the IOP (Video 13-13). After the cataract is removed, a blunt instrument, viscoelastic, and/or forceps are used to tease the iris off the TM. Goniosynechialysis is more effective when performed in combination with cataract surgery and when PAS formation is more recent.

VIDEO 13-13 Goniosynechialysis.
Courtesy of Chandrasekharan Krishnan, MD.

Azuara-Blanco A, Burr J, Ramsay C, et al; EAGLE Study Group. Effectiveness of early lens extraction for the treatment of primary angle-closure glaucoma (EAGLE): a randomised controlled trial. *Lancet.* 2016;388(10052):1389–1397.

Rodrigues IA, Alaghband P, Beltran Agullo L, et al. Aqueous outflow facility after phacoemulsification with or without goniosynechialysis in primary angle closure: a randomised controlled study. *Br J Ophthalmol.* 2017;101(7):879–885.

Cataract Surgery in Conjunction With Trabeculectomy or Tube Shunt Surgery

Often, patients who require incisional glaucoma surgery also have a visually significant cataract. If appropriate, cataract surgery prior to tube shunt surgery or trabeculectomy is indicated to decrease the amount of postsurgical inflammation at the time of tube implantation or trabeculectomy. When glaucoma surgery is more urgent, the surgeon may determine that the best approach is to remove the cataract at the time of glaucoma surgery, especially given the increased rate of cataract progression after glaucoma surgery.

AGIS (Advanced Glaucoma Intervention Study) Investigators. The Advanced Glaucoma Intervention Study: 8. Risk of cataract formation after trabeculectomy. *Arch Ophthalmol.* 2001;119(12):1771–1779.

Cataract surgery and plate-based tube shunt implants

There is a high rate of cataract progression after plate-based tube shunt surgery. Thus, for glaucoma patients with visually significant cataracts, consideration should be given to removing the cataract at the time of tube shunt implantation. Deepening the anterior chamber by cataract extraction allows for more posterior placement of the tube in the anterior chamber or the possibility of implantation in the ciliary sulcus, reducing the risk of corneal decompensation.

Cataract surgery and trabeculectomy

When removing a cataract concurrently with trabeculectomy, the surgeon can perform a single-site surgery (inserting the phaco handpiece underneath the trabeculectomy flap) or a 2-site surgery (creating a corneal wound separate from the trabeculectomy flap). Outcomes are thought to be similar.

Studies evaluating the effect of cataract surgery after trabeculectomy have mixed results: some have shown no effect on IOP, while others have demonstrated a slight rise in IOP or an increase in the number of medications needed for IOP control. If cataract surgery is planned to be done after trabeculectomy, delaying cataract surgery for 6–12 months may improve long-term trabeculectomy survival and IOP control.

Gdih GA, Yuen D, Yan P, Sheng L, Jin YP, Buys YM. Meta-analysis of 1- versus 2-site phacotrabeculectomy. *Ophthalmology.* 2011;118(1):71–76.

Husain R, Liang S, Foster PJ, et al. Cataract surgery after trabeculectomy: the effect on trabeculectomy function. *Arch Ophthalmol.* 2012;130(2):165–170.

Other Glaucoma Surgeries

Minimally Invasive Glaucoma Surgeries

Minimally invasive glaucoma surgery (MIGS), also called *microinvasive* or *microincisional glaucoma surgery,* refers to procedures that enhance preexisting pathways for aqueous outflow. Approaches include decreasing trabecular meshwork resistance to aqueous flow, improving aqueous flow through Schlemm canal, and/or creating a low-resistance pathway for aqueous flow between the anterior chamber and the suprachoroidal space. Despite the name, MIGS procedures are incisional surgeries, are invasive, and carry risk. However, significant complications occur less frequently with MIGS than with traditional glaucoma surgeries.

Because MIGS aims to increase flow through preexisting pathways, the efficacy of most of the procedures (other than those that shunt aqueous to the suprachoroidal space) is limited by the episcleral venous pressure (EVP) and distal outflow resistance. In most patients, the EVP is 6–9 mm Hg. Typically, MIGS procedures lead to IOPs in the mid to high teens.

MIGS procedures fall into 3 general categories:

- stents to Schlemm canal
- TM disruption
- stents to the suprachoroidal space

Indications and contraindications

Angle-based MIGS necessitates a gonioscopic view of the anterior chamber angle during surgery. Developing appropriate eye-hand coordination with a blunt-tipped instrument (such as a cyclodialysis spatula) while visualizing the angle with a gonioprism is useful in attaining the dexterity required to perform angle-based MIGS.

Postoperative management involves the use of steroids and antibiotics. For procedures that require TM disruption, pilocarpine is also used. Complications include hyphema, postoperative IOP spikes, prolonged postoperative inflammation, obstruction of the device by iris tissue, improper insertion of the device, cyclodialysis, iridodialysis, corneal decompensation, and hypotony.

Patient selection

There is limited evidence to guide the use of these devices in advanced glaucoma, and they are not well suited for eyes that require a very low target IOP. MIGS procedures are often performed in conjunction with cataract surgery. Indications for MIGS include

- patients with mild to moderate glaucoma who require additional IOP reduction
- patients who would benefit from a reduction in medication burden

Trabecular bypass devices

Trabecular bypass devices are designed to create a low-resistance pathway between the anterior chamber and Schlemm canal.

iStent The *first-generation iStent* (Glaukos Corporation) has an L-shaped design (Fig 13-19A). The sharp tip of the iStent is designed to pierce the TM tangentially. There are several retention rings on the outer aspect of the hollow body of the iStent, which are designed to keep the stent in place.

The *second-generation iStent (iStent inject)* has a different design, with a "head" located in Schlemm canal, a "thorax" that is lodged in the trabecular meshwork, and a flange that remains in the anterior chamber (Fig 13-19B). Two iStent inject devices are implanted in the same eye.

TECHNIQUE An incision is made in the temporal cornea, and the eye is filled with a cohesive viscoelastic. The patient's head is tilted away from the surgeon, and the microscope is adjusted appropriately. The angle is visualized with a direct gonioscope.

With the first-generation iStent, the device tangentially approaches the trabecular meshwork, and the tip of the iStent pierces the TM and is advanced into Schlemm canal. When the device is in appropriate position, it is released from the handpiece with the push of a button (Video 13-14).

VIDEO 13-14 iStent implantation.
Courtesy of Shakeel Shareef, MD.

With the second-generation device (iStent inject), the preloaded handpiece is introduced into the eye and the protective sleeve is retracted, exposing the delivery device tip.

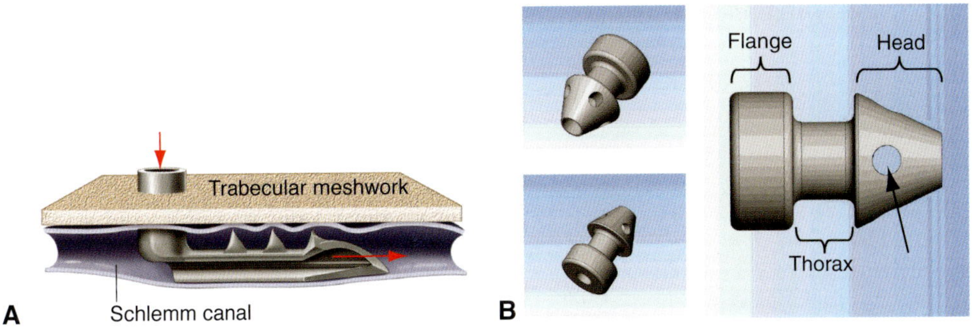

Figure 13-19 Illustration of the iStent. **A,** In the first-generation iStent, the tip pierces the trabecular meshwork (TM), allowing the device to slide into the Schlemm canal. Retention rings hold the device in place. The snorkel is open to the anterior chamber, allowing aqueous to flow through the device into Schlemm canal. *Arrows* indicate aqueous flow. **B,** The head of the iStent inject contains 4 equal-size and evenly spaced ports for fluid passage *(arrow)*. The head is connected to a narrow thorax that attaches to a wider flange region. An inlet port runs the entire length of the iStent inject. *(Part A illustration courtesy of Mark Miller; part B courtesy of Bahler CK, Hann CR, Fijeld T, Haffner D, Heitzmann H, Fautsch MP. Second-generation trabecular meshwork bypass stent (iStent inject) increases outflow facility in cultured human anterior segments.* Am J Ophthalmol. *2012;153(6):1206–1213.)*

The tip is embedded into the TM and a button is pushed to deploy the stent. A second preloaded stent is inserted 2 to 3 clock-hours away (Video 13-15).

VIDEO 13-15 iStent inject.
Courtesy of Wayne Tie, MD.

EFFECTIVENESS A 2-year study comparing cataract surgery combined with implantation of the first-generation iStent and cataract surgery alone found that patients receiving the iStent were more likely to achieve a 20% reduction in unmedicated IOP (53% vs 44%), though this was not statistically significant. iStent patients were statistically more likely to have an unmedicated IOP ≤21 mm Hg (61% vs 50%).

In a similar 2-year study of the iStent inject device, patients underwent a medication washout at baseline and at the conclusion of the study. In the microstent group, mean diurnal IOP reduction was greater (7.0 ± 4.0 mm Hg vs 5.4 ± 3.7 mm Hg; $P < .01$), and there was a higher likelihood of achieving a 20% reduction in unmedicated IOP (76% vs 62%).

Craven ER, Katz LJ, Wells JM, Giamporcaro JE; iStent Study Group. Cataract surgery with trabecular micro-bypass stent implantation in patients with mild-to-moderate open-angle glaucoma and cataract: two-year follow up. *J Cataract Refract Surg.* 2012:38(8):1339–1345.

Hydrus The *Hydrus* implant (Ivantis) is similar to the iStent in that the Hydrus is designed to traverse the TM. However, this device is also designed to dilate the Schlemm canal over approximately 3 clock-hours.

TECHNIQUE The initial steps are similar to those for iStent. The inserter containing the Hydrus stent is introduced into the anterior chamber, and the tip of the cannula perforates the trabecular meshwork, allowing for delivery of the Hydrus into Schlemm canal (Video 13-16).

VIDEO 13-16 Hydrus.
Courtesy of Iqbal "Ike" Ahmed, MD.

EFFECTIVENESS A 2-year study comparing cataract surgery combined with implantation of the Hydrus device versus cataract surgery alone found that patients who received the Hydrus were more likely to achieve a statistically significant 20% reduction in unmedicated IOP (80% vs 46%). Mean diurnal IOP reduction was greater in the Hydrus group as well (9.4 mm Hg vs 7.4 mm Hg).

Pfeiffer N, Garcia-Feijoo J, Martinez-de-la-Casa JM, et al. A randomized trial of a Schlemm's canal microstent with phacoemulsification for reducing intraocular pressure in open-angle glaucoma. *Ophthalmology*. 2015;122(7):1283–1293.

Trabecular disruption

These procedures are designed to disrupt or remove the inner wall of Schlemm canal and TM, opening the canal and downstream collector channels directly to aqueous outflow. In addition to topical steroids and antibiotics, pilocarpine is used to prevent the development of PAS.

Trabectome The *Trabectome* (MicroSurgical Technologies) is used to ablate the TM and inner wall of Schlemm canal. The device consists of a handpiece with a tip that ablates the tissue by means of a bipolar 550 kHz electrode. There are also irrigating and aspirating ports to dissipate heat, remove debris liberated during the procedure, and maintain anterior chamber stability.

TECHNIQUE A temporal clear corneal incision is created, and a gonioscopy lens is used (Video 13-17). Unlike other angle-based procedures, viscoelastic is not employed during the surgery because of concerns that gas bubbles resulting from ablation could be trapped in the viscoelastic and obscure the view of the trabecular meshwork. The TM and inner wall of the Schlemm canal are removed by the ablating tip of the handpiece. Up to 180° of TM is excised during the procedure. Postoperatively, viscoelastic may be placed in the eye to prevent blood reflux from the exposed collector channels.

VIDEO 13-17 Trabectome: setup and procedure.
Courtesy of Sameh Mosaed, MD.

EFFECTIVENESS No prospective randomized trials have yet compared the efficacy of the Trabectome to that of cataract surgery alone.

Polat JK, Loewen NA. Combined phacoemulsification and Trabectome for treatment of glaucoma. *Surv Ophthalmol*. 2017;62(5):698–705.

Kahook Dual Blade Conventional goniotomy (see Chapter 11) is most effective in primary congenital glaucoma; however, it has been attempted in other forms of glaucoma as well.

The *Kahook Dual Blade* (New World Medical) is a device designed to allow the surgeon to perform an excisional goniotomy by removing of a strip of tissue from the TM and inner wall of Schlemm canal (Video 13-18).

VIDEO 13-18 Kahook Dual Blade goniotomy.
Courtesy of Iqbal "Ike" Ahmed, MD.

TECHNIQUE An incision is created in the temporal cornea, and the eye is filled with a cohesive viscoelastic. The nasal angle is visualized using a direct goniolens. The device tip is embedded into the trabecular meshwork, and the TM and inner wall of Schlemm canal are stripped and excised.

EFFECTIVENESS No prospective randomized controlled studies have evaluated goniotomy with the Kahook Dual Blade.

Sieck EG, Epstein RS, Kennedy JB, et al. Outcomes of Kahook Dual Blade goniotomy with and without phacoemulsification cataract extraction. *Ophthalmol Glaucoma.* 2018;1(1):75–81.

Gonioscopy-assisted transluminal trabeculotomy *Gonioscopy-assisted transluminal trabeculotomy (GATT)* is similar to ab externo 360° suture trabeculotomy (see Chapter 11), except that the suture is introduced into Schlemm canal through an intracameral approach (Videos 13-19, 13-20). An alternate term for GATT is *360° ab interno suture trabeculotomy*. An advantage of GATT over the ab externo procedure is that it spares the conjunctiva.

VIDEO 13-19 GATT and ab interno canaloplasty.
Courtesy of Iqbal "Ike" Ahmed, MD.

VIDEO 13-20 Ab externo trabeculotomy.
Courtesy of Lauren Blieden, MD.

TECHNIQUE Two paracenteses are created: 1 for intracameral surgical manipulations and the other for entry of a suture or illuminated microcatheter. The eye is filled with a cohesive viscoelastic. A goniotomy blade is used to create a 1–2-mm goniotomy in the nasal angle. A suture or microcatheter is introduced into the Schlemm canal through the goniotomy site. The device is passed 360°, and the distal and proximal ends of the suture are grasped and used to cheese-wire the TM/Schlemm canal complex, creating a 360° trabeculotomy. The chamber is partially filled with viscoelastic to mitigate postoperative bleeding.

EFFECTIVENESS No prospective comparative studies have been performed. A retrospective study of 198 eyes showed an average reduction in IOP of 9 mm Hg in POAG patients and of 14 mm Hg in secondary open-angle glaucoma patients at 24 months after GATT. In addition, patients were on 1–2 fewer medications at 24 months.

Grover DS, Smith O, Fellman RL, et al. Gonioscopy-assisted transluminal trabeculotomy: an ab interno circumferential trabeculotomy: 24 months follow-up. *J Glaucoma.* 2018;27(5):393–401.

Ab interno canaloplasty *Ab interno canaloplasty (AbIC)* uses a specially designed illuminated microcatheter that is introduced into Schlemm canal via an internal approach. Viscoelastic is injected through the microcatheter into Schlemm canal to viscodilate the canal and, possibly, the downstream collector channels.

TECHNIQUE The procedure is similar to that of GATT; however, viscoelastic is injected while the catheter is advanced into the canal, and a goniotomy is not performed unless specifically desired (see Video 13-19).

EFFECTIVENESS No prospective trials have evaluated AbIC.

Aqueous shunt into the suprachoroidal space

Currently, there are no devices approved by the US Food and Drug Administration (FDA) to shunt aqueous into the suprachoroidal space. The *CyPass Micro-Stent* (Alcon), a tube-shaped device placed in the anterior chamber angle to create a conduit from the anterior chamber to the suprachoroidal space, was formerly available. In a 2-year prospective randomized controlled trial, CyPass combined with cataract surgery demonstrated an additional IOP reduction of 2.0 mm Hg below baseline compared with cataract surgery alone. Despite its efficacy, the device was recalled by the FDA in 2018 because increased endothelial cell loss was observed during extended observation of patients in the pivotal clinical trial.

Vold S, Ahmed II, Craven ER, et al; CyPass Study Group. Two-year COMPASS trial results: supraciliary microstenting with phacoemulsification in patients with open-angle glaucoma and cataracts. *Ophthalmology*. 2016;123(10):2103–2112.

Short Aqueous Stent to Subconjunctival Space

The *XEN Gel Stent* (Allergan) and *PreserFlo Microshunt* (formerly called *InnFocus Microshunt;* Santen Inc.) are 2 devices that shunt aqueous humor to the subconjunctival space. Unlike traditional plate-based tube implants, these devices do not have a plate attached to the subconjunctival portion of the tube.

In *XEN Gel Stent* implantation (Video 13-21), a clear corneal incision is created in the inferior cornea. The eye is filled with viscoelastic, and a goniolens is placed on the eye to visualize the superior angle. The injector is introduced into the eye, and the superior TM is pierced by the injector. The needle is driven through the sclera, exiting 3 mm posterior to the limbus into the subconjunctival space. The device is carefully injected into the subconjunctival space, and the needle is retracted. MMC is used to reduce postoperative fibrosis.

VIDEO 13-21 XEN implantation.
Courtesy of Wayne Tie, MD.

In the pivotal study for the FDA, 75% of patients had ≥20% reduction of IOP at 12 months, 32% required postoperative transconjunctival needle revision, and 25% had transient hypotony. Potential complications are similar to those of trabeculectomy and tube shunt, including choroidal effusion, tube erosion, prolonged hypotony, and infection.

Of note, there was no comparator arm in this trial. In 2 retrospective studies, there was no significant difference in success rates between trabeculectomy and XEN Gel Stent surgery.

The *PreserFlo Microshunt* is an externally placed, nonplated tube implant currently undergoing FDA evaluation. A 4-year nonrandomized study showed that 80% of eyes attained an IOP <14 mm Hg from a baseline of 25 mm Hg.

Grover DS, Flynn WJ, Bashford KP, et al. Performance and safety of a new ab interno gelatin stent in refractory glaucoma at 12 months. *Am J Ophthalmol.* 2017;183:25–36.

Nonpenetrating Glaucoma Surgery

Nonpenetrating glaucoma procedures are incisional glaucoma surgeries that do not enter the anterior chamber; their goal is to lower IOP while avoiding some of the complications of trabeculectomy. These nonpenetrating procedures include *deep sclerectomy, viscocanalostomy,* and *canaloplasty* (Video 13-22). In both viscocanalostomy and canaloplasty, a deep sclerectomy is augmented with injection of viscoelastic into Schlemm canal. In viscocanalostomy, a cannula is used to inject viscoelastic into a limited section of Schlemm canal. In canaloplasty, a flexible illuminated catheter is utilized to inject viscoelastic into the full 360° of Schlemm canal and to pass a suture through it; the suture is then tied under moderate tension, leaving the canal stretched. For these 3 procedures, the surgeon creates a fornix-based conjunctival incision and then a superficial scleral flap. Deeper sclera and peripheral cornea are removed underneath this flap, leaving only a thin layer of sclera and Descemet membrane. This allows aqueous to percolate through Descemet membrane into a scleral lake formed by removal of the deep scleral flap.

VIDEO 13-22 Canaloplasty.
Courtesy of Steven Vold, MD.

These surgeries are indicated for OAG. Currently, there are limited long-term data from prospective randomized trials comparing these newer procedures with trabeculectomy. Although nonpenetrating surgery may avoid some of the complications associated with trabeculectomy, they are technically challenging; and most results suggest that IOP reduction with these procedures is less than that obtained with trabeculectomy. They also cause conjunctival scarring, which may limit future surgical options. In addition, the surgeon may need to convert intraoperatively to trabeculectomy. Postoperative Nd:YAG laser goniopuncture of Descemet membrane may be needed to increase aqueous flow. Complications include Descemet detachment and infection.

Chai C, Loon SC. Meta-analysis of viscocanalostomy versus trabeculectomy in uncontrolled glaucoma. *J Glaucoma.* 2010;19(8):519–527.

Gilmour DF, Manners TD, Devonport H, Varga Z, Solebo AL, Miles J. Viscocanalostomy versus trabeculectomy for primary open angle glaucoma: 4-year prospective randomized clinical trial. *Eye (Lond).* 2009;23(9):1802–1807.

Lewis RA, von Wolff K, Tetz M, et al. Canaloplasty: circumferential viscodilation and tensioning of Schlemm canal using a flexible microcatheter for the treatment of open-angle glaucoma in adults: two-year interim clinical study results. *J Cataract Refract Surg.* 2009;35(5):814–824.

Special Considerations in the Surgical Management of Elderly Patients

When deciding whether to perform surgery in an elderly patient, the surgeon must consider several issues specific to this population. Considerations include the severity of the glaucoma and the risk of functional vision loss in relation to the patient's life expectancy, as well as the presence of any major systemic disease that could affect the outcome. The surgeon must also assess the patient's ability to adhere to medical therapy. For example, a patient who has poor medication adherence preoperatively (because of memory loss, poor vision, tremor, or arthritis) is likely to be nonadherent in the postoperative phase as well, which could jeopardize the outcome.

Once the decision has been made to proceed with surgery, the surgeon should determine which procedure is most likely to be adequately successful in reducing IOP with the fewest possible complications. The surgeon should consider the patient's ability to return for multiple follow-up visits. If a patient is not mobile or lacks easy transportation options, a nonpenetrating surgery, MIGS, or cyclodestructive procedure may be preferred, as these procedures require fewer postoperative visits than does a trabeculectomy or tube shunt surgery. If a trabeculectomy is selected, a limbus-based conjunctival flap might be considered, as it is less likely to leak than a fornix-based flap. The patient's use of anticoagulants and antiplatelet medications should also be evaluated, as these drugs increase the risk of serious complications from intraocular hemorrhage; however, stopping them is associated with a risk of vascular events. Finally, the surgeon must factor in compromised healing in elderly persons and be cautious about the use of antifibrotics in this group, as their tissues tend to be thinner and more fragile compared with those of younger patients.

Additional Materials and Resources

Related Academy Materials

The American Academy of Ophthalmology is dedicated to providing a wealth of high-quality clinical education resources for ophthalmologists.

Print Publications and Electronic Products

For a complete listing of Academy products related to topics covered in this BCSC Section, visit our online store at https://store.aao.org/clinical-education/topic/glaucoma.html. Or call Customer Service at 866.561.8558 (toll free, US only) or +1 415.561.8540, Monday through Friday, between 8:00 a.m. and 5:00 p.m. (PST).

Online Resources

Visit the Ophthalmic News and Education (ONE®) Network at https://www.aao.org/glaucoma to find relevant videos, online courses, journal articles, practice guidelines, self-assessment quizzes, images, and more. The ONE Network is a free Academy-member benefit.

Access free, trusted articles and content with the Academy's collaborative online encyclopedia, EyeWiki, at aao.org/eyewiki.

Get mobile access to the *Wills Eye Manual,* watch the latest 1-minute videos, and set up alerts for clinical updates relevant to you with the AAO Ophthalmic Education App. Download today: Search for "AAO Ophthalmic Education" in the Apple app store or in Google Play.

Basic Texts and Additional Resources

Allingham RR, Damji KF, Freedman S, Maroi SE, Rhee DJ. *Shields' Textbook of Glaucoma.* 6th ed. Lippincott Williams & Wilkins; 2010.

Anderson DR, Patella VM. *Automated Static Perimetry.* 2nd ed. Mosby; 1998.

Kahook MY, Schuman JS, eds. *Chandler and Grant's Glaucoma.* 5th ed. Slack; 2013.

Levin LA, Nilsson SFE, Ver Hoeve J, Wu SM, Kaufman PL, Alm A. *Adler's Physiology of the Eye: Clinical Application.* 11th ed. Saunders/Elsevier; 2011.

Schacknow PN, Samples JR, eds. *The Glaucoma Book.* Springer-Verlag New York; 2010.

Stamper RL, Lieberman MF, Drake MV, eds. *Becker-Shaffer's Diagnosis and Therapy of the Glaucomas.* 8th ed. Mosby; 2009.

Weinreb RN, Mills RP, eds. *Glaucoma Surgery: Principles and Techniques.* 2nd ed. Ophthalmology Monographs 4. American Academy of Ophthalmology; 1998.

Requesting Continuing Medical Education Credit

The American Academy of Ophthalmology is accredited by the Accreditation Council for Continuing Medical Education (ACCME) to provide continuing medical education for physicians.

The American Academy of Ophthalmology designates this enduring material for a maximum of 10 *AMA PRA Category 1 Credits*™. Physicians should claim only the credit commensurate with the extent of their participation in the activity.

To claim *AMA PRA Category 1 Credits*™ upon completion of this activity, learners must demonstrate appropriate knowledge and participation in the activity by taking the posttest for Section 10 and achieving a score of 80% or higher.

This activity meets the Self-Assessment CME requirements defined by the American Board of Ophthalmology (ABO). Please be advised that the ABO is not an accrediting body for purposes of any CME program. ABO does not sponsor this or any outside activity, and ABO does not endorse any particular CME activity. Complete information regarding the ABO Self-Assessment CME Maintenance of Certification requirements is available at https://abop.org/maintain-certification/cme-self-assessment/.

To take the posttest and request CME credit online:

1. Go to www.aao.org/cme-central and log in.
2. Click on "Claim CME Credit and View My CME Transcript" and then "Report AAO Credits."
3. Select the appropriate media type and then the Academy activity. You will be directed to the posttest.
4. Once you have passed the test with a score of 80% or higher, you will be directed to your transcript. *If you are not an Academy member, you will be able to print out a certificate of participation once you have passed the test.*

CME expiration date: June 1, 2023. *AMA PRA Category 1 Credits*™ may be claimed only once between June 1, 2020, and the expiration date.

For assistance, contact the Academy's Customer Service department at 866.561.8558 (US only) or +1 415.561.8540 between 8:00 a.m. and 5:00 p.m. (PST), Monday through Friday, or send an e-mail to customer_service@aao.org.

Study Questions

Please note that these questions are not part of your CME reporting process. They are provided here for your own educational use and identification of any professional practice gaps. The required CME posttest is available online (see "Requesting Continuing Medical Education Credit"). Following the questions are answers with discussions. Although a concerted effort has been made to avoid ambiguity and redundancy in these questions, the authors recognize that differences of opinion may occur regarding the "best" answer. The discussions are provided to demonstrate the rationale used to derive the answer. They may also be helpful in confirming that your approach to the problem was correct or, if necessary, in fixing the principle in your memory. The Section 10 faculty thanks the Resident Self-Assessment Committee for drafting these self-assessment questions and the discussions that follow.

1. What is the second leading cause of blindness worldwide?
   a. cataract
   b. diabetic retinopathy
   c. glaucoma
   d. trauma

2. According to the Goldmann equation, what is the ratio of the increase in intraocular pressure (IOP) to the increase in episcleral venous pressure in millimeters of mercury (mm Hg)?
   a. 1:0.5
   b. 1:1
   c. 1:1.5
   d. 1:2

3. What type of tonometer uses the Imbert-Fick principle for measurement of IOP?
   a. Perkins tonometer
   b. pneumatonometer
   c. rebound tonometer
   d. Schiøtz tonometer

4. How is uveoscleral outflow affected by pressure, age, and cycloplegia?
   a. pressure sensitive, decreases with age, decreased by cycloplegic agents
   b. pressure insensitive, decreases with age, increased by cycloplegic agents
   c. pressure sensitive, increases with age, decreased by cycloplegic agents
   d. pressure insensitive, increases with age, increased by cycloplegic agents

5. Which parameter of the modified Goldmann equation cannot be directly measured clinically and must be calculated from the other parameters of this equation?
   a. aqueous humor formation rate
   b. episcleral venous pressure
   c. outflow facility
   d. uveoscleral outflow rate

6. What layer of the optic nerve can be better visualized with the ophthalmoscope using the red-free (green) filter?
   a. laminar region
   b. nerve fiber layer
   c. prelaminar region
   d. retrolaminar region

7. A patient with a history of 2 piggyback intraocular lenses (IOLs) in the left eye, both placed within the capsular bag, is referred by a local optometrist for evaluation of elevated IOP in that eye. Endothelial pigment deposition is noted on slit-lamp examination. What gonioscopic finding might be expected in this scenario?
   a. peripheral anterior synechiae (PAS)
   b. posterior embryotoxon
   c. Sampaolesi line
   d. widened ciliary body band

8. When considering examination of the anterior segment, which modality allows one to best visualize the ciliary body and ciliary processes?
   a. anterior segment optical coherence tomography (AS-OCT)
   b. anterior segment ultrasound biomicroscopy (UBM)
   c. B-scan ultrasonography
   d. dynamic gonioscopy

9. A patient presents with narrow angles and findings suspicious for iris and/or ciliary body cysts. What is the best imaging modality for further investigation?
   a. anterior segment UBM
   b. AS-OCT
   c. B-scan ultrasonography
   d. computed tomography (CT) scan of the orbits

10. A patient has a unilateral glaucoma in the right eye with an IOP of 35 mm Hg on maximal medical therapy. The IOP in the left eye is 13 mm Hg. The external examination of the right eye discloses proptosis, dilated, arterialized conjunctival vessels, and chemosis. What is the most likely finding on further examination?
    a. anterior chamber cells
    b. blood in Schlemm canal
    c. rubeosis iridis
    d. sectoral iris atrophy

11. In a nonglaucomatous optic disc, what quadrant of the neural rim is generally the thickest?
    a. inferior
    b. nasal
    c. superior
    d. temporal

12. From primarily where is the arterial blood supply for the anterior optic nerve derived?
    a. central retinal artery
    b. circle of Zinn-Haller
    c. pial arteries
    d. short posterior ciliary arteries

13. What is the average rate of change in the average thickness of the peripapillary retinal nerve fiber layer in healthy subjects over time?
    a. −0.25 μm/year
    b. −0.50 μm/year
    c. −0.75 μm/year
    d. −1.0 μm/year

14. What optic disc characteristic is most specific for glaucoma?
    a. exposed lamina cribrosa
    b. focal notching of the rim
    c. nasal displacement of vessels
    d. peripapillary atrophy

15. What type of visual field testing varies the stimulus intensity while keeping the stimulus size constant?
    a. automated static perimetry
    b. frequency-doubling technology (FDT)
    c. kinetic perimetry
    d. tangent screen testing

16. What pattern of visual field defect is most typical of glaucoma?
    a. arcuate scotoma
    b. blind spot enlargement
    c. centrocecal scotoma
    d. hemianopic defect

17. A glaucoma suspect patient demonstrates superior and inferior defects on perimetry in the left eye with a reliable baseline visual field test (Swedish Interactive Threshold Algorithm Standard 24-2). What is the next best course of action?
    a. Begin medical therapy with a prostaglandin analogue.
    b. Obtain imaging of the optic nerve head.
    c. Order neuroimaging.
    d. Repeat visual field testing.

18. When is a false-positive error recorded in perimetry?
    a. when, on retesting, the patient does not respond to a stimulus that was previously seen
    b. when the patient falsely responds to a visual stimulus presented in the blind spot
    c. when the patient moves his or her eyes from the central fixation point
    d. when the patient responds even though no visual stimulus was presented

19. In the Collaborative Normal-Tension Glaucoma Study (CNTGS), what was the IOP reduction target?
    a. 10%
    b. 20%
    c. 30%
    d. 40%

20. What percentage of patients with primary open-angle glaucoma (POAG) present with an IOP below 22 mm Hg?
    a. 0%–25%
    b. 30%–50%
    c. 50%–75%
    d. 75%–100%

21. What was the finding of the Baltimore Eye Survey with regard to the impact of aging on glaucoma?
    a. Impact of perfusion pressure on glaucoma increases with age.
    b. Prevalence of glaucoma increases with age.
    c. Rate of conversion from ocular hypertension to POAG increases with age.
    d. Rate of glaucoma progression increases with age.

22. What is a Sampaolesi line?
    a. pigment deposition anterior to the Schwalbe line
    b. pigment deposition at the lens equator
    c. pigment deposition on the corneal endothelium
    d. pigment deposition on the surface of the lens

23. An 89-year-old woman presents with eye pain in her right eye. She reports that the vision in her right eye has been poor for years, due to complications from a retinal detachment. On examination, the IOP in her right eye is 40. Her exam is significant for a white cataract with a wrinkled anterior capsule. On gonioscopy, ciliary body is visible in all quadrants. Cell and flare is noted in the anterior chamber, but no keratic precipitates are observed. What is the most likely diagnosis?
    a. lens particle glaucoma
    b. phacoantigenic glaucoma
    c. phacolytic glaucoma
    d. phacomorphic glaucoma

24. Which topical agent should be avoided in patients with uveitic glaucoma?
    a. carbonic anhydrase inhibitors
    b. miotic agents
    c. α-agonists
    d. β-blockers

25. A 50-year-old woman presents with an IOP of 27 in the right eye and 12 in the left eye. On examination, an abnormal corneal endothelium is noted in the right eye; the left eye is normal. The anterior segment exam is otherwise unremarkable. On gonioscopy, PAS to the Schwalbe line are noted in 1 clock-hour. What is the most likely diagnosis?
    a. Chandler syndrome
    b. Cogan-Reese syndrome
    c. essential iris atrophy
    d. Fuchs dystrophy

26. What is the most common cause of blindness related to glaucoma in the Chinese population?
    a. primary open-angle glaucoma
    b. secondary open-angle glaucoma
    c. primary angle-closure glaucoma
    d. secondary angle-closure glaucoma

27. What is the mode of inheritance of Axenfeld-Rieger syndrome?
   a. autosomal dominant
   b. autosomal recessive
   c. sporadic
   d. X-linked

28. A patient with primary congenital glaucoma asks the ophthalmologist's advice regarding family planning. Notably, she has no relatives with primary congenital glaucoma. What is the likelihood of her having a child affected with primary congenital glaucoma?
   a. 0%–25%
   b. 25%–50%
   c. 50%–75%
   d. 75%–100%

29. A 1-year-old boy is brought in for an eye examination because of persistent tearing. What corneal diameter measurement should trigger concern for glaucoma?
   a. greater than 11.5 mm
   b. greater than 12.0 mm
   c. greater than 12.5 mm
   d. greater than 13.0 mm

30. What finding on examination of a patient with congenital glaucoma can continue to change and indicate progressive glaucoma even though the IOP appears to be controlled?
   a. axial length
   b. corneal thickness
   c. gonioscopic findings
   d. myopia

31. Which class of ocular hypotensive agents is associated with the development of apnea in infants and young children?
   a. carbonic anhydrase inhibitors
   b. cholinergic agonists
   c. nonselective β-antagonists
   d. α_2-selective adrenergic agonists

32. What were the findings of the Zhongshan Angle Closure Prevention (ZAP) trial?
   a. Laser peripheral iridotomy (LPI) had no impact on the course of progression to any type of angle closure.
   b. LPI significantly reduced the incidence of the development of acute angle closure.
   c. LPI significantly reduced the incidence of the development of primary angle closure.
   d. LPI significantly reduced the incidence of the development of POAG.

Answers

1. **c.** The prevalence of blindness for all types of glaucoma was estimated at more than 8 million persons, with 4 million cases caused by primary open-angle glaucoma (POAG). Glaucoma was theoretically calculated to account for 12.3% of cases of blindness; it is therefore the second leading cause of blindness worldwide, following cataract. Diabetic retinopathy and trauma are less common causes of blindness worldwide.
2. **b.** According to the Goldmann equation, $P_0 = (F - U)/C + P_V$, where P_0 is the intraocular pressure (IOP) in millimeters of mercury (mm Hg), F is the rate of aqueous humor production, U is the rate of aqueous humor drainage through the pressure-insensitive uveoscleral pathway in microliters per minute (L/min), C is the facility of outflow through the pressure-sensitive trabecular pathway in microliters per minute per mm Hg (L/min/mm Hg), and P_V is the episcleral venous pressure in mm Hg, IOP rises by 1 mm Hg for every 1 mm Hg of rise in episcleral venous pressure. Patients with Sturge-Weber syndrome, carotid-cavernous sinus fistulas, cavernous sinus thrombosis, and thyroid eye disease (partial increase) have increased episcleral venous pressure from obstruction of venous return to the heart or from shunting of blood from the arterial to the venous system. Episcleral venous pressure is normally relatively stable, ranging from 6 to 9 mm Hg, as measured with special equipment. Increased episcleral venous pressure can increase outflow resistance by collapsing Schlemm canal and may alter uveoscleral outflow.
3. **a.** Like the Goldmann tonometer, the Perkins tonometer is an applanation tonometer and, as such, is based on the Imbert-Fick principle. The Imbert-Fick principle relates the pressure inside a dry, thin-walled sphere to the force required to flatten a specific area. The Goldmann applanation tonometer and the Perkins tonometer use the same measurement tip, which balances the surface tension of the tear film with the rigidity of the cornea to approximate a dry, infinitely flexible, thin-walled sphere for eyes with corneal thickness of 520 µm. Rebound tonometry, the pneumatonometer, and the Schiøtz tonometer do not rely on the Imbert-Fick principle.
4. **b.** Uveoscleral outflow is the nontrabecular outflow of the eye. It is pressure insensitive, and the predominant mechanism is one of aqueous passage from the anterior chamber into the ciliary muscle and then to the supraciliary and suprachoroidal spaces, exiting the eye through an intact sclera or along the nerves and the vessels that penetrate it. It can account for up to 45% of the total aqueous outflow. Uveoscleral outflow decreases with age and in patients with glaucoma. It is increased by prostaglandin analogues and by cycloplegic and adrenergic agents and cyclodialysis clefts early on. The opposite effect is observed with miotics. Outflow for the uveoscleral pathway cannot be measured clinically and is therefore calculated by the Goldmann equation.
5. **d.** Direct measurement of uveoscleral outflow rate is an invasive process that involves perfusion of a tracer into the anterior segment of the eye, followed by estimation of the tissue distribution of the tracer. Thus, in humans, uveoscleral outflow rate must be calculated by using the Goldmann equation and the parameters IOP, aqueous humor flow rate, outflow facility, and episcleral venous pressure. By contrast, aqueous humor formation rate is measured with fluorophotometry; episcleral venous pressure, with venomanometry; and outflow facility, with tonography. All of these procedures are noninvasive.

6. **b.** The nerve fiber layer is a useful finding with regard to normal optic nerve appearance. Axons in the nerve fiber layer of the normal eye may best be seen with red-free illumination. The nerve fibers travel as bundles of axons from the peripheral retina to converge at the optic nerve head and look like fine striations. This is the layer that atrophies in glaucoma; thus, the clinician can see a reduction in nerve fiber layer brightness (either focally or diffusely) in a glaucoma patient with thinning of the retinal nerve fiber layer (RNFL). Normally, the brightness and striations are more easily seen in the superior and inferior poles versus the temporal and nasal regions. When there is RNFL loss, the difference in brightness between the vertical and horizontal regions decreases. The ophthalmologist should try to appreciate the nerve fiber layer with the green filter in healthy persons and glaucoma patients. The more normal findings one sees, the better one can appreciate abnormal findings.
7. **c.** Interlenticular opacification and iris chafing are possible complications seen with implantation of piggyback intraocular lenses (IOLs) within the capsular bag. Iris chafing can result in a pigment dispersion syndrome and associated elevated IOP, presumably from obstruction of the trabecular meshwork by pigment granules. Findings associated with pigment dispersion syndrome include pigment deposits on the corneal endothelium (Krukenberg spindle), midperipheral iris transillumination defects, pigment deposits of the lens capsule at the insertion of the zonular fibers (Zentmayer ring or Scheie stripe), heavy uniform pigmentation of the trabecular meshwork, and pigment speckling at or anterior to the Schwalbe line (Sampaolesi line). The other findings are not associated with pigment dispersion syndrome.
8. **b.** Anterior segment ultrasound biomicroscopy (UBM) enables visualization of the ciliary body and ciliary processes. Anterior segment optical coherence tomography (AS-OCT) allows high-resolution imaging of the anterior segment, including the anterior chamber angle (see Fig 4-13 in this volume), but unlike UBM, it does not permit visualization of the ciliary sulcus and ciliary body. As with UBM, AS-OCT does not always yield images that allow reliable identification of angle landmarks. Furthermore, neither modality can differentiate between appositional and synechial angle closure—a distinction possible only with dynamic gonioscopy. AS-OCT is noncontact and can be performed relatively rapidly, whereas gonioscopy and UBM require corneal contact. B-scan ultrasonography is used to image the posterior segment at a lower frequency than UBM.
9. **a.** UBM is the best way to image the ciliary body and anterior choroid. It can help diagnose plateau iris syndrome, ciliary body cysts, and ciliary tumors. AS-OCT does not have enough penetration to adequately image the ciliary body. B-scan ultrasonography is not ideal for imaging anterior structures. Computed tomography (CT) scans do not provide detailed imaging of anterior segment structures.
10. **b.** The complex of external findings in this case combined with ocular hypertension points to a diagnosis of carotid cavernous fistula. IOP elevation associated with increased episcleral venous pressure can occur in the setting of thyroid ophthalmopathy, arteriovenous malformations, carotid-cavernous fistulas, or dural sinus fistulas. In these patients, a reflux of blood into Schlemm canal may be visible on gonioscopy. Depending on the etiology, proptosis, ocular pulsations, and an orbital bruit may also occur. Anterior chamber cells can be found in the setting of uveitic glaucoma. Rubeosis iridis is found in neovascular glaucoma. Sectoral iris atrophy can be seen in herpetic disease. In rare instances, signs of ocular ischemia or venous stasis may be present.

11. **a.** The physiologic neural rim is typically the broadest inferiorly, followed by the superior, nasal, and temporal rims. This is commonly referred to as the ISNT (*i*nferior, *s*uperior, *n*asal, *t*emporal) rule. Inferior (or often also superior) rim thinning in the absence of field loss should be considered suspicious and might represent early glaucoma. Any violation of the ISNT rule should be considered as a potential indicator of early glaucoma or glaucoma suspect, but the clinician should keep in mind that violation of the ISNT rule is not highly specific and may be seen in normal eyes as well.
12. **d.** The arterial supply of the anterior optic nerve is derived entirely from branches of the ophthalmic artery via 1–5 posterior ciliary arteries. Typically, between 2 and 4 posterior ciliary arteries course anteriorly before dividing into approximately 10–20 short posterior ciliary arteries prior to entering the posterior globe. Often, the posterior ciliary arteries separate into a medial and a lateral group before branching into the short posterior ciliary arteries, which penetrate the perineural sclera of the posterior globe to supply the peripapillary choroid, as well as most of the anterior optic nerve. Some short posterior ciliary arteries course, without branching, through the sclera directly into the choroid; others divide within the sclera to provide branches to both the choroid and the optic nerve. Often a discontinuous arterial circle, the circle of Zinn-Haller, exists within the perineural sclera. The central retinal artery, also a posterior orbital branch of the ophthalmic artery, penetrates the optic nerve approximately 10–15 mm posterior to the globe. The central retinal artery has few, if any, intraneural branches, the exception being an occasional small branch within the retrolaminar region, which may anastomose with the pial system. The central retinal artery courses adjacent to the central retinal vein within the central portion of the optic nerve. Arterioles also branch from the short posterior ciliary arteries and the circle of Zinn-Haller and course posteriorly to supply the pial arteries. These pial arteries often contribute to the laminar region.
13. **b.** Longitudinal studies have found mean rates of change of approximately –0.50 µm/year in average retinal nerve fiber layer (RNFL) thickness in healthy subjects followed over time. High rates of false-positive detection of progression may occur when progression is considered to have occurred merely if a statistically significant negative slope of change is present (ie, a slope that is statistically significantly different from 0 with $P < .05$). For instance, with 5 years of annual testing, up to 25% of normal eyes can be falsely identified as having progressed if such a criterion is used for RNFL thickness change.
14. **b.** Glaucomatous cups are associated with both generalized and focal ophthalmologic signs. General signs include large optic cup, asymmetry of the optic cups, and progressive enlargement of the cup. Focal signs include notching of the rim, vertical elongation of the cup, cupping to the rim margin, RNFL hemorrhage, and nerve fiber layer loss. Less specific signs are also observed, including exposed lamina cribrosa, nasal displacement of rim vessels, baring of circumlinear vessels, and peripapillary atrophy.
15. **a.** Automated static perimetry keeps the stimulus size constant and varies the stimulus intensity in testing. Static testing presents a stationary stimulus at various locations, varying the brightness. Frequency-doubling technology (FDT) measures the patient's ability to distinguish changes in contrast. In kinetic (Goldmann) perimetry and tangent screen testing, a target is moved into an area only until it is seen (automated or manual).
16. **a.** Patterns of visual field loss in glaucoma correspond to the RNFL anatomy. Glaucomatous visual field defects include arcuate scotoma, paracentral scotoma, nasal step, altitudinal defect, temporal wedge, and generalized depression. An arcuate scotoma is an

arc-shaped defect that occurs 10° to 20° from fixation; a complete arcuate defect arches from the blind spot to the nasal raphe and is wider and closer to fixation on the nasal side. This defect is a result of nerve fiber bundle damage at the superotemporal or inferotemporal disc, common areas of damage in glaucomatous optic neuropathy. Blind spot enlargement is more often seen in papilledema and chorioretinal inflammatory conditions such as multiple evanescent white dot syndrome and acute idiopathic blind spot enlargement. It can also be seen in tilted myopic discs. A centrocecal scotoma involves both the blind spot and the point of fixation and is seen in conditions such as toxic optic neuropathy, nutritional optic neuropathy, and Leber hereditary optic neuropathy. Hemianopic defects are caused by retrochiasmal disease.

17. **d.** Visual field testing is a subjective examination, and different responses may be obtained each time the test is performed or even during the same test. Such fluctuation can confound the detection of disease progression. To detect true visual field progression, the clinician needs to evaluate whether the observed change exceeds the expected variability for a particular point or area. The Humphrey perimeter provides Guided Progression Analysis (GPA) software to assist in detection of visual field progression. The software presents an event-based method that is based on the pattern deviation plot and, therefore, adjusts for the potential confounding effects of diffuse loss of sensitivity from media opacities. New or progressing worsening visual field defects are identified by comparison to a pair of baseline tests; therefore, it is critical to have reliable baseline examinations. Often, the patient experiences a learning effect, and the second visual field may show substantial improvement over the first. To address this phenomenon, the clinician should perform at least 2 visual field tests as early as possible in the course of a patient's disease. If the results are quite different, a third test should be performed. The software automatically selects the first 2 available examinations as the baseline tests. However, one can easily override this selection to a more suitable time point (eg, change in therapy after progression), or to avoid initial learning effects (which could reduce the sensitivity to detect progression). The software then compares each follow-up test to the average of the baseline tests. It identifies points that show change greater than the expected variability (at the 95% significance level), as determined by previous studies with stable glaucoma patients. If significant change is detected in at least 3 points and repeated in the same points in 2 consecutive follow-up tests, the software will flag the last examination as *Possible Progression*. If significant change is detected and repeated for the same 3 or more points in 3 consecutive follow-up tests, the GPA software will flag the last examination as *Likely Progression*.

    In this scenario, it is best to obtain at least 1 more visual field test to determine reproducibility of the scotoma before initiating treatment. The defect, if in a typical glaucomatous pattern matching optic nerve appearance, will not usually require neuroimaging. Imaging of the optic nerve head is important in diagnosis and management of glaucoma, but repeating the visual field test would be the most appropriate next step to confirm a defect and obtain a baseline.

18. **d.** A false-positive error occurs when the patient presses the button when no visual stimulus is presented. The first scenario represents a false-negative error. The second is fixation loss as detected by the Heijl-Krakau method. The third scenario is fixation loss detected by infrared gaze tracking.

19. **c.** The Collaborative Normal-Tension Glaucoma Study (CNGTS) was a multicenter trial wherein patients were randomized to either no treatment of IOP reduction of 30%. The

study found that reducing IOP by 30% decreased the 5-year progression risk from 35% to 12%, after adjusting for the effect of cataract.

20. **b.** Elevated IOP is a significant risk factor for the development of glaucoma. However, several studies have shown that between 30% and 50% of patients with glaucoma present with an initial IOP measurement below 22 mm Hg. In addition, IOP can vary considerably over a 24-hour period. As such, IOP alone cannot be used to establish a diagnosis of glaucoma.

21. **b.** The Baltimore Eye Survey found a significant increase in the prevalence of glaucoma with aging, particularly among African American individuals. In this group, the prevalence was 11% in people over the age of 80. Ocular perfusion was not studied in the Baltimore Eye Survey. The Ocular Hypertension Treatment Study found an increase in risk of conversion from ocular hypertension to glaucoma as patients aged. The Collaborative Initial Glaucoma Treatment Study found that visual field defects (ie, glaucoma progression) were much more likely to progress in patients over the age of 60 versus patients younger than 40.

22. **a.** A Sampaolesi line refers to pigmentation anterior to the Schwalbe line and is found in patients with pseudoexfoliation and pigmentary glaucoma. Pigment deposition at the lens equator is referred to as a Zentmayer line (or Scheie stripe). Pigment deposition on the corneal endothelium in a spindle pattern is referred to as a Krukenberg spindle. Zentmayer lines and Krukenberg spindles can be seen in patients with pigmentary glaucoma. Pigment deposition on the surface of the lens is called Scheie stripe.

23. **c.** The most likely diagnosis is phacolytic glaucoma, caused by the leakage of high-molecular-weight proteins through microscopic openings of an intact lens capsule of a mature cataract. These proteins block the trabecular meshwork, resulting in elevated IOP. Lens particle glaucoma occurs as a result of lens material retention after cataract surgery or ocular trauma. Phacoantigenic glaucoma occurs as a result of sensitization of the eye to native lens protein, causing a granulomatous reaction. The absence or presence of keratic precipitates helps differentiate phacolytic glaucoma from phacoantigenic glaucoma. Phacomorphic glaucoma is induced by a relatively large lens pushing the iris forward, causing angle closure.

24. **b.** Miotic agents should be avoided in patients with uveitic glaucoma. Pupillary constriction and paralysis can lead to the formation of central posterior synechiae, and miotic agents can also exacerbate inflammation. Topical carbonic anhydrase inhibitors, α-agonists, and β-blockers are all effective medications in the treatment of uveitic glaucoma.

25. **a.** Chandler syndrome, Cogan-Reese syndrome, and essential iris atrophy constitute the iridocorneal endothelial (ICE) syndrome. All are marked by an abnormal corneal endothelium, leading to progressive peripheral anterior synechiae (PAS) and elevated IOP. ICE syndrome is unilateral in most cases. In Chandler syndrome, there are minimal anterior segment changes other than high PAS. Cogan-Reese syndrome is marked by pedunculated nodules or pigmented lesions on the anterior iris surface. Eyes with essential iris atrophy demonstrate heterochromia and corectopia. Fuchs dystrophy causes endothelial changes similar to those observed in ICE syndrome, but these changes are typically bilateral and are not associated with PAS.

26. **c.** Primary angle-closure glaucoma is the most common cause of blindness related to glaucoma in the Chinese population. It has been estimated to be responsible for more than 90% of glaucoma-related blindness in the Chinese population.

27. **a.** Axenfeld-Rieger syndrome is an autosomal dominant disorder and presents with a variety of phenotypes.

28. **a.** This patient has sporadic primary congenital glaucoma. Such patients very rarely have affected children (approximately 2%).

29. **c.** A normal corneal diameter for a newborn is between 9.5 and 10.5 mm. By age 1 year, the normal corneal diameter increases to 11 to 12 mm. A measurement greater than 11.5 mm in a newborn or greater than 12.5 mm in a child above the age of 1 year suggests glaucoma.

30. **a.** In children younger than 3 years, the sclera is elastic and will stretch if IOP is not well controlled. This can result in increased axial length despite good pressure during examination under anesthesia. Corneal thickness decreases as corneal edema resolves and, once stable, is often less than the average central corneal thickness. The angle can further develop as a child ages, but this does not indicate poor pressure control. Myopia in congenital glaucoma is not necessarily an axial myopia.

31. **d.** α_2-Selective adrenergic agonists have been reported to cause severe, life-threatening apnea, central nervous system depression, and bradycardia in infants and children. These agents can cross the blood–brain barrier, particularly in infants. They are contraindicated for use in young children and should be avoided in nursing mothers.

32. **c.** The Zhongshan Angle Closure Prevention (ZAP) trial identified 889 primary angle-closure suspects. One eye of each subject was randomized to laser peripheral iridotomy (LPI), while the contralateral eye served as a control. At 6-year follow-up, control eyes were more likely to develop primary angle closure, largely on the basis of developing PAS. However, there was no statistically significant increased risk of the development of acute angle closure or POAG, and the incidence of these outcomes was low in both the treated and untreated eyes.

Index

(*f* = figure; *t* = table)